*Fitness from
Six to Twelve*

Books by Bonnie Prudden:

Basic Exercise #1
Is Your Child Really Fit?
Bonnie Prudden's Fitness Book
How to Keep Slender and Fit After Thirty
Testing and Training for Physical Fitness
Improve Your Body
Improve Your Physical Fitness
How to Keep Your Child Fit from Birth to Six (revised 1986)
Quick Rx for Fitness
Teenage Fitness
Physical Fitness for You: A Talking Book for the Blind
Fitness From Six to Twelve (revised 1987)
Teach Your Baby to Swim
How to Keep Your Family Fit and Healthy
Exersex
Pain Erasure: The Bonnie Prudden Way
Myotherapy: Bonnie Prudden's Complete Guide to Pain-Free Living
Bonnie Prudden's After Fifty Fitness Guide

Fitness from Six to Twelve

Bonnie Prudden

Photographs by Suzanne Szasz

Ballantine Books · New York

Copyright © 1987 by Bonnie Prudden, Inc.
Copyright © 1972 by Bonnie Prudden
Photographs copyright © 1987 by Suzanne Szasz
Illustrations copyright © 1986, 1987 by Holly Johnson

All rights reserved under International and Pan-American Copyright Conventions. Published in the United States by Ballantine Books, a division of Random House, Inc., New York, and simultaneously in Canada by Random House of Canada Limited, Toronto.
This is a revised edition of this title, which was originally published by Harper & Row Publishers, Inc. in 1972.

Library of Congress Catalog Card Number: 86-92100

ISBN: 0-345-33302-0

Text design by Holly Johnson

Manufactured in the United States of America

First Ballantine Books Edition: October 1987
10 9 8 7 6 5 4 3 2 1

CONTENTS

Foreword		ix
Chapter One:	The Starting Line	1
Chapter Two:	Tests Tell Truths	12
Chapter Three:	A Stitch in Time	25
Chapter Four:	How Good Are You . . . Really?	31
Chapter Five:	Girls and Their Muscles	62
Chapter Six:	The First Step—Warm-Ups	65
Chapter Seven:	Standing Exercises	81
Chapter Eight:	Kneeling, Sitting, and Lying Exercises	90
Chapter Nine:	Flexibility Exercises	97
Chapter Ten:	Across-the-Floor Progressions	107
Chapter Eleven:	The Russian Series	121
Chapter Twelve:	Tumbling	128

Chapter Thirteen:	Equipment	145
Chapter Fourteen:	Exercises on the Equipment	151
Chapter Fifteen:	Making and Using Weight Bags	189
Chapter Sixteen:	Pipes, Ropes, and Rings	197
Chapter Seventeen:	The Garage or Basement Gym	216
Chapter Eighteen:	Dance	228
Chapter Nineteen:	Tennis	249
Chapter Twenty:	The Family—Together	260
Chapter Twenty-One:	The Fathers	270
Chapter Twenty-Two:	The Mothers	275
Chapter Twenty-Three:	A Union for Parents	280
Chapter Twenty-Four:	Backyard Track Meet	286
Chapter Twenty-Five:	Running	298
Chapter Twenty-Six:	Swimming	307
Chapter Twenty-Seven:	Riding	321
Chapter Twenty-Eight:	Skiing	334
Chapter Twenty-Nine:	Figure Skating	351
Chapter Thirty:	Summer Camp	362
Chapter Thirty-One:	Helping the Handicapped	378
Chapter Thirty-Two:	The Citadel	394
Chapter Thirty-Three:	Ammunition PTA	406
Chapter Thirty-Four:	Myotherapy: A Way to Get Rid of Pain	411
Chapter Thirty-Five:	How to Help a Friend	439
Sources		445
Exercise Index		449
General Index		459

ACKNOWLEDGMENTS

This book was written about children and for children. In many ways it was written *by* children.

No two children are exactly alike, and each brings to experience a different physical and mental makeup. A teacher does not merely present a given subject to a class, but rather engages in an *exchange* with several people at one time. Fifty children will see and hear fifty versions of the same lesson, and each of those versions will be treated differently once absorbed. When the work involves movement, there will then follow fifty different physical *translations*. The teacher must observe these translations and deal with them.

In one single exchange there are at least two hundred units of presentation, acceptance, translation, and observation involved. All of that takes place before the final stage, which calls for many degrees of correction, reinforcement, and praise. Success will depend not only on the teacher's ability to present *to* the children, but on the art of taking and learning *from* the children. Children have taught me many things about teaching, the most important of which are:

• *The subject must have* true value *for the pupil. Children will not accept counterfeit, and the younger the child, the harder he or she is to deceive.*

• *Children insist on* simplicity. *True value does not need confusing language or complicated form. Faced with either, children slip back into dreams and close the door.*

• *The teacher must* believe *in the subject,* feel *the subject, and* live *the subject. Children recognize the honest teacher at once and the dishonest one just as quickly . . . even when that is the parent.*

If you believe in what is to be taught . . . if it has true value and if you can teach it simply . . . children will learn.

If this book is helpful to children, then they should be grateful to other children. In that wonderful miracle of learning, I have been that most privileged of pupils . . . a teacher.

FOREWORD

You whose children are between the all-important years of six and twelve, or who are working with children traveling between those two mileposts, should know that *it is already half past midnight.* The new day is not far off, and that day must be met by those children, ready or not. The thought that such young children are about to be assaulted by life would have been unacceptable only a few years ago, but the drug scene has changed all that. The world is no longer a children's garden of song and verse. The night begins to lower earlier and earlier.

No child is ever a true *tabula rasa*. The slate already bears a full set of tendencies, and from day one these tendencies are reinforced or diminished by the things that happen to and around the child. The born follower starts incredibly soon to follow another's lead. Unless someone spots this weakness and works to strengthen the child's sense of worth and independence, the only hope will lie in luck. Lucky indeed is the child who finds a *good* leader to follow, since the odds are overwhelmingly in favor of the other kind. Inborn violence erupts first in the nursery, and to neglect that weakness is to abandon the helpless. One day, holding one's breath will not be enough, and holding someone else's is not beyond the realm of possibility.

Having looked around at the world, you may be willing to accept that things are not what they used to be (if they ever were), but what, you wonder, has physical activity and fitness to do with it one way or another? The answer lies in the fact that the *physical* level is that level on which young children are most comfortable and where they function most easily. It is also a wide-open field under a noon sun that welcomes children and grown-ups *equally*. It is without shadow and permits both children and grown-ups to welcome each other without reservation. On that field there is no "generation gap." Communication is instant and quite clear. Everybody starts out even. The warmth of the sun and the prickling chill of first raindrops feel the same to all. Small or great victories thrill each in the same pleasant way, and defeat is bearable when it is shared. There is honesty in physical action, and that honesty breeds pride, tolerance, and friendship.

None of the above emotions happens automatically. Filial love, even as a reassuring myth, is long gone. Children do not love their parents simply because of that highly suspect relationship. Love, liking, and tolerance come (or do not come) because of what goes on day after day at home. Teachers also stand in the full blaze of light and, for the price of a good look, can see themselves mirrored in the eyes of their pupils. The younger the eyes, the clearer the image.

There are many things a child must learn before the battle of life is joined, and for good or not so good, it is up to parents *and* teachers to get the basics across. If either depends on the other to do the whole job, the child will lose, but not only the child. One good look at what is going on in our land today will tell you that hell has many levels and a lost child never goes there alone.

Since the job of teaching basics to children is not all that easy (nor, God forgive me, *fun*), the wise teacher or parent will seize every last opportunity when he or she can legitimately—bidden, welcome, and belonging—to enter the child's world. From six to twelve the key to the gate is *physical* activity, from a walk in the woods to the most sophisticated sport. The nice thing about kids is that they really don't care which; they are just delighted to have you around. Don't wait another moment—even if it's raining. Grab your chance today, because before you know it, the gate will close. Even while you are reading this page, the sun of the next generation's day is climbing higher below the horizon. When it reaches first light . . . your chance will be gone.

CHAPTER ONE
THE STARTING LINE

Before you can design a program for a child, you need to know some special things about that child. Each has different strengths and weaknesses, preferences and problems. We all become so accustomed to the children in our houses that we are apt to overlook the very things that need emphasis because they have value or that need correction because they do or will cause trouble in the future.

Some children habitually snort and snuffle through stuffy noses. Some have teeth that push and crowd each other in narrow jaws. A few *never* walk down the stairs without holding on to the banister and they wouldn't climb a tree even if it grew right up through the living room floor. There are children who constantly turn their heads as if listening for mice in the chimney and others who strut on their toes whenever they are barefoot. Some poke their tummies out, some turn their toes in, and some have chapped lips even in summer.

We tell the stuffy noses to blow, and eventually we get braces for the crowded teeth. The banister holders get glasses, and we move the ones who don't hear well up to the front row. We keep shoes on the toe walkers and get wedges for the pigeon-toed. We girdle the protruding abdomens and put cream on the cracked lips. But we miss all the *reasons* until it is too late to do the most or the best. Early is the bird that catches the worm, and early is the time to spot a problem and fix it. Start your wonderful work with children by *looking at them*. Then you will know what you are *looking at* because you know what you are *looking for*. Let's all get started.

Keep a notebook for each of your children, and keep it as though your child's life depended on it. Someday it may. The most trivial things cause trouble, and you cannot imagine how useful it is when a doctor takes a case history and you can say that you know exactly when the difficulty started. As people go through life, they forget things that happened in childhood; even parents forget. But if it's all down in a notebook and a wise, searching person is looking for clues, the answer to the problem may be right there in black and white. The backache, the nutritional deficiency, the stiff neck, and even the painful arthritis often send up flares before children can say, "It hurts here." Then, too, coming events do cast their shadows before them. Sometimes by watching the physical habits of children you are able to direct them into training that will give them the tools for life.

AGE

The three best years for building an excellent body, patterns, and attitudes come between birth and three. In those years all that a person will be is formed. Many people working with children take exception to this, but studies show that in this respect children can be likened to furniture. When you decide to build a chair, you must start from the first moment building a *chair*. Its purpose is decided. After its form is laid down and glued together, it is a chair, not a table, not a dresser, not a lamp—a chair. That parallels the first three years for children. You can then paint the chair, upholster it, add a cushion, casters, even wheels. It is still a chair. You can similarly educate children, give them goals, a profession, all kinds of skills, but the initial person underneath is still the one put together in those first years. The optimist, the pessimist, the unsure, the timid, the outgoing, and the skeptic are all formed early.

At this moment, looking at an uncontrollable screamer, a self-willed producer of tantrums, a monster of destruction of seven, you may be inclined to join the cop-outs. You might feel similarly about the no-neck roly-poly who spends each waking moment either at the fridge or in his room with the TV. In both cases you know something is wrong. If age three is the deadline, what else is there to do? The screamer has the strength of ten and that's a plus. He is also without question the most stubborn individual you know, and he needs to be first so badly he even cheats at "Old Maid." Strength can be channeled, and so can the will to do and the drive to be first. They often add up to a good game of tennis, which has its own ways for making cheating a bore.

Roly-poly people are really *instead-of* people. They eat instead of what they would like to do. Sometimes (mostly) children get to be roly-polies because of their parents' eating habits. *They* can't do what they would like to do, so they eat *instead of* in a vicious cycle. Nobody can ever really like other people until he can like himself. Roly-polies and screamers *never* really like themselves, so your first job is to shine up the likable qualities. The earlier you can start, the better will be the results, and know in advance that everything your child has developed to this point *can be used to his benefit*—because now he can understand what you will be doing together.

HEIGHT AND WEIGHT

It is never too early to teach concern for the body your child lives in. If *you* are interested in the child's height and weight, the child will be interested. You should also be interested in your own. I remember very well being sent off to Sunday school one unpleasant wintry day. My mother was still in bed, and I asked her why I had to go and she didn't. Her answer could not have been very reassuring because it was after that Sunday that I started playing hooky. *You* set the example.

Weight is something that should matter always, since it is a road map. If you know where you are (and the scale is very truthful) and you know where you want to go, *if you keep track*, you can see how successful your present course of action is. Many adults weigh themselves only occasionally and are taken unawares by the accumulation over the years. Children can accumulate too much in a matter of months.

Height can be an aid in achieving good nutrition. Most boys want to be tall and most girls do not want to be small. You can say with truth that milk builds height. After World War II the Japanese, always considered small people, added milk to their children's lunches in school. To everyone's surprise and delight, the generation with this advantage grew an average of four inches taller than their parents. This bit of information may help to keep your children on milk and off soda, which rates zero in nutrition but is quite high in tooth destruction and fat production. A word of warning: Fat is always dangerous, especially in a sedentary society, so give your children skim milk. It is not only easy but desirable to add nonfat dried milk to the skim milk. The addition will give the milk more body, make it taste better, and also add nutrients. The trapped fat in homogenized milk soon gets trapped in your children.

BUILD

Build is important, and knowing something about the subject is very helpful, more as a warning than anything else. People who study body builds have come up with three divisions, which are especially helpful when applied to children: The *ectomorph* is the thinnish, nervous type, who runs to length; the *mesomorph* is considered to be athletic and is mostly bone and muscle; the unfortunate *endomorph* can best be described as fat, and the dictionary adds "good-natured" without the very necessary qualification "seems to be."

Unfortunately, people get bogged down in the descriptions and forget to *do* anything about it. They also forget to look back into the lives of their subjects to find out just when the build was built. The genes *plus nutrition* contribute to tallness, slenderness, and "nervousness," but training and opportunity decide whether the young ectomorph will be a four-minute miler or a scarecrow. The mesomorph, confined to playpen, stroller, and TV set, can turn into a confirmed endomorph in a very short time. If one parent is fat, a child has a 40 percent chance of being fat. If both parents are fat, obviously the odds go up.

Instead of letting "nature take its course," which in its true sense is an impossibility in most of the civilized world today, it is necessary to *do* something about build. There are basics that apply to all animals (and that includes children): proper nutrition, rest, and exercise. There are also some specials that apply to each of the builds, specials that the builds cry out for. Provide them early and you mold a delightful, efficient plant for your child. Ignore them and you limit potential. If the ectomorph has the basics and then gets the special skills that go with being slender, long-muscled, tallish, and "nervous," you may develop a very skilled happy-about-it runner, tennis player, or squash player. That doesn't mean that other fields are not open to the ectomorph or that other builds are excluded. It's just that if you look over the field, you will find that the ones who seem to love those sports most are tall, slender, and "nervous."

If you give your mesomorph the chance, you usually develop someone who is excellent in contact sports, a child whose school marks and joy in living reflect the satisfactions of self-confidence. Block the way and you can develop quite another personality.

The endomorph is not fated to be a fatty. Most fat people are both flexible and graceful, but they rarely get the chance either to enjoy these qualities or to exhibit them. Given the basics, the tendency to fat can be controlled. Given the attractive body, the drive to overeat can be conquered. Given the outlet, whether it be a sport or the active art of dance, the need to make up for something wanted and denied can be satisfied.

Look your child over and decide which way the tendency runs. After you have provided the basics, try out the specials. There is such a wide choice that something will ring a bell. When it does, you will have placed a very powerful friend in your corner as well as your child's.

FAT

Since so many young children in America are fat, this needs a special section. There are no such qualifications as baby fat, chubby fat, adolescent fat; there is just fat, and no, it will not just go away. Very often the diet provided for children is so loaded with fat and carbohydrates that they get overweight long before they can protect themselves, as so many teens and adults are doing today, with dieting regimes. Except for the seriously diseased (of which there are very few), people cannot get fat if they eat properly and get enough exercise. You will never see a child raised in a family deeply concerned with nutrition who is either fat or fatigued. I remember when I first spoke to groups interested in natural foods. I wondered why many of these so-called food faddists looked so worn and tired. If their ideas were correct, they should be great examples of observable health. Many were not. That is, many adults were not. But the children—oh, the children were lovely. Their skin was clear, their teeth beautiful, and their eyes bright; their hair shone, and they were both slender and straight. It was some time before I realized that many of the adults had come to natural foods only after illness had robbed them of beauty. They were slowly repairing themselves, but the same regime was *preventing* illness and ugliness in their children. By the same token, fat, pimply, tired children are participants in quite another kind of diet.

If your child is overweight, say to yourself, "My child is ill, my child's happiness is in danger, my child's health is in danger, my child's *life* is in danger." Then with all the honesty that those who have made such a statement must apply, ask yourself how it happened. Do you allow cookies, candy, soda, potato chips, pies, cakes, and gum? Is it easier to say yes than to fight through a no? Are *your* addictions such that you have already built addictions into your child? It is as dangerous to be a "foodoholic" as it is to be an alcoholic, and often one moves with ease from the former to the latter.

Make a pair of calipers by covering the tips of your scissors with Scotch tape. Then take a roll of fat at your child's waist and hold it between thumb and forefinger. Measure the width with the tips of the scissors and lay the tips along a ruler. Make a note of the size of the roll at the waist, the top of the thigh, and the back of the upper arm. Explain what you are doing and why, because in the coming weeks and months you are going to need all the help you can get from the child whose happiness and life you are trying to save. The slightest improvement is cause for a celebration. Go somewhere exciting, but don't reward with food—not ever again.

BONES

Bones can tell you a lot about the diet you are providing. If you are shy on vitamins, bones will tell you at once. It is a rare thing to find rickets today, since children are getting enough milk, but even rickets do show up from time to time. Much more often we see unattractive children, which means the same thing on perhaps a smaller scale. Look at your child's chest. Is it flat or caved in or do the bottom ribs flare out? Check the face. When the diet is right, the eyes are well spaced (even if Uncle Arthur's weren't). The jaw is wide enough for all the teeth without crowding, and the roof of the mouth is well domed (not narrow and not in the form of an inverted U or pointed, which prevents good sinus drainage). The chin is strong, not "weak" and receding. The forehead is well made and neither sloped back nor bulging. If your child's face reflects any of these troubles, look to the diet, not heredity.

Ten years from now it will be more important that you fed yourself and your family a good diet than that you lived in an expensive neighborhood. You can save thousands of dollars in the next few years if you provide the food that will prevent the necessity for teeth braces. If not knowing these things has already caused bones to develop poorly, start at once to rectify matters. In three years there will be a great difference in all of you.

SKIN, MOUTH, HAIR, AND NAILS

The first person to spot a deficiency is usually the dentist. Spongy red, swollen gums speak most eloquently even before cavities appear. If your child is beginning to have tooth problems, start right this minute to think about the food you are providing. If you know it's good because you really know about proper nutrition—which immediately knocks out all the no-no stuff and replaces it with fresh vegetables, fruit, and skim milk—(see page 264), wonder what's going on outside your home and prevent it if it is harmful.

Skin, too, reflects diet *and exercise.* If it is dry and scaly or broken out, check the diet for vitamins, minerals, and enzymes. You only have to list daily activities to find out about exercise.

Are the tongue and lips a healthy pink? Is the tongue coated or a bright raspberry color? Look at your own. You, too, may be suffering from a vitamin deficiency. What about the lips: Are they chapped and scaly with painful cracks in the corners? Diet again. A vitamin deficiency.

Hair and nails are like Little Sir Echo. When the skin is clear and the mouth is healthy, so are the hair and nails. If one looks seedy, so will the others. If your child or you exhibit any unhealthy signs, look first to diet.

FEET

What is the condition of your child's feet and how do they behave? Feet not only carry us from here to there, they are tension indicators.

When we were testing hundreds upon hundreds of schoolchildren, I found that when we had them remove their shoes in the morning, their socks seemed to fit their feet. By late afternoon the mounting tension, caused by prolonged sitting without the relief of physical activity, could be seen in their socks. The constant wiggling of little toes had pushed the sock ends out into wads. Later in life, after people have tensed their feet over and over again, the muscles tighten and shorten. They become rigid and often painful.

There was a saying when I was little, "They used to kiss my little feet, but they wouldn't do it now." Cared-for feet are kissable at any age, as are cared-for hands. It's the callused, horny, lumpy, bumpy ones that are not . . . *and they didn't start out that way.* Appearance isn't the only revealing thing about feet; they shout of poor function as well. Do they turn in, which is called *pigeon toes?* Do they turn way out, which is referred to as a *duck waddle?* Are they pancake flat or are the leg muscles spasmed so tight that the little person must tiptoe around the house? All of these conditions will interfere with running and play skills. The poor player is a liability to the team, and the child will get his heart stepped on when somebody says, "Aw, you take him. Our team had him yesterday." Flat, weak, overturned feet walk funny, and since they are the support for the rest of the body, they often set the little person up for poor posture and inadequate function from the moment erect stance is achieved.

Then there is a condition called *the long second toe.* It is a hereditary condition suffered by one or both parents and fully described on page 435. What it amounts to is a structurally poor foot. It is known by several names, and the nicest (and most useful to you) is *the classic Greek foot.* Take the child who has one to any museum boasting a sculpture section and examine the Greek statues.

All of them have overlong second toes. Look at your own foot and see if you, too, are slightly "classic." You need not have a protruding second toe to have the problem. I have a foot that looks almost as square as Huck Finn's river raft, but the "Greek" structure is there nonetheless. See page 435 so that you can determine the state of every foot in the family. Then note what to do about it in order to get the most from your muscles and avoid foot, leg, and back pain, sprained ankles and knees, and even arthritic hips. It's worth the effort and is called "the $1.80 cure."

PAIN: TO BE AVOIDED

In 1976 we found a way to get rid of 95 percent of all muscle pain—and most pain is muscle related. Most children have pain at one time or another, and some children have a lot of pain. They may start out with headaches resulting from birth. That can lead to colic from swallowing air as they scream for hours on end with the head pain. Children may have pain when they're teething, pain when they suffer from colds and grippe. Asthmatics have pain as they struggle for air. Accidents of a hundred kinds cause children pain, as do operations and disease. When children suffer, so do their parents, and you will be glad to know that starting on page 411 is the information that can stop most pain and that you the parent or teacher will be able to do it yourself.

POSTURE

Posture is a dead giveaway when it comes to mood and even attitude. The defeated person usually slumps. The timid, frightened person usually pulls the shoulders forward in a self-protective motion. The person with fatigue (sometimes caused by poor nutrition) seems barely able to stand and begins to fold at various spots in the spine. Since attitudes and patterns are set quite early, so is posture, and it is folly to hope that a girl will stand straight and lift her chest "once she starts to develop." It will be quite the opposite: She will round her shoulders even more. Nor will a boy stand any taller simply because he adds inches. There will just be more of him leaning at that precarious angle. *Check posture now,* and do something about it while habits and bones are green, soft, and pliable.

ROUND BACK

In its extreme form, round back is called *kyphosis.* Look first at the shoulders. Are they straight and thrust back or are they stooped and rounded? Is the upper back flat and wide or do the wings poke out? Diet of course has much to do with posture, since well-fed muscles and bones usually fall into proper alignment. Later in life, when posture is affected by the constant pressures from various occupations, shoulders may be pulled out of line. The dentist and the violinist are prime examples. They are forced to round so much that the chest muscles shorten. With children this *should* be rare indeed, but unfortunately, childhood round backs are all too frequent. If you feel the urge to say "Stand up" half a dozen times a day, your child has the problem. If *you* have the problem, you may not notice it in the child. For help in this ask a friend who has good posture how *you* stand and how your child stands. When you give your family the tests in chapter 2, you will find that the round-back cannot spread his elbows very well in test 4.

If the shoulders round, it follows that there will be other unfortunate and unattractive roundings. The *forward head* is one of these. The rounding spine carries its line right up to the head. Try it yourself. Round your shoulders and your head will bow. In that position, however, you will not be able to see very far in front of you, so you will have to raise your head to lift your eyes. This can be done only if your neck stretches forward, which gives you and everybody else with the problem the look of a turtle emerging. The forward head then leads to stiff and painful shoulders and neck, and headaches. Correct the round back, and the head will come back into line of its own accord (see page 54).

At the other end of the round-back curve is the protruding abdomen, and it is unattractive no matter what size abdomen protrudes, even one as empty of fat as an old sack.

SWAYBACK

This condition seems to show up more often on little girls, although boys are not immune. The angle of the pelvis is accentuated, and a deep curve appears in the back just at the waist. This pushes the buttocks back and the tummy seems to curve outward in front. Very often the child will compensate for this awkwardness by turning the toes out into a ten-past-ten position. It interferes with motion, and eventually the strain can lead to backache.

FLAT BACK

This is not seen as often as the swayback, but it does exist and it does cause back pain. In the flat back the angle of the pelvis is not deep enough—just the opposite of the sway. The back appears to be unusually straight at the waist. It is difficult to get pants and skirts to stay up, and the back looks a little like a flat board.

PROTRUDING ABDOMEN

This can pair with the swayback or it can have the stage all to itself. When a baby is born, his abdominal muscles are very relaxed and its back muscles are stretched as a result of the fetal position. The abdominal muscles must be stretched and strengthened, and it is not childhood that produces the melon tummy, but inactivity. (See the Sources section for my book *How to Keep Your Child Fit From Birth to Six*.) If your child's tummy pokes out, don't count on growth and adolescence to bring it in. Exercise daily.

KNOCK-KNEES

There is still time to correct bone problems, and knock-knees seem to go with being overweight and undervitaminized. They rarely appear on properly fed and exercised children, which immediately gives the clue to correction. Not only is it important to eat as little as possible of foods that do nothing for the body, but it is highly important to provide the builders (see page 264). Strengthen the leg muscles that can provide your child with straight legs only if proper food and exercise are made available.

BOWLEGS

We don't see bow legs often anymore, but occasionally the diet is especially low in vitamin D. An excellent source of vitamin D is sunlight. The trick is not so much getting the sun to the child; if children play outdoors several hours a day, it will find them. Many mothers don't know that vitamin D is caught by the oil on the skin. If faces are washed well with lots of soap, oils are washed away. Then, if they are not replaced with a good skin oil, the vitamin can't find its element. Furthermore, if the sun finds the child and the vitamin D settles down in the oil, it still takes time for the skin to absorb the vitamin D into the body. If one bathes before the several hours needed for the absorption, the vitamin is lost. With this in mind, give sunbaths *after* water baths and *after* applying oil. Then allow several hours to pass before the next cleanup session. That would go for the hot, soapy shower following an hour at the beach. Give the vitamin D a little working time.

DROPPED SHOULDER

If you notice that one of the child's shoulders droops lower than the other, don't assume that it was caused by carrying a briefcase. He hasn't got a briefcase. That theory evolved because the usual time for noticing posture problems is in high school, when they have finally become so bad that even the folks at home see them. *There is nothing so invisible as something you see every day.* The briefcase or the daily stack of books going home for homework may exacerbate the condition causing the unequal shoulders, but it is highly unlikely to have been the primary cause. Sometimes the problem is not so much a dropped shoulder as a raised one. In either case we must look for the spasm in one or more muscles that causes the anomaly. You will find the answer to the child's posture problems as well as your own in the chapter on Myotherapy.

In order to be of value to the child you must now become an observer. *Look for trouble now, while it is still in its beginning stages.* Watch your family with educated eyes. Be aware that the human body is never really "finished" as long as it lives. It changes daily depending on

The Starting Line

the growth stage, the environment, and the level of stress. In addition there are variable influences such as nutrition and exercise, fatigue, and self-image. For these six years your influence will carry weight. Now is the time to make that influence felt.

SCOLIOSIS

Scoliosis means one or more lateral curves in the spine, and there are many causes. Diseases like polio, and accidents, can destroy muscle function, and so can bad habits: The child who continually sits on one foot throws the spine out of line. When we tested the muscles of children in schools where they spent the whole school day in the homeroom, we found more than the usual number of posture problems. It seemed that the light always coming in over the same shoulder forced the children to maintain the same posture all day as they worked at their desks. Ideopathic scoliosis is the usual diagnosis, and *ideopathic* really means "nobody knows why." If you get a note from school saying that your child has scoliosis and must see a doctor at once, don't be alarmed. For most such cases the answer is again muscle spasm, and what to do about that is on page 428.

CHAPTER TWO
TESTS TELL TRUTHS

Any child can fake good posture for the few seconds it takes to snap a posture picture in front of a graph, and it is surprising how quickly they learn what it is you want—shoulders back, tummy flat, seat under, feet parallel, head up. The children at the Posture Clinic at the Presbyterian Hospital in New York City were past masters at complying, and the doctors felt they needed some sort of posture detective. So they developed the Kraus-Weber Test for Minimum Muscle Strength and Flexibility. It is medically valid, takes just ninety seconds to give, is easy to record, and is a cinch to compute—also, it tells the truth.

Years ago when I started exercise classes for my two daughters (success was guaranteed by inviting ten of their friends to join the "class"), I used the test so that I would know if I was doing the right things with the children. It didn't take very long for the original ten children to bring their friends to class, and the friends brought friends. It was important to have not only a test that worked but one that took little time away from classwork and one that pointed unerringly to the deficient area so that I could fix it quickly. Once a deficient area was fixed, I found that everything else improved as well. In time I discovered that there were many extra things the test reported if you had eyes to see with *and if you cared about children.* If you are a parent giving the test, you won't be able to pick up your children's tensions so easily because they know you well and you are not a new experience to them. But if you are a teacher, you will be able to learn things about the children you never suspected. You will be able to help them in ways that will count all the rest of their lives.

THE KRAUS-WEBER TEST

You will need a pillow and a ruler for your testing. Be sure to draw the following test card in your notebook. Teachers will find test sheets for working with a whole class on pages 59–61. The names given to these tests designate areas, not specific muscle groups.

K-W Test Card

A.	Date	A+	A−	P	UB	LB	BHF	B.	Signs	
									Sub.	
									Lead	
									Arch	
									Uneven	
									Curve	

TEST 1: ABDOMINALS PLUS PSOAS (A+)

Purpose: To test the strength of the abdominal muscles plus a muscle *inside* the pelvis called the *psoas* (hip flexors).

Position of Child: Lying supine, hands clasped behind head. Hold the feet down on the table (or floor).

Command: "Keep your hands behind your head and try to roll up to a sitting position." If the child sits up, no matter with what sort of contortions, the test is passed. Put a check under "A+" in box A. If the test was at all difficult, add a small *c* to the check. If the child could not sit up, enter a 0 in the box. Illness and bed rest will turn a *c* into a 0, so do correctives (pages 25–29) whenever you had to add *c* to the check.

There are two clues a child may give you while doing this. The first one is called *substitution.* When you say, "Roll up," you mean just that. The head should come off the table first; then, with a rounded back, the rest of the torso follows. Most children today who have never seen the old-fashioned (very bad) straight-back sit-up will roll up *if they can.* If they come up with a stiff, straight back, usually accompanied by a hitching jerk, it is because some area of muscle is not functioning. Try again and make it very clear that you want a nice *round* roll-up. If the straight sit-up is repeated, put a check next to "Sub." (substitution) in box B. Make a mental note to work endlessly with exercise 1.

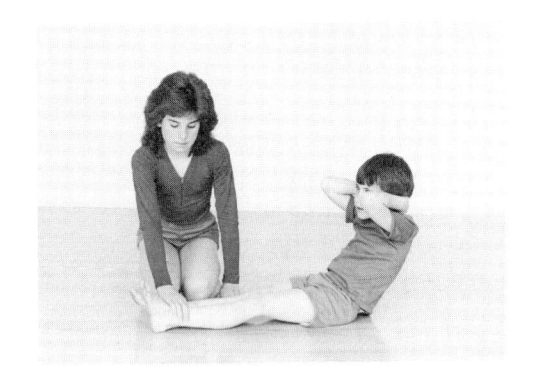

The second clue is called *lead.* As the child rolls up, one elbow may lead and the other follow. This indicates another imbalance caused by another "lazy" area. Put the letter *L* for a left-elbow lead or *R* for a right-elbow lead next to "Lead" in box B. Have your child do exercise 1, but for the present *with the other elbow in advance.* When you get an even sit-up, you will know the weak area has been strengthened.

TEST 2: ABDOMINALS MINUS PSOAS (A−)

Purpose: This is a further test for the abdominals. First, slide feet toward *seat.* The bent-knee position lessens the assisting power of the psoas, throwing most of the strain on the abdominals.

Position of the Child: Same as for test 1, but with knees bent.

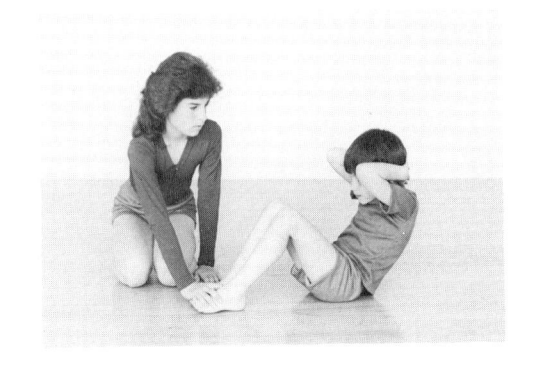

Command: "Keep your hands behind your neck and roll up into a sitting position." If the child can sit up, put a check under "A – " in box A. If it was difficult, add a small *c.* If it was impossible, enter a O.

Watch for the same clues as in test 1 and also watch for a leading elbow as the child goes back down onto the table.

TEST 3: PSOAS (P)

Purpose: To test the strength of the psoas or hip flexors. This area is developed by running, skipping, and jumping.

Position of Child: Same as for test 1.

Command: "Keep your knees straight and lift your feet up to here [indicate a point about 10 inches above the table] while I count." The count is ten seconds. Using a stopwatch is inadvisable, since checking a watch necessitates taking your eyes from the child and contact is lost. Just add a three-syllable word after the number (such as "*one*-chim-pan-zee, *two*-chim-pan-zees," etc.); this is quite reliable.
Ideally the child's spine should remain flat on the table or very slightly arched. The pelvis should remain fixed.

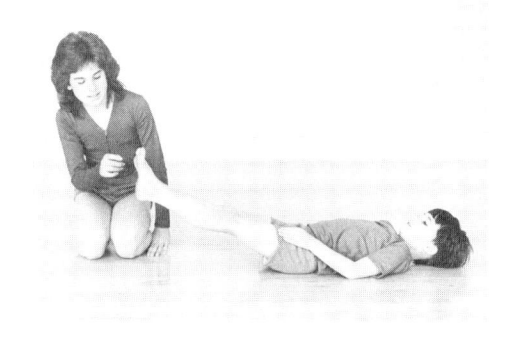

If the child must either hitch the pelvis or force the back up into a strong arch in order to lift the legs, the test may be passed, but the clue to weakness is there. Enter a check next to "Arch" in box B. If the child can hold for the ten-second count, put a check under "P" in box A. If it is difficult, add a small *c.* To correct failure or "arch," do exercise 2.

TEST 4: UPPER BACK (UB)

Purpose: To test the strength of the upper back muscles.

Position of Child: Lying prone with a pillow or rolled towel under the hips. This gives the body the appearance and function of a seesaw, which, if weighted at either end, would be able to hold the other end in the air. Hands are clasped behind the head, and feet are held down by pressure over the calves.

Command: "Put your hands behind your head and raise your chest, head, and shoulders like a plane taking off. Hold while I count." With young children it helps to place one hand on a shoulder and pull upward to give them direction. Don't let the child arch unduly, or you will bring other muscles into play. The count is ten seconds as in test 3.

While the child holds the position, search for clue number four, uneven development in the two ridges of muscle that flank the spine. Cup your free hand over the muscles at the waist, first on one side of the spine, then the other. Move up and repeat at mid and then upper back. If an imbalance exists, you will be able to feel it. Enter the letter for right or left indicating the thicker side,

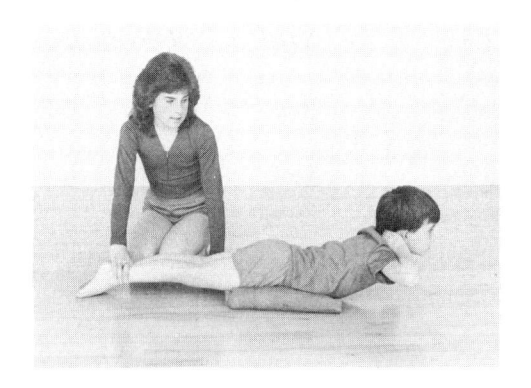

next to "Uneven" in box B and make a mental note to check the back clue carefully when you get to test 6. Put a check under "UB" for pass and a 0 if the lift was not maintained for ten seconds. To correct, do exercise 3.

TEST 5: LOWER BACK (LB)

Purpose: To test the strength of the lower back.

Position of Child: Prone over the pillow as in test 4, head resting on arms and back held down by pressure on the upper back.

Command: "Lift your legs up, but don't bend your knees. Hold legs up while I count." Again the count is for ten seconds. Passing rates a check under "LB" and failure a 0. The corrective is exercise 4.

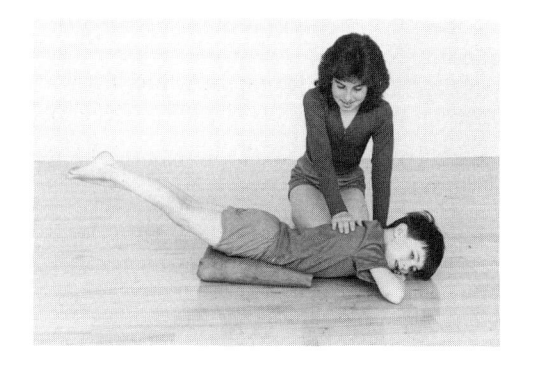

TEST 6: FLEXIBILITY OF BACK AND HAMSTRINGS (BHF)

Purpose: To test the flexibility of the back and hamstring muscles. This is the only one in the battery of tests that tests flexibility—which, incidentally, seems to be the greatest problem American children have. Since flexibility relates to stress and tension, it is important to check for its absence and provide it as quickly as possible.

Position: Standing erect in socks or bare feet, feet together, legs straight, and arms at sides.

Command: "Keep your knees straight and lean over *slowly*. See how close you can bring your fingertips to the floor. Stay down there while I count." This time the count is only three seconds. *Do not allow bouncing or permit any warm-up.* The farthest point reached without bouncing and held for three seconds is the marking point. Use the ruler to determine exactly how far the fingertips are from the floor. Touching is a pass and rates a check under "BHF" in box A. If the child failed to touch, enter the minus distance. To correct, use exercise 6 (page 30). The Back and Hamstring Flexibility Test should then be done a second time. The first time you were looking for flexibility; the second time you will be screening for scoliosis. If you stand behind the child as he or she *slowly* leans down to touch the floor, you will be able to spot a scoliosis at once if one is present: One side of the back will be higher than the other at some time during the descent. If it is, don't panic; it is easy to fix. Turn to page 428 in the chapter on Myotherapy and take it from there.

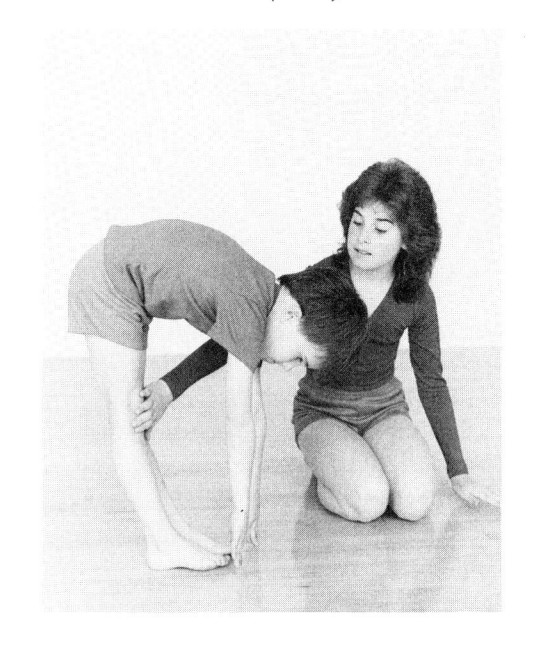

The K-W test is a *minimum* test, and everyone, even Great-grandpa, should be able to pass it if he is to get along comfortably in simple everyday living. Of course the minimum would never be enough for a child who wanted to be a good dancer or athlete, just as it would never be enough for the woman who expects a baby or the man who wants to play golf or tennis over the weekend. Once the test is passed, you'll want to go on from there. Minimums are all very well, but they will not be enough for you. Refer to the Prudden Supplement (PS) Test for Optimum Performance on page 31.

In 1945 I started to test many children over the course of each year, and I found that when some of them came to my classes for the first time in September, they performed miserably. They failed the test that the doctors said any healthy child could pass. By spring of the following year, after we had worked on both specific areas and a general program, most went home with a passing mark. It didn't seem to matter what they did over the summer—stay home, visit cousin Emily, or go to camp—they lost ground during those three months. When we tested again in the fall, we found they had lost both strength and flexibility. But the return to normal was much quicker in their second year, and on the test for optimums they improved quickly. By the following spring all but 4 percent of the children could pass—and pass easily. Then came the miracle. The second summer, no matter what they did, they kept their gains, and many even improved. It seemed that once the major weaknesses in *the key posture areas* are corrected, the rest of the body can use any daily activity to build strength, flexibility, and coordination.

While doing a series of tests on newcomers, the following autumn I discovered that the failure rate for the group was 58 percent. I had always been concerned with individuals before and had never bothered to compute a group as a whole. I was horrified. Had I been giving the tests wrong? After all, doctors had assured me this was the minimum for health—but 58 percent of the children flunked! I called the hospital, and a check the following week showed that the tests were being given correctly; something was certainly wrong with the children.

At the request of the doctors I set up testing teams and started to check on not only children but adults in every walk of life. We tested the children in both public and private schools, whole towns and cities. We went to nursery schools, parochial schools, Sunday schools, and schools for the handicapped, the disturbed, and the delinquent. We checked out colleges and universities, prisons, camps, and even homes for the elderly. We separated people into sports groups and work groups, rural, suburban, and urban. Nobody escaped, not even policemen. We then went to Italy, Switzerland, Austria, and Guatemala. Some of my colleagues tested in Japan and Scandinavia, and people interested in physical education sent in reports from India, Australia, New Zealand, Great Britain, and Canada. The YMCA sent representatives to my institute to be trained in the test procedures and began testing in every state in America. The results make nervous reading.

Adults could pass the test with greater regularity than young people, especially the floor-touch test for flexibility. Boys everywhere were worse off than girls, and the same went for grownups. Europe was in much better shape than America as far as public school children were concerned; Europeans had an 8.7 percent failure compared to our 57.9 percent failure. Right behind us came Canada and Great Britain. The test results from India, which showed a 39 percent failure, told us that even hunger was not as bad as lack of exercise. In Guatemala—where I had hoped to find even better figures than I'd found in Europe, because Guatemalans were closer to nature and were even more dependent on their muscles for their daily living—I found that food did play a part. Lacking in protein and other nutrients, many had what is called *compression lordosis,* an extreme swayback. The weight of burdens carried on little heads supported by poorly fed bodies forced their backs to bend so far that they lost as much as five inches in height. They had sprue and numerous intestinal parasites, but the failure rate was still only 27 percent. The failure rate in Japan was reported as only 15 percent. The question kept coming up: Why is it so terrible here?

I began a study of our way of life—how it differed from other parts of the world and even how it differed from place to place here. There was still room for children to roam in the rural areas, and the failure rate in Vermont was the lowest I found in public schools.

In one study where there were no school buses we found that the children living in the valley (the school was on a high plateau) had a lower failure than the children living on the plateau—but it was the only place we found children lucky enough to be without buses.

When we checked on very young children, we found only two groups with perfect scores, a day care center in Guatemala City and one in southern Austria. Both groups had good diets and played out of doors all day every day. There was no question that exercise and food played important roles.

Economics had something to do with it too. Six-year-olds coming into public schools had a 53.7 percent failure, while their peers entering private schools were up to 58.3 percent. What a sad commentary on American childhood. European youngsters entered school with a failure of 7.8 percent. Certainly nobody could blame that enormous discrepancy on the inactivity associated with school days. It had to start at home, and a quick survey of what went on in homes bore this out.

The American baby comes home from the hospital in pretty fair shape. Home is usually clean, and mother has read all the books. Baby is popped into a crib, usually well wrapped in many layers to avoid drafts. The baby's days are spent in singular inaction (a puppy would rebel at once; our children wait until later). When it's time for solid food, the baby is put in a highchair, then onto a toidy seat. Then, well wrapped, he is parked in the yard (if there is a yard) in a carriage. At noon the baby is unwrapped, washed, oiled, powdered, rewrapped, stuffed into the highchair, stuffed full of lunch, stuffed onto the toidy seat, and then popped into bed for "rest." The question should come right now: Rest from what?

After the nap the baby is dressed in warm clothes (his mother feels the cold) and stuffed into a stroller. At the supermarket he rides in a basket, and if he is noisy (he soon learns to be noisy), something tasty and highly caloric is stuffed into his mouth. At the checkout counter the baby and the groceries are stuffed together into the stroller, and home they all roll. He is then unwrapped, as are the groceries. The groceries go into the cupboard, and the baby goes into the playpen. He immediately sets up a wail and his mother freaks out; she has been reading what somebody said Freud said. Freud said that many adult neuroses have their roots in early childhood. The interpreters said that children can be destroyed by unhappiness in childhood, and it was every mother's duty to keep children happy—to provide love and a climate conducive to growth and individual development. The wailing child is obviously not happy. Why should he be? He is a small growing animal like a puppy or a kitten and needs action. So far he hasn't done one thing all day that an eighty-year-old man with arthritis couldn't do better.

The mother, however, hasn't made this deduction. For some reason she thinks it's perfectly natural for a child to throw all his toys out of his playpen while he rocks back and forth like a frantic lion at the zoo. What scares her are the tears splattering on the bib: The baby is unhappy. The right thing, of course, would have been to burn the playpen in the fireplace, put a gate on the door, and turn the baby loose with a bunch of boxes, blocks, and pots to bang. It would have helped if she had exercised the baby's arms and legs every time she changed his pants and let him "swim" in the tub. It would make all the difference if that baby, once on his feet, had to walk a few blocks on those sturdy little legs. But these sensible answers to stress caused by inaction never entered her thinking. Instead she turns on the TV right over the baby's head (she's in the kitchen, so it has to be loud as well as lousy) and feels content that neurosis has been held at bay.

This all sounds pretty extreme, and not all of it happens the same way to the same baby every day. However, enough of it does happen and to enough babies to inhibit their development of even minimum strength and flexibility. Since coordination is made up of strength and flexibility in proper timing and intensity, a lot of trouble is brewing for more than half the children in America.

I was raised by physical educators. First there was a black-eyed, always tanned lady at DeWitt Clinton No. 9. She taught us to stand straight, turn sharp corners when we marched, right-dress, do "setting-up exercise" in the classrooms between classes, and play dodgeball to win even if a shoe fell off.

Then there was Herr Schmidt. He taught down at the Turn Verein where my best friend went. By the time I got there, I thought I was pretty hot stuff. He showed me I wasn't, but that maybe, with terribly hard work, I might get to be passable.

Miss Sullivan followed. She was the first one to tell me that growing up was a difficult business, and it had been for her, too.

Agnita Powell, the English hockey coach, told me I played the most scientific game she'd ever seen, I was always where the ball was. Herr Schmidt had made us run our lungs out from the time we were eight. I really didn't know much about hockey, but I sure could run—that's why I was where the ball was.

Miss Gulick taught me to hold my temper and to look for the one thing a student could do well—and to say so. I really learned most of my teaching from Miss Gulick.

Ruth Jones opened the door to modern dance and got me my first real teaching job at Camp Tegawitha. She expected a great deal of me, and I learned that if much is expected, one usually finds the strength to produce.

Physical educators were often the only family, friends, and hope I had. When test scores showed that something was very wrong with the bodies of the children, I went to the physical educators to find out why physical education wasn't fixing it.

The first thing I found out was that 91 percent of our elementary schools did not have gyms. Way back in the 1920s we had gyms—what happened? It turned out that what had happened was a combination of the Depression, the population explosion, and some more of those helpful interpreters, this time John Dewey's. Dewey said education should have more scope, that it should have more imagination and less authoritarianism. Someone interpreted that to mean that in physical education we should give up all those nasty authoritarian commands like "Attention!" "Right face!" "Hands on hips . . . place!" Instead of unimaginative calisthenics that didn't do anything *but build bodies*, we could have games that built self-confidence and good sportsmanship. Besides, said the interpreters, children love games (true of some children), and they'll be happy, which Freud says they have to be. Along with being happy they'll all get healthy playing. The trouble was it didn't work out that way.

Play was substituted for work; that happened all right, and it was even called "play." Well, you couldn't very easily dignify "play" as a subject, so pretty soon "play" didn't even appear on report cards. Then came the Depression. When committees met to decide where school expenditures should be made, "play" got short shrift: "My kids need an education—they can *play* at home." My friends, the great teachers who had once taught me the basics of life and living, would have been horrified. The last hired was the PE teacher—and he or she was also the first fired when the going got rough.

To round out the whole sad story we had a population explosion. The Depression had put classrooms and labs ahead of gyms; the population explosion turned the few existing gyms into classrooms and labs. Phys. ed. was relegated to the playground (where the new American mother, reared on protecting children rather than preparing them, soon put a stop to any real action) and was more often taught by the classroom teacher, who obviously had more than enough to do without *that*.

Just how devastating this turn of affairs was showed up in the tests. Since "play" was the order of the day, that's what the children got, even when the unwilling perpetrator of the crime was a perfectly well-trained teacher of the old school. To begin with, in order to teach, you must have a place in which to teach, and as we have seen, most schools didn't have such places. The "all-purpose room" (which I call the "no-purpose room") is certainly not an answer to anything. The teacher couldn't get going until all the buses had arrived, and had to get out by eleven thirty so that the cooks could get set up for lunch. The afternoon was often interrupted for band practice, the class play, the orchestra, and meetings every other Tuesday. Besides, it was right next to the study hall, and quiet was never first cousin to physical activity. On top of all these small irritations, there wasn't a single piece of apparatus (basketball nets are not apparatus), the floor was tile over cement (which is very resistant to bones, especially skulls), and the ceiling was so low that the only "play" activity no longer considered un-American, a ball game, was out of the question. What was left? Square dancing.

Then there was the question of getting the time in which to teach. Since physical education had been reduced to "play," it had very little status. If there were sixty children of assorted sizes and abilities without anything specific to do, they were sent to physical education. If there was a rehearsal or a makeup exam, it was no trouble to "get them out of physical education." Principals, who have enough trouble trying to meet state requirements, were absolutely delighted when there were none (in most states) for phys. ed.; it gave them a chance to juggle schedules. It also drove many of the best PE teachers out of the field. Nobody minds working hard and long if there are great results. Nobody worth a plug nickel stays on a job that requires merely that they be there, take the roll, and throw a ball out on the floor—and it showed up on the tests.

The children in first grade failed at 54 percent, and by the time they reached fourth grade they still had 54 percent failure. The private schools did a bit better; probably because more time was allotted to PE, they had gone down from 58 percent to 43 percent failure. However, the Europeans had an 11 percent failure rate in fourth grade.

Junior high is a very important place, and those years are very important years. For one thing, you usually go to a new school, studies get harder, and things start to happen to your body and your emotions. If there is one thing you really need at this point in life, it's physical outlets. First off, you still *like* physical outlets; then, too, sitting all the time is such a drag. I checked with friends who taught in junior high. One of them had two hundred in a class. When I asked what she could teach two hundred kids at one time, she exploded: "*Teach!* Who *teaches?* I take the roll—that's how we know who's in school."

Then I checked on the school one of my daughters was attending. I sat there in the gym and watched. They were very proud of the gym at that school. It was big and polished—but empty. Not a single piece of apparatus cluttered its gleaming floors. Thirty little kids rushed into the locker room, and I timed them—from the moment they got there, took off school clothes, wriggled into gym clothes, dashed (not terribly fast: there's a rule about running) up to the gym, stood in line, took the roll, and decided what they would play, they had used up ten minutes. They had to do the same in reverse, so there were twenty minutes left. Since the game was basketball, only ten could play at a time; the other twenty sat on the floor and watched. Three groups into twenty minutes gives each child about six and a half minutes on the floor. Twice a week this adds up to thirteen minutes. *Thirteen minutes a week* in which to build the bodies that will support the brains—and make no mistake: It is the body that supports the brain and even puts a limit on it. Thirteen minutes a week in which to prepare for life, for a battlefield, for the delivery room, for the daily grind that goes with nine to five in the office (but three hours getting there and back). What teacher can teach French in thirteen minutes, or English, physics, chemistry, history, or in fact anything? No teacher can do that job.

My friend Ruth Jones is dead, and her loss as a teacher cannot be adequately appreciated unless you realize that she reached even the least likely pupil when it came to physical activity. But even she could have done very little in the time and under the conditions allotted to physical education today. The tests for junior high showed that 62 percent of the children coming up from the elementary grades flunked the minimum test. Now in most schools, if there is a time when PE starts for real, it's in junior high, but so do the new things that happen to young bodies about that time and the tension that goes along with it. In the two junior high years the failure rate climbed to 65 percent. In the private schools where parents paid tuition and asked about PE and teachers had a chance to really work children, things were better; they went from 40 percent failure to 33 percent. The difference was not only in time spent but in program. If you have time, you can work up a program—if you don't, you are stuck with a sort of fill-in recreation. In Europe the failure rate dropped from 10 percent to 8 percent. Knowing what we do now about the part the body plays in brain function, I can only feel how lucky those children were—and are. Studying comes so much easier when the body is fit.

High school is the *dernier cri* for most kids. It's the last possible chance to get the most for the least effort when it comes to anything physical. There's still time, you feel pretty good, and you like movement. A couple of years after graduation most people are bogged down one way or another. If they have to go to work, there is usually not much energy left over in the evenings, and if they haven't developed a motor skill in childhood, they don't find getting started quite so easy. It depends a lot on what your friends do, but the tests say more than half of them don't do much of anything. If you get pregnant, life is going to be a round of baby chores and weariness unless you are in shape for it, and 58.6 percent are not. If you go to college, studies take up a lot of time. I can remember the head of the physical education department at Vassar asking me what could be done to motivate girls to take part in sports. I felt like saying, "It is too late—it should have been done in elementary school," but I didn't.

The tests had showed that 60 percent

of the thirteen-year-olds flunked the test in public schools while 31 percent of the private school kids flunked. Ten percent of the Europeans failed. In their first year in public high school the youngsters worsened until they failed at the rate of 63 percent. I asked one desperate friend who taught those classes for girls why 55 percent of them couldn't do a single sit-up, and she waved a fistful of notes under my nose. Every last one of them had been written by mothers asking to have their daughters excused because of menstrual cramps. "If I could get past the mothers long enough to exercise the girls, they wouldn't *have* cramps."

And it wasn't only the mothers of girls writing those notes. The boys had excuses too, everything from asthma to dizzy spells. Most of the notes were transparent frauds written by mothers still under the spell of Freud's interpreters: "Keep them happy, keep them happy."

Inflexibility is intricately tied up with tension, and tension signs mean that stress is piling up, that there isn't enough outlet to support healthy living. What, then, does it mean to you when the tests on thirteen-year-old boys show that 75 percent cannot touch the floor, as in test 6? Forty-one percent of the private school boys had the same problem, but only 15 percent of the European boys were that tense.

When the youngsters were graduated at sixteen from public schools, 52 percent were still failing, and when I asked one of the best physical education men in the system why so much time was spent on teams when so many other kids were in desperate shape, he answered me very sadly, "Because coaches have to eat." It seems that if a man is hired for a high school, he is expected to get out a winning team. If he spends his time on *all* the boys, the team suffers, and when the team loses, parents begin to call up. He may get away with it one year, but not two, and soon he is looking for another job. Nobody asks what he was able to do for *all* the boys—only what his record of wins was. If he repeats the same thing in a second town, his chances of getting a job in the third are slim indeed. *He* knew what to do for the kids, and he wanted to do it. It was parent power that stood in the way. Now, my question to you is this: Is your son on the team, and if not, what is *he* getting at school and what are *you* doing to back up the coach who wants to do a job? If such a coach is not at your school, do you know about it? The kids do—ask them.

And now it's 1987. Things should be better, shouldn't they? You will be distressed to hear that they are much worse. Whereas back in the forties and fifties little children coming into school failed at 54 percent, today they range between 85 and 100 percent failure. The overall failure rate is way up and so are blood pressure, cholesterol levels, and obesity. Ninety-eight percent of the children have at least one risk of a heart attack—*and these are children!*

Yes, you need this book. More than ever.

CHAPTER THREE
A STITCH IN TIME

One of the troubles with tests is that while they tell you which children don't measure up, they don't always tell you either why they don't or what to do about it. The Kraus-Weber test told you exactly where the trouble is (and if everybody in your family passed, wait a minute—we'll get to them).

The following exercises are correctives for the areas pointed out by the tests. If your children (or you) had difficulty with any area, be sure to make a project of these exercises. Not only will passing be possible, but performance in general will improve.

ABDOMINALS

Failure or even difficulty in tests 1 or 2 means that the all-important abdominal area is weak. You and the child should do the following series *several times a day* until passing is possible. Then continue with exercise 1C (page 27) for the rest of your life.

1. BENT-KNEE SIT-UPS

1A.

• Start lying supine with bent knees, feet held down, and arms extended on the floor above the head. *Throw* the arms forward and allow the momentum to carry the body to the sitting position. If the child (or you) cannot effect even one such sit-up, then start in the sitting-*up* position and roll *slowly* down with chin on chest and arms extended forward. Get up any way possible and repeat five times daily. When a sit-*up* can be done with ease, move on to exercise 1B.

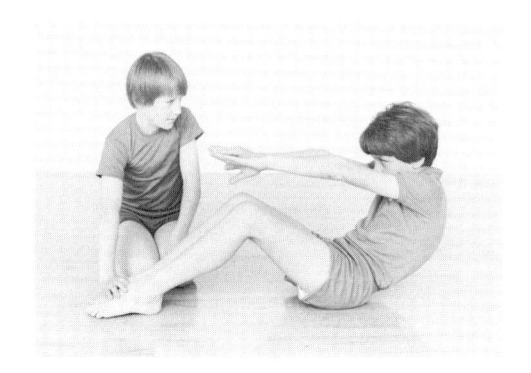

If there is a check next to "Sub." in box B on the K-W test card, see that the head stays down and the back *rounded* on both sit-ups and roll-downs. At first you may have to provide some help for the last third of the roll-down. It may take a little time for the vacationing muscles to resume their responsibilities.

1B.

• *Cross the arms over the chest and roll up to the sitting position. If this is too difficult, sit* up *with arms extended and roll down* slowly *with arms across the chest.*
• *Do this several times a day, working toward a roll-*up *with the arms crossed. If you put an R or an L in the space next to "Lead" in box B, have the child* lead *with the following side when doing the roll-downs and later the roll-ups.*

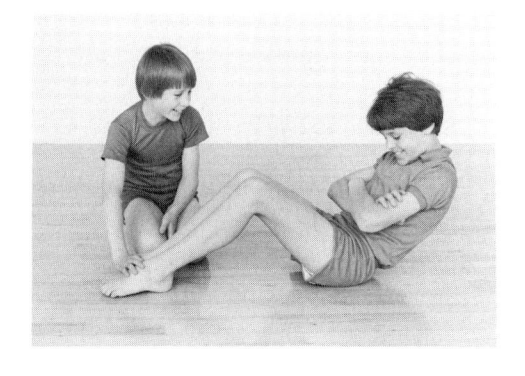

1C.

- *Place the hands behind the neck, as in tests 1 and 2 (page 14), and roll down slowly.*
- *Roll up with arms folded across the chest. Repeat several times a day until rolling up with the hands in back of the neck is possible. Remember to* round the back, *and if one elbow led in the test, lead with the opposite until an even sit-up can be done with ease.*

PSOAS

If the child (or you) failed test 3 for psoas, or hip-flexor, strength (page 15), it means that not enough time has been spent running, skipping, jumping, and climbing. Add these activities to your lives as often as possible.

2. SPINE-DOWN STRETCH

- *Start supine with bent knees and spine pressed tight to the floor. That is the* rest *position.*
- *Next, stretch the legs straight up toward the ceiling at right angles to the body.*
- *Return to the* rest *position.*
- *In the second extension, drop the legs about six inches closer to the floor while checking the back.* The back must stay tight to the floor.
- *Return to the* rest *position.*
- *On the third extension, drop the legs still lower and return.*

At some point you will notice that the back has left the floor; that means you have gone too far for the strength of the psoas.

- *Return to the level of the last successful extension in which the back was able to stay on the floor, and do five.*

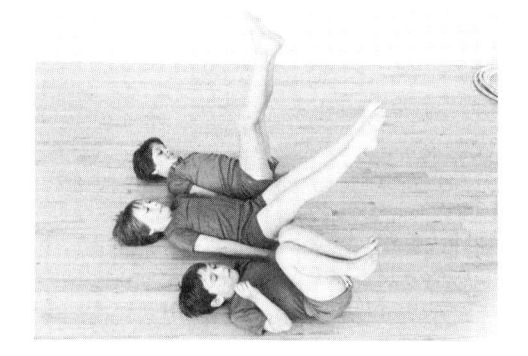

As the strength of the psoas improves, you will be able to go lower and lower. *Never do straight leg lifts from the floor until you can do an extension an inch above the floor with the spine held down.* The spine-down stretch is also used for correction of swayback and for the clue "Arch" in box B.

3. UPPER-BACK LIFT

If the child (or you) had difficulty with test 4 for the upper back, (page 15) do this exercise first with both legs flat on the floor (note the child on the right in the picture).
- *Lie prone with arms extended straight ahead on the floor.*
- *Lift first one arm and set it down, then the other and set it down.*
- *Alternate arms for 8.* Do not roll your chest from side to side. *Even if you had no trouble with tests 4 or 5, do the exercise as a preventive.*

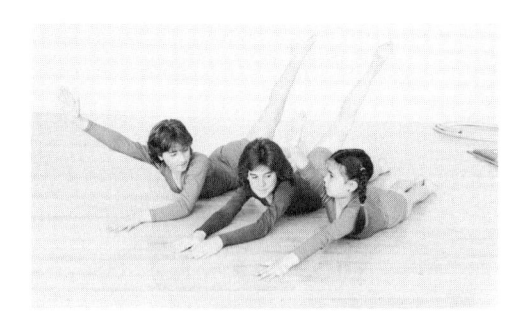

4. LOWER-BACK LIFT

This is the corrective for test 5 (page 16).
- *Stay prone, like the child in the middle of the trio.*
- *Stretch your arms forward as for exercise 3.*
- *Raise first one leg and then the other. Alternate for 8 counts and then go back to exercise 3.*
- *Alternate for eight counts with the arms and follow with exercise 4 again.*

5. DIAGONAL PULL-BACK LIFT

- *Extend both arms and legs.*
- *Raise the right arm and the left leg.*
- *Lower; raise the left arm and right leg.*
- *Start with 8 and work up to 16.*
- *As strength improves, finish each 8 with two lifts, in which both legs and both arms are raised all at once.*

The last of the tests, and therefore the last of the correctives, tells more than any of the others (except perhaps test 2, the one for the abdominals minus the psoas). While failure in that test points to less than the minimum abdominal strength for simple, daily living, failure to pass test 6 (page 17), the one for back and hamstring flexibility, means even more. Abdominal weakness assures poor athletic performance in youth and is an almost infallible augury for back pain in adulthood, if not before. Inflexibility also predicts back pain. In addition, it prevents the development of an athlete's potential and predisposes to injury, *and* it has a secret to divulge: *It is a sign of stress.* Babies are not born with inflexible bodies; that happens later when the child is exposed to stress *and is not provided with the physical outlets to defuse that stress.*

Poor coaching can cause inflexibility, but it is the rare American child—other than swimmers, divers, gymnasts, and dancers—who is exposed to well-rounded coaching. Coaches of those sports know that flexibility *must* be maintained for success—not only the child's but also their own.

The excuse once offered for inflexible basketball teams—that the boys had long legs and short arms—holds no water at all, as proven by the underwear and airplane manufacturers who measured many thousands of boys and men. If your child, or your team, is inflexible, put the excuses away and get to work providing that all-important combination: Remember—*strength plus flexibility in the proper timing and intensity yields coordination.* Coordination is the stuff of success.

There is something else you need to know about flexibility and the exercise used to achieve it. It comes best through coaxing, not by determination. As usual with the body, the muscles respond best to the rhythms found in music rather than a voice counting "One, two, three, four." For centuries dancers, who have always been noted for their flexibility and flowing motions as well as for their incredible strength and control, used what is now called *ballistic stretch.* This means improving flexibility through *gentle*, rhythmic bouncing. That much the "ancients" had right. Where they were wrong, however, was in *when* they did their stretch. They started off their practice sessions with stretch, which is asking for injury. A cold muscle needs to be warmed up with the kind of rhythmic exercise that calls for no extreme effort or stretch at all.

In the early 1930s physical education took a turn for the worse in America. Girls, who were erroneously reputed to be fragile, were disenfranchised, and the first sign was a change in exercises. Someone in physical education discovered that pubescent and postpubescent girls developed glands on their upper torsos and that these glands, called breasts, *could* be heavy, certainly heavier than those on boys. Suddenly girls were not expected to do a normal push-up, but must do "modified" push-ups, from their knees. That was the start of a different kind of thinking, the Make-It-Easier School. And it went downhill from there. Next came chin-ups which were to be done on a slant with heels on the floor. That was followed by half knee-bends. Full knee-bends were outlawed because they had hurt some football players and weight lifters. No one seemed to understand that *the knees of players engaging in such activities were injured by those sports, not by full knee-bends.*

Then ballistic stretch came under scrutiny, and a huge effort was made to replace it with something called *static stretch*, which was inspired by the importation of yoga. In static stretch, the stretch is carried to its ultimate (inside the bounds of pain) and held for forty to sixty seconds. As with the "ancients," no consideration was given to warming the cold, tight muscles before making this effort. One trouble with yoga in America is our cold climate. In much of India the temperature is 120 degrees F in the shade, and everyone is warm most of the time. Not so in the United States, outside of the Sun Belt. Secondarily, but not unimportant, are the types of personalities in the two countries. In India much attention is given to introspection and the achievement of serenity. Not so in America. We are a tense, driving, often violent people, who need strong physical outlets for our tensions.

To find out which of the two stretch systems got the better results was easy. All one had to do was pay a visit to a PE class using static stretch and another to a dance class using ballistic stretch. Students in the former were tight and lacking in flexibility in every joint. Pupils of the dance master were flexible, lithe, and coordinated.

The outcome of the stretch controversy will make you comfortable with all the stretch exercises in this book. Something "new" has been discovered: It is called *pulsing*. What is it? It is simply ballistic stretch with a brand-new name. Later in the book you will discover other "new" activities that have evolved as our exercise pendulum takes wide swings year after year. One thing you may want to use is common sense—the use of that commodity really is "new" in our country.

6. BACK AND HAMSTRING STRETCH

• *Stand with feet well apart, knees straight, hands clasped behind the back, and head up.*
• *Lean forward from the hips and, keeping the head up,* bounce the upper body downward 8 times. *A pull will be felt behind the knees.*
• *Next, allow the upper body to relax and fall downward toward the floor in 8 easy bounces. Be sure that everything is relaxed—head, neck, torso, shoulders, arms, and hands.*
• *Repeat to both right and left, and once more to the center.*

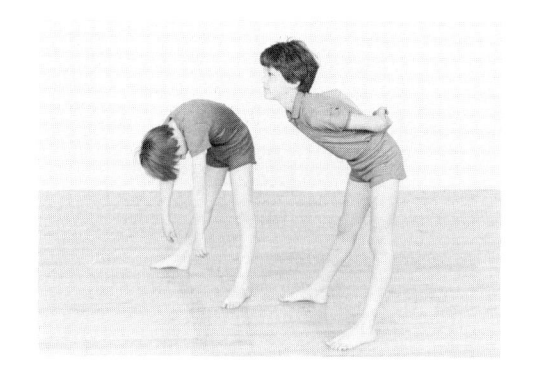

CHAPTER FOUR
HOW GOOD ARE YOU ... REALLY?

THE PRUDDEN SUPPLEMENT TEST FOR OPTIMUM PERFORMANCE

Passing a minimum test isn't enough. That is barely the beginning. Now you go on to the next step, and the next step, like the first one, should involve the whole family.

The P-S test, like the K-W, is simple, requires little time to administer, and is easily recorded and computed. Most important, it yields useful data. It differs from the K-W test in that it is designed to test for optimum performance.

It, too, involves key posture muscles, but adds arm and shoulder girdle strength and tests legs for explosive power.

School people are very prone to seek norms in tests. Individuals can test themselves against norms, but norms have a way of giving a sense of confidence where, as in the United States, it may be wholly undeserved. Technically advanced nations such as ours must realize that our way of life has weakened us to the point where "norms" for us are the norms of a *physically* inferior people.

In the United States there has even been a trend toward lowering requirements when large numbers of students are unable to pass a given test. Two notable examples of this shortsighted action were "modified" push-ups and chin-ups for girls and the total exclusion of flexibility tests (in which American children make a very poor showing).

The P-S is meant for self-competition, but there is no reason why it cannot also be used for family and group competition.

Make another test card in your notebook and label it "Optimum Test."

P-S for Optimum Performance

Date	Push-up	Sit-up	Chin-up	Broad Jump	Flex.

TEST 1: PUSH-UPS

Start in the prone position *flat on the floor*, toes curled under, the backs of your arms on the floor at your sides. This is called the starting position, and *you return to it between each push-up*. This means that you will have to lift your body weight from the floor each time, and it is the initial lift which is the most difficult; the half push-up is no real test. Next, place your hands flat on the floor just outside your shoulders. *Keeping the body rigid*, push up from the floor until the arms are straight. Then let the body down *slowly*, taking three seconds for the descent. Come to rest at the starting position. That is one push-up. Continue in this manner for as many as possible. (Note: Push-ups for girls are the same as for boys. Modification should not even be considered.) Enter the number under "Push-up."

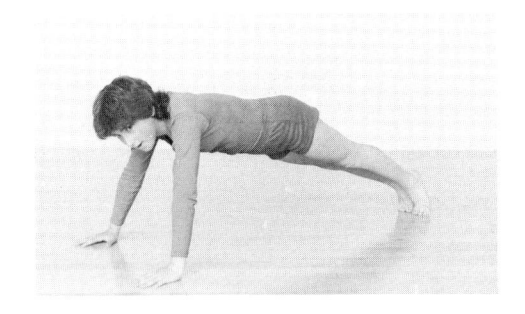

To increase the number of push-ups, do half the number achieved during the test both night and morning. After a month, retest and then do half the new number.

How Good Are You . . . Really?

7. LET-DOWNS FOR PUSH-UPS

If you were unable to do even one push-up, don't be discouraged.

• *Take the position at the top of the push-up but with legs spread wide. Be sure to keep the body rigid. There must be no sway in the back (neither the child's nor yours).* Yes, you should do this exercise too, whether you are a teacher or a parent. Fitness is for everyone, and children learn by example, not from being *told* what to do. If you are in shape and can be a good example for them, they will copy you. If you are a good example of someone trying to *become* a good exerciser, they will cheer you, help you, and *also* copy you. Of the two examples, the second is the more valuable to the struggling child.

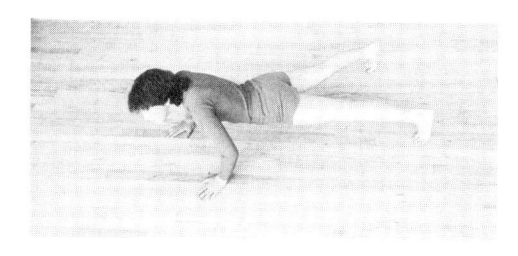

• *From the top of the push-up, lower yourself* slowly *to the floor, trying to take 5 seconds for the descent. Get up to the top of the push-up any old way, and descend again. Do 3 night and morning, and in a month test again. You will then be able to do at least 1 push-up, as will the children.*

When you test for optimum strength of the abdominals, keep in mind that testing to exhaustion by repetition is not only the hard way, it's the *wrong* way, and it will cost you later in life. Any injury to the coccyx or the muscles in that area can lead to back pain as well as spasm in the floor of the pelvis. Such spasm can cause everything from menstrual cramps to impotence in later years. The best way to get a good picture of the optimum strength of the subject, whether that subject be a child, a teacher, or a parent, is by the use of weight bags (see page 190).

A set of weight bags is made up of two five-pounders, two two-pounders, and two one-pounders. They add up to sixteen pounds—more than enough to test the average person.

TEST 2: WEIGHTED SIT-UPS

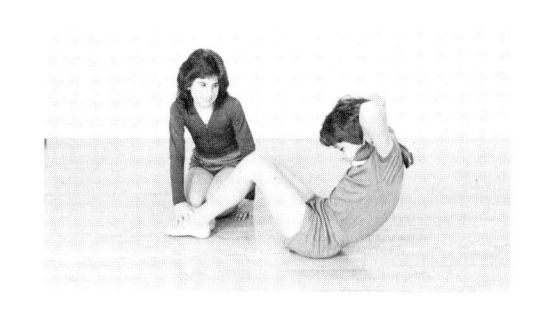

Have the child take the bent-knee sitting position with hands behind the head and feet held down. Place a 1-pound weight bag in the child's hands. The child rolls down to the lying position, sits up once and rolls down again. Replace the 1-pounder with a 2-pound bag. The child sits up holding the heavier weight. Keep adding a pound with each sit-up until it is not possible to sit up with the last added weight. Enter the last weight carried on the test card. *The child then does 5 sit-ups morning and night, carrying one-half the heaviest weight carried successfully to the sit-up position.* Use half the successful lift twice daily and retest in a month.

The weight-bag system is the most accurate and safe way, but if bags are not available, any appropriate weight can be used for repetitions. A child could use a light book, an adult a fairly heavy one— one guaranteed not to permit a starting score of more than 10 sit-ups. Keep a record of what was used for the test. Use that same weight twice daily, but for half the number achieved in the test. Retest in a month with a heavier book.

TEST 3: CHIN-UPS

Hang from a bar (if you get a chinning bar in a sports store, reinforce it with two small brackets, even if the directions say you don't need to) with arms at full stretch and palms facing *away* from the body. Slowly and evenly pull the body upward until the chin is above the bar. Lower slowly, as in the push-up test, taking a full three seconds to reach complete arm stretch.

Drop from the bar and reverse the hold so that the palms face *toward* the body. Repeat the chin-up and three-second descent. Alternate in this fashion for as many chin-ups as possible. There should be no modification of this test for girls.

To improve, do half the optimum number daily. If the score is zero, start to improve these muscles by hanging with the chin *above* the bar and doing a slow ten-second letdown. At first you will be lucky if you can slow it down to three seconds. When you or the child can do five slow letdowns, a chin-up will be possible.

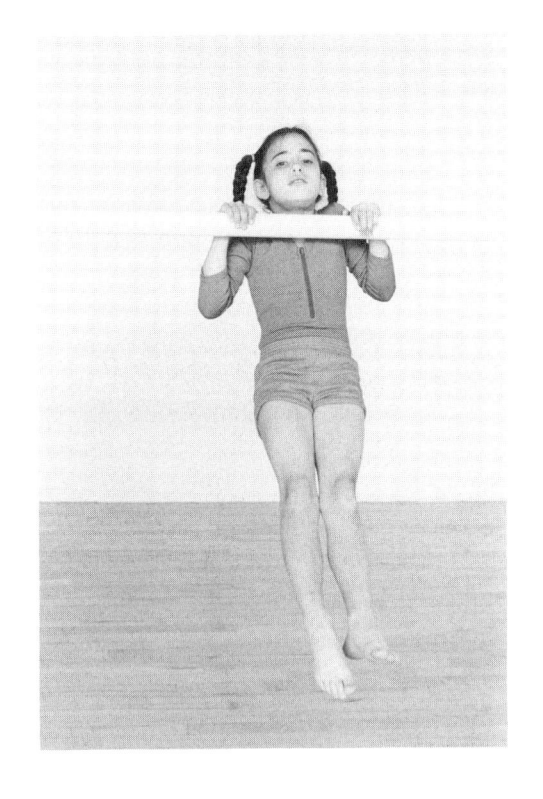

TEST 4: BROAD JUMP

This test can be done indoors on wood, tile, or cement. Be careful of carpets; they slip. If possible put down a permanent jumping area with either paint or colored tape so that children will be encouraged to practice often. (To set up a good outdoor jumping pit, see page 287.)

The jumper stands behind the starting line with feet parallel and apart for balance. The jump is made *from* both feet, and the landing is made *on* both feet. The measurement is taken from the starting line to the heel nearest the starting line. Should you or the child fall backward, the score is taken from that part of the body touching the ground nearest the line. *Don't* fall backward.

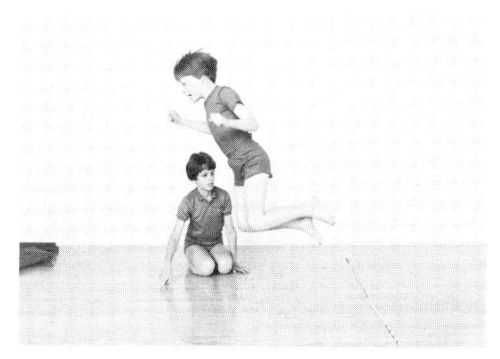

Each jumper gets three tries, and the best score is entered under "Broad Jump." To improve—*jump*. Retest in one month.

TEST 5: FLEXIBILITY

The K-W test was passed if the fingers could just touch the floor. But flexibility is so important to every sport that we should ask for much, much more. In order to measure improvement, there is a better way:

Have the child stand on a box or a stair and see how much further down the side of the platform the fingers can reach. To improve, use exercise 6 daily.

If you are a teacher and have many children in your care, watch for any changes in flexibility. Shortening of the back and hamstrings usually means one of two things. Either the child is under extreme stress or the physical outlets provided are insufficient to balance everyday stresses. Muscles often shorten just before an illness reaches the full-blown stage, a time when emotions take a dip and irritation is on the rise. This is the time when the disease is sneakily infectious—*before* the fever or spots.

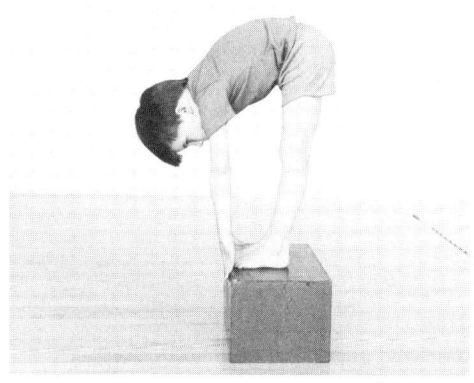

VITAL CAPACITY

Vital capacity is extremely important, especially today, when air pollution is so prevalent and running areas so limited. Your child may not breathe well owing to posture habits or the lack of opportunity to develop good lungs. Check vital capacity now and every month after you have begun the program. Have the person being tested blow out all the air and measure the size of the chest in its deflated state. Then ask the child to inhale as deeply as possible. Take the measurement of the inflated chest and note the difference in inches as the child's *vital capacity*. Singers and mountain climbers can measure as much as 5 inches. Three inches would be excellent for a child, ½ inch a disaster. Lungs are built by running, swimming, biking, and any other sport requiring endurance. You will find all of these activities discussed in this book. Just keep in mind that running builds heart and lungs; sitting destroys both. Refer to the chapter on Myotherapy.

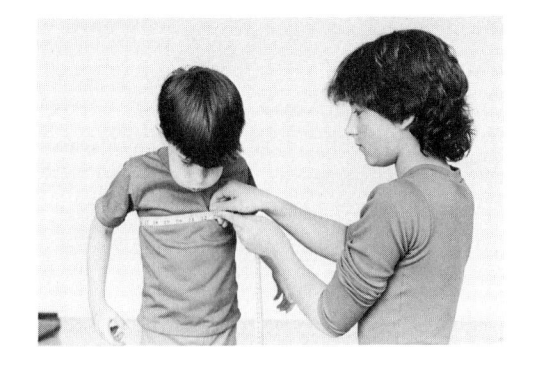

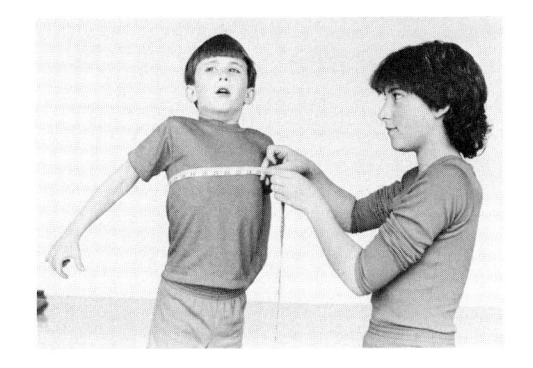

WHAT DOES YOUR FAMILY WEIGH?

Again we come back to the business of example. If you are interested and concerned about *your* weight, your children are going to pick it up. If you check yours daily, so will they. You should have a family weight graph or an individual graph for each person. The graphs should be taped to the wall near the scale and a pencil kept within reach.

Enter the starting weight on the line and then use the chart as a graph, testing once a week. (It wouldn't hurt to weigh yourselves every day, however.) For those needing to lose, set the starting line high on the graph. For those wishing to gain (or, as in the case of children, sure to gain) set the starting line lower.

How Good Are You . . . Really?

Individual Weight Graph

Date:

Starting

Weight

THE SHAPE OF THE SHAPE

If your child has a weight problem, more than a scale should be consulted. Fat weighs less than muscle and is also far less attractive. If your program replaces fat with muscle, weight loss may not be significant and the young or older athlete may be discouraged. To prevent this, measure and enter your findings on the figure measurement chart.

Figure Measurement Chart

Date												Difference
Neck												
Right Arm												
Left Arm												
Chest												
Waist												
Abdomen												
Hips 1												
Hips 2												
Right Thigh												
Right Knee (above)												
Right Knee (below)												
Right Calf												
Right Ankle												
Left Thigh												
Left Knee (above)												
Left Knee (below)												
Left Calf												
Left Ankle												

ARMS

Measure each arm in a relaxed position about 3 inches from the armpit.

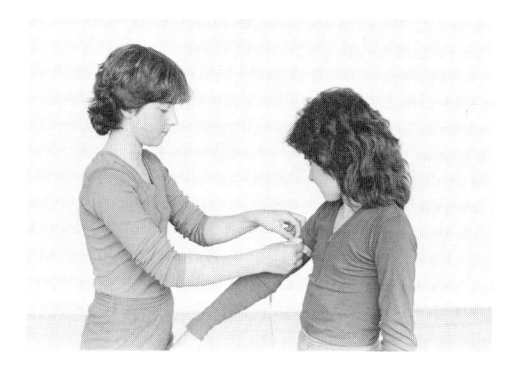

CHEST

Measure with lungs holding a normal amount of air. Understand at the outset that girls differ vastly in their thirteenth year. The athlete and dancer often have no bosom at all. Some girls have already outdone their mothers. It can be a touchy subject for a girl, just as a boy's height can be.

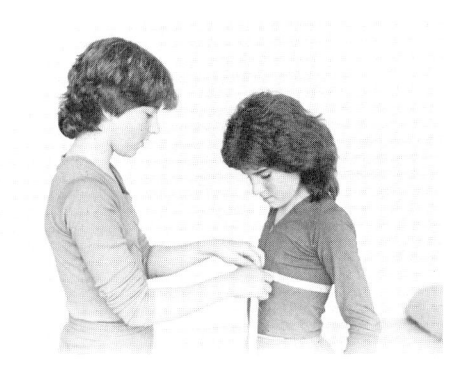

WAIST

The waist is easy to find, but remind the child not to pull in. You want to know facts. Then, as the measurement improves, there will be considerable satisfaction for everyone.

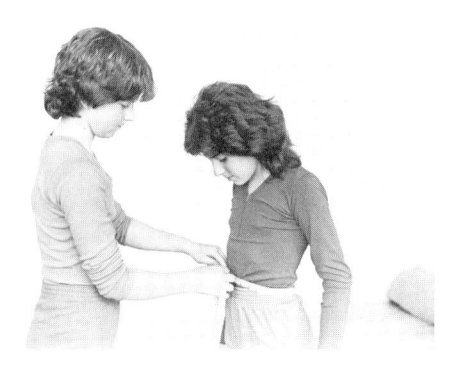

ABDOMINALS

It is never too early to make children aware of this measurement. It matters for many reasons all through life. For girls, a strong, flat abdominal wall means better fit in clothes; for the pregnant woman, it means an easier birth. For the athlete, another sign of fitness. For a boy, it's a sure sign of fitness, and for a man, it is the life line. A too-big life line can mean a shorter life. For everyone it signals freedom from backache. Measure just below the navel and try to keep the tape level.

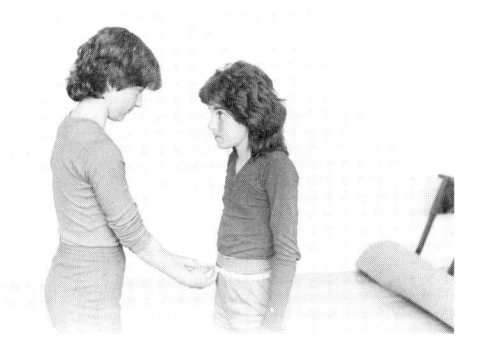

HIPS 1

On adults and even slightly overweight children there are two bulges on the outsides of the hips. These unattractive protuberances are called *saddle bags*. It is important to spot them *before* they settle in.

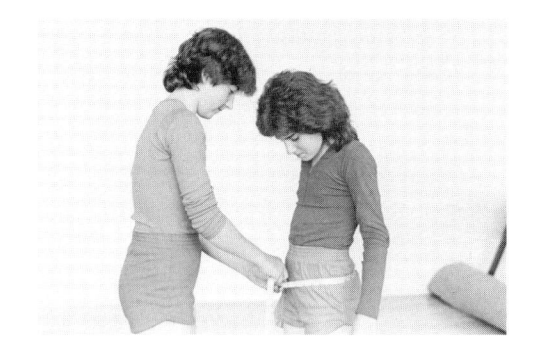

HIPS 2

This is the measurement taken around the widest point of the hips.

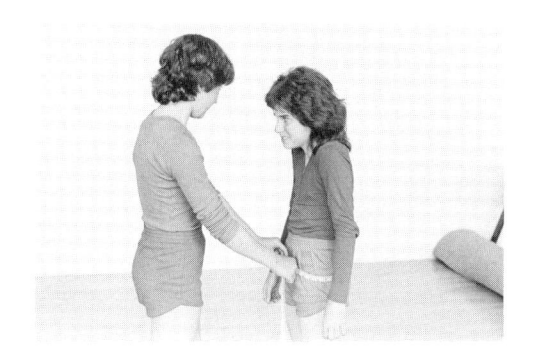

THIGHS

Measure the thighs at their widest points. (Be sure to unweight the leg for *all* leg measurements.)

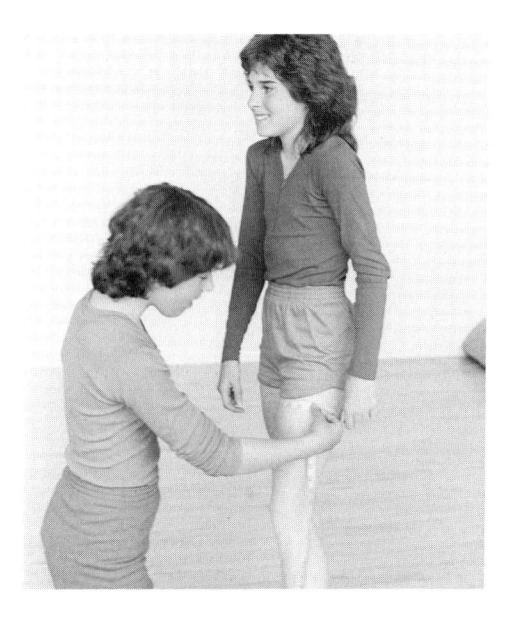

KNEE (ABOVE)

Measure just above the knee on the relaxed leg.

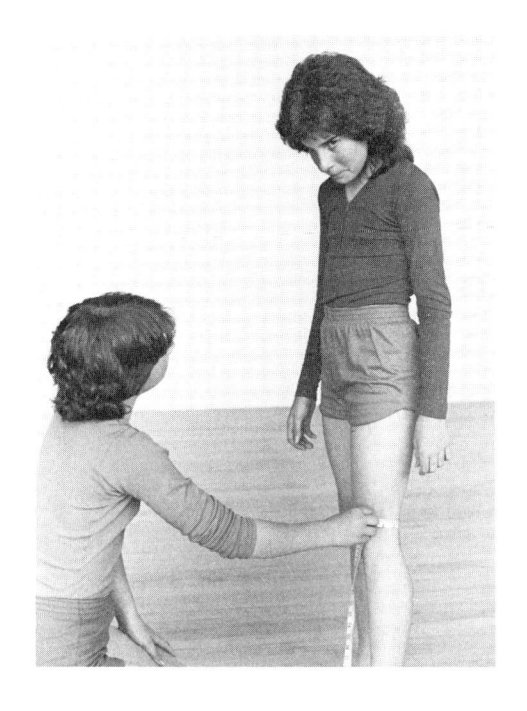

KNEE (BELOW)

On obese children there will be a fat pad just below the inside of the knee. It will fade away with exercise and attention to diet. That usually means abstaining from junk food.

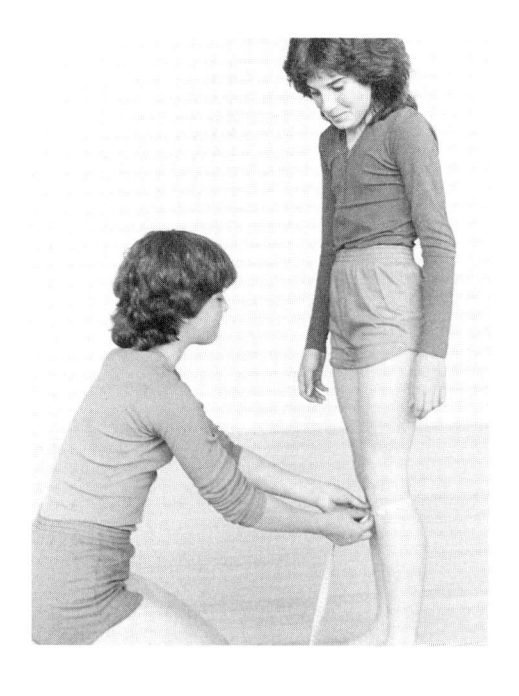

CALF

Measure the calf at its widest point. Be sure the leg is unweighted and the muscle relaxed.

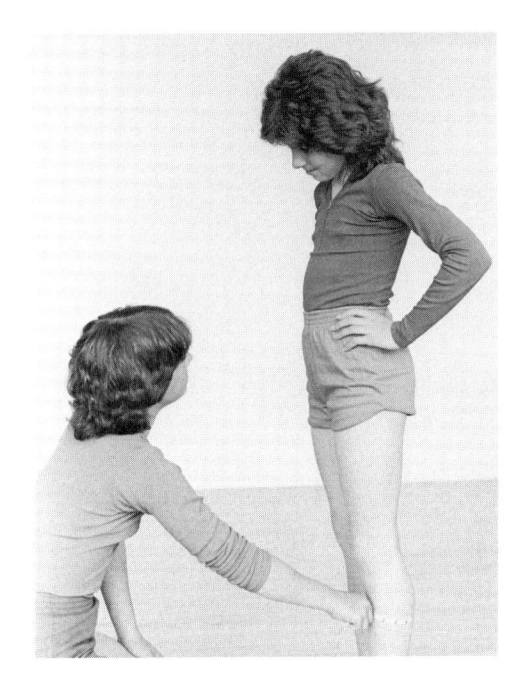

ANKLE

If the ankles are heavy or give the impression of swelling, by all means measure them. Refer to the chapter on myotherapy for injuries to the extremities. Swelling at wrist or ankle, even without pain or loss of function, may be a sign of injury higher up in the leg. This measurement is very important if the child is diabetic.

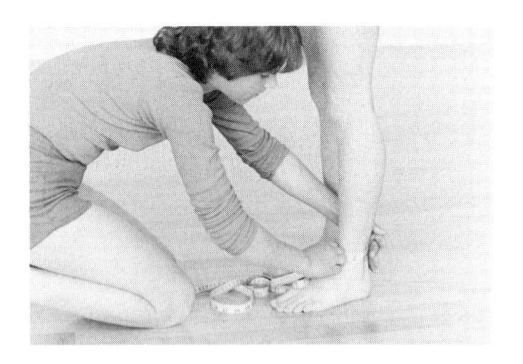

EAT SHEET

If you or your child has a weight problem, it is very helpful to keep "eat sheets." It is easy for the unwary to overeat and never notice it. However, if you keep track of everything that goes into your mouth (including the tastes you taste while tasting the taste of the dinner you are preparing) you find out where the weight came from and you will be more careful. Example plays a part here. If you are honest and accurate with *your* sheet, so will your child.

Daily Eat Sheet for the Week of _____

	Sunday	Monday	Tuesday	Wednesday	Thursday	Friday	Saturday
Breakfast							
Break							
Lunch							
Snack							
Dinner							
Snack							

TESTING GROUPS

This next section is for those of you who work with groups, any groups at all. Let's say you are a Scout leader, or perhaps beginning as I did as the neighborhood Pied Piper. Perhaps you plan to add fitness to the Sunday school program, or want to lead an hour at your club.

It is also for teachers. If you give the Kraus-Weber test to your class in September, you will know not only who is weak or inflexible (and how to fix it) but also where some of the anxieties lie. If you use the Prudden Supplement for Optimums, you won't ever have to worry what to do with the class again on a rainy day. Perhaps you have a friend across the hall who would like to set up a little interclass competition, or perhaps you can interest the principal in testing the whole school. There is much a principal can learn from a school testing. The class that has the most failures is the class that is going to have the most academic failures, too, and the most kids sent to the office with behavior problems. Much of this could be helped with a good physical program.

If you test in September and then put in a real program, you will bring the failure rate way down by Christmas. The children who pass the flexibility test before vacation and flunk it when they get back to school probably had a rough time over the holidays. You might want to give them a little extra kindness. We found in our testing that public school, day school, and boarding school children passed the strength tests quite soon after a program was instituted. The boarding school youngsters passed the flexibility tests too, quite soon. The public school and private day students had a much harder time, and some never did pass. Daily family stress tells.

If the group you are working with is very small and easy to keep track of, you can keep all your records of tests, improvement, and which child needs what kind of special help in one notebook. However, if you have a big group to work with, then you will need a system to make the job easier and more efficient. The Physical Evaluation Test Card has it all, but you may want to use only part of it. If you intend to give only the K-W test, mimeograph only the K-W test in boxes A and B. The posture problems should be included against the day you might have time, or somebody might have time to try to help.

If you intend to carry the testing *and program* further, then add the P-S part of the card. If no program is to be forthcoming, it is a waste of time to use the P-S—and frustrating to the children. The K-W is useful always, even if only to point out to "the powers" how bad things are in the hope that you will be given some help in making improvements.

It was our report to President Eisenhower on the comparative fitness of American and European children that caused the formation of the President's Council on Youth Fitness way back in 1955. At least we were able to make people aware of the danger. The fact that six-year-olds now enter school with higher than 85 percent failure does not necessarily mean it will never get any better, even though the government has known of this danger for thirty years and, so far, it hasn't helped.

It was today's generation of parents that was tested in the 1950s. Those of you who were six then and just entering first grade had a failure rate in that *minimum* fitness test of 54 percent. Today, your oldest child is probably around twelve and whatever could have been done to give him or her a good start physically has already been done or left undone.

Those of you who were at the all-important boundary between eleven and twelve back then had a failure rate that had *risen* to 65 percent while you were in school supposedly getting physical education to offset the time spent sitting in classrooms. Your first children are between seventeen and eighteen, and you *know* that what they are going to be they already are. Your influence is probably at its all-time low.

Those of you who were sixteen and seventeen and just getting out of high school had a failure rate then of 52 percent. That meant that over half of you would suffer from back pain. At forty-six, your first children are in their twenties, and some have given you grandchildren. What about those children and grandchildren? What has been done to correct the errors visited on *your* generation? How are things now?

Children entering school today have a failure rate that ranges between 85 and 100 percent. That would be hard to turn around even if there were a good physical program in the schools, but what has happened there? If you know, then you will be watching your child's physical condition and taking steps to rectify it either in school or out, through the PTA or your own efforts.

Sixty-five percent of the twelve-year-olds tested in the 1950s flunked the minimum test, and the flunking meant that life, which is hard enough when you have everything going for you, would be harder for them. Too many developed back pain, and since they were not trained in things physical, they lacked the physical outlets that relieve stress. The stress reliever for your generation was alcohol. Today teenagers are making headlines with different drugs—cocaine and crack. Back pain, shoulder pain, headaches, and what will be labeled arthritis for your generation in five or ten years will be epidemic. If one is to believe the TV advertisements, those things are epidemic already—and could have been prevented between the ages of six and twelve.

Your kids, all of them, have been born into "interesting times." You are there, too. When you were children, people didn't know much, if anything, about fitness. They didn't know much about nutrition either. They had passed up both discipline and education to keep in step with the "new modes" called "progressive." Now their piper is being paid by you. Who will pay yours? Those children you decided to have. Can you blame anybody? Not really, it happened the same way erosion happens. The trick will lie in recognizing the erosion and fighting it. *You* will have to do something about it, now, while there is still time for *your* children. For if you can give the world children who are really prepared to *do* something about its problems, not just protest the problems (which in today's world is both "in" and easy), you will have justified your own life.

If you have not already started to wonder why you are here, what life really is all about, if what you are doing is all there is to it—a job, kids, the daily grind, the bills, the sickness, the heartaches—the questions will not be long in coming. For the sake of your happiness you must have the answer. If you drift on just wondering, it can only end badly for you *and* your children, who will be the victims of the victims of the victims. It is time to stop running, time to turn and take a stand. It is well after midnight.

If you plan to test lots of youngsters, say a whole school, it is best to prepare the way and so make it easier all around. You first sell the other teachers on the idea. If you know the physical weak spots and have an opportunity to fix them, children will feel better, study better, and behave better. You might want to carry it a step further, as we did in the Greenacres School in Scarsdale, New York. We told the teachers that if they would do the two-minute program (page 149) before each class *with* the children, *they* would lose their backaches, stiff necks, headaches—and even a few inches where teachers almost always have extra inches. It was the truth, and not only did the teachers benefit, but the children felt better, had better concentration, and grades improved.

Enlist a few volunteers to make up testing teams, and allow about half an hour to brief them on the K-W test.

Don't worry too much about their finding posture problems; that takes more training. Anyone can tell when a child can sit up or not or when she leads with one elbow. If they get those facts for you, *you* will know from the test cards where the weaknesses lie, and it is weakness that leads to poor posture. Repair the deficiencies and you avoid the poor posture ahead of time.

Set aside a testing day and testing space. You will need one strong table per testing team and each team should have a tester and a recorder. The only equipment necessary is a ruler and a pillow for each table.

Have the children come to you by classes, and as they arrive, they should remove their shoes. Allow ninety seconds for each child on the table. Since they will be watching each other go through the battery, you won't have to do much explaining. Each child should bring a pre-filled-out card. The recorder then enters the K-W findings as uncovered by the tester. *Always* do the tests in the order set out on page 12. Keep the card and send the youngster on his way with a kind word; it may be the only one he hears that day.

As the group to be tested begins to dwindle, send for the next class so that there is no delay. Testing is hard work, and you will be tired after the morning's activity. Allow yourself plenty of rest at the noon hour, and by all means wear comfortable shoes.

Computation of K-W tests is very simple:

   1. Divide the cards of one group by sex.

   2. Divide all the cards by age.

How Good Are You . . . Really?

Physical Evaluation Test Card

Date _____

Name _____ Sex _____ Age _____ Class _____

Kraus-Weber

	A+	A–	P	UB	LB	FLX
First Testing						
2nd Testing						
3rd Testing						

Box A

Box B

Substitution	
Lead	
Arch	
Uneven	
Curve	

Prudden Supplement

Dates										
Chin-ups										
Push-ups										
Broad Jump										
Weighted Sit-ups										
Flexibility										

3. Start with the youngest on a scratch sheet and enter the following headings:

Scratch Sheet

Age	Total Tested	OK	Deficient	Incid. of fail.	Flexibility	Weakness	Abdominals	Backs	Psoas	2	3	4
6	30	15	15	23	10	13	6	3	4	4	2	0
7												
8												
9												

4. Let's take the cards for thirty boys age six. First separate the failures from the passing, or OK, cards.

5. Enter the OKs. Suppose there were fifteen.

6. With a red pencil, note on each card the nature of the failure.

A—for either or both A+ and A−
B—for either or both UB and LB
P—for psoas
F—for flexibility

You may find some tests failed in combinations as well as singly. *AF* is the most common and indicates abdominal failure *and* flexibility failure, an almost surefire cause of adult backache. *AP* stands for abdominal and psoas failure. Sometimes the failures come in threes, for example *ABP*, or abdominal, back, and psoas failure. It has been our impression that when a child exhibits multiple deficiencies, the physical outlets are so limited that there cannot help but be emotional difficulties as well. One nun in a parochial school, when viewing a table full of cards showing multiple failures, exclaimed, "Why, those are all the *characters!*" Indeed, children who are loaded with tension and unrelieved anxieties or hostilities do behave like "characters."

7. Now, with no attention to combinations, count all the *F* (flexibility) failures and enter the number under "Flexibility." Let us say there were ten.

8. Count all the *A*'s for abdominal failures and enter them under "Abdominals." Let's say there were six.

9. Count all the *B*'s for back failures and enter them under "Backs." Three.

10. The psoas failures number four and are entered under "Psoas."

Now that you have the basics, put them together.

11. Add all the "weakness" failures together—abdominals, backs, and psoas—and enter them under "Weakness."

12. Add the "flexibility" failures to the "weakness" failures and enter them under "Incidence." In this case they add up to twenty-three and represent the number of *tests* failed. It is important to know the difference between the number of *children* failing and the number of *tests* failed, because when there is a considerable difference, it indicates that there is a high number of "characters" or children under much pressure with far too few outlets.

13. Add up the number of failing *cards* and enter them under "Deficient." In this case there are fifteen, and "Deficient" represents the number of children failing.

14. Count up those failing two tests and enter under "2." Remember, "A+" and "A−" count as only one test failed, "Abdominals." The same applies with "UB" and "LB" for upper and lower back. They count as just one test failed, "Backs."

15. Count up the triple failures and enter them under "3." In this case there are two.

16. Count the cards registering four failures and enter them under "4." Hopefully, you will not find any such sad little creatures among those who come into your hands, but I have. One day while testing in a big city I found one and asked the teacher what she knew about him. She told me he was a terrible problem and she didn't know *what* was

How Good Are You . . . Really?

the matter with him. The year before, he could read and write just fine. Now he wrote all his *E*'s, *P*'s, and *F*'s backward, wet his pants, and told terrible lies: "Ever since his father deserted the family, he's been the worst child in the class." I wondered how that little body would function in a happy, secure situation—and with it his eyes, brain, bladder control, and satisfaction with the truth.

The following are counterchecks on the test:

17. Add the "OK" cards to the "Deficient" and you get thirty, the number of children tested.

18. Does the total number of "Weakness" failures (thirteen) plus the "Flexibility" failures (ten) add up to "Incidence" (twenty-three)?

19. Do "Abdominals" (six), plus "Backs" (three), plus "Psoas" (four), add up to the number of "Weakness" failures (thirteen)?

20. Does the difference between "Deficient" (fifteen), and "Incidence" (twenty-three), in this case eight, equal the number of double failures (four), plus the triple failures (two times two)?

21. Note that the column for "OK" entries has been omitted from the tally sheet on page 50. You won't need it there.

22. Figure the percentages and enter in red in the columns provided on the tally sheet.

If you are working only with your class or group, you will want the "Individual Failing Scores" sheet so that you can have it handy for daily exercises. The few minutes each day spent with each child doing the special exercise needed to earn a passing rate will be amply repaid.

If you persuaded other teachers in the school to go along with you on the testing, it is only fair to provide them with the same thing.

The following tally sheets will give an excellent check on your progress and, put into graph form, the best argument you will ever have for more time, space, and equipment for physical education.

Individual Failing Scores

Name	A+	A−	P	UB	LB	Flex

Tally Sheet Forms

Boys

Age	Total Tested	Deficient		Incid. of fail.		Flexibility		Weakness		Abdominals		Backs		Psoas		Two		Three		Four	
		No.	%	No.	%	No.	%	No.	%	No.	%	No.	%	No.	%	No.	%	No.	%	No.	%
5																						
6																						
7																						
8																						
9																						
10																						
11																						
12																						
13																						
14																						
15																						
16																						
17																						
18																						
Total																						

Girls

Age	Total Tested	Deficient		Incid. of fail.		Flexibility		Weakness		Abdominals		Backs		Psoas		Two		Three		Four	
		No.	%	No.	%	No.	%	No.	%	No.	%	No.	%	No.	%	No.	%	No.	%	No.	%
5																						
6																						
7																						
8																						
9																						
10																						
11																						
12																						
13																						
14																						
15																						
16																						
17																						
18																						
Total																						

Boys and Girls

Age	Total Tested	Deficient		Incid. of fail.		Flexibility		Weakness		Abdominals		Backs		Psoas		Two		Three		Four	
		No.	%	No.	%	No.	%	No.	%	No.	%	No.	%	No.	%	No.	%	No.	%	No.	%
5																						
6																						
7																						
8																						
9																						
10																						
11																						
12																						
13																						
14																						
15																						
16																						
17																						
18																						
Total																						

Muscular Fitness Test Tally Cover Sheet

School _____ Date _____
Address _____

	Total		Boys		Girls	
	No.	%	No.	%	No.	%
Total Tested						
Deficient						
Incidence of Failure						
Flexibility Failures						
Weakness Failures						
Abdominal Failures						
Back Failures						
Psoas Failures						
Combination of Two						
Combination of Three						
Combination of Four						

Signature _____

Incidence = Number of tests failed. Two, Three, and Four = Number of children failing two tests, three test, or four tests.

If you are a classroom teacher with "play" or "recreation," or "recess," or "PE" written on your daily schedule, you will need some important information. Since the average American child is incapable of meeting even the minimum requirements of fitness needed to get through the day comfortably and happily, you need some encouragement, and here it is.

In France, where the education of children from six to twelve is extremely demanding in hours, subject matter, and discipline, a very important experiment was conducted some years ago . . . long enough to prove the efficacy of the results. To begin with there were some children who were below the "norms" for French children. For those children, as for too many of our own, the future looked bleak. They, too, weren't "going anywhere." They were saddled with poverty and fifth-rate destinies. It all began in the city of Lyon, in the department of the Seine Suburbs in Paris, many years ago, under the direction of one man, Dr. Latarjet.

The doctor was concerned with deficiencies largely confined to the children in the working-class quarter of the city and couldn't imagine why those children needed the very demanding French education for the work that would be available to them. He decided to experiment. First, he selected the medically weakest eleven-year-olds in a girl's primary school. The children suffered from hereditary defects, bad housing, and malnutrition. He chose the thirty worst cases in the school as judged by retardation, growth, and intellectual standards. These he formed into a single class.

The doctor's next move was a masterstroke. He chose a highly intelligent and *active* teacher who also had good physical education qualifications. The daily schedule for intellectual study was reduced by two hours. These hours were given over to physical education activities . . . *European* physical education, not "play."

From the very first month a noticeable change was evident in height and weight. Later, when the children were compared with a comparable group being used as controls, it was found they had surpassed them morphologically and physiologically. They had also made gains in vital capacity, which indicated an increase in nutrition to the entire body, including the brain.

What was even more surprising was the attendance record. There were a total of fifty-three absences in the eighteen months of the experiment. The control group toted up 1,113! Intellectually, too, the "health class" showed improvement, or at least no deterioration as a consequence of giving up two hours a day of academic work.

French children go to school 259 days out of the year, whereas American children go only 180. Each week they are subjected to twenty-three and one-half hours of intellectual work plus five hours of physical exercise consisting of three hours of recreation (games, walks, etc.) and two hours of physical exercise (calisthenics, etc.). To these are added ten hours of homework . . . for children ages twelve and thirteen.

There were interesting results. First, Dr. Latarjet was able to interest his fellow doctors. As a member of the faculty of medicine at the University of Lyons, he had noted the overload of intellectual study in French education and been in a position to initiate the study. He claimed that a child needs nine to eleven hours of sleep depending on the age; two hours for play *plus a properly conducted physical education program.* (You teachers need not be concerned about your training in PE; the program you need is right here in this book, and you will find it easy as well as fun.) The doctor also set aside two hours a day for meals and one hour for hygiene. By that he meant personal care, baths, shampoos, sunbaths, tooth care, dressing and undressing, and so on. He held that children need recreation beyond organized physical education *for the purpose of thought and intellectual relaxation.* None of those hours were designed to include mind-numbing TV. Dr. Latarjet felt the above needs must be met first and *then* one could set up a study program—not as we do it, the other way around. If you are the parent rather than the teacher, think about those things. There are no hard-and-fast American rules; there are only habits. Those, you *can* control.

Suddenly headmasters were interested, since they felt (saw) that 90 percent of the intellectual work that was done between 1:30 and 4:30 in elementary school was lost. The medical and educational people got together and launched an attack on the Ministry of Education, and the Vanves experiment was on its way.

The class selected for this next phase became a milestone in French public education. It consisted of thirty-two children, average age eleven and one-half. The control group was set up in another school in a town some miles away. These children pursued the "normal" regime.

THE AIM

A. To reduce to a minimum the hours *needed* for intellectual school subjects and at the same time allow more time for physical exercise *with a view to obtaining better physiological development and consequently better intellectual efficiency.* This study was going on in France at precisely that time when America was cutting back on time allotted to things physical.

B. To compare the two groups, not only in regard to the intellectual and cultural factors, but also the state of health, physical development, sports performance, and certain moral qualities as well. Today this would apply also to the use of drugs.

The first Vanves experiment was followed by others in the Paris region in Tours, Lyons, and Montauban. Medical reports based on extensive individual examinations of all the pupils showed tremendous improvement in sports such as swimming. That was to be expected, but there were other plusses.

1. There was considerable improvement in overall physique—height, weight, and total lung capacity. In this country that would be cause for rejoicing since that and that alone (aerobics) is thought to be important at this time.

2. Posture improved markedly, including reductions in kyphosis (round back) and scoliosis (lateral curvature of the spine). While self-image was not reported, it most certainly improved. Any prepubescent, pubescent, and postpubescent young person cares about his or her looks—and posture can contribute or detract.

3. There was a lessening in minor diseases such as colds and digestive disorders. This of course contributed to the improved attendance.

4. There was better psychological and emotional balance: more assurance, loyalty, and cheerfulness. Keep in mind that low self-esteem, depression, and a feeling of uselessness often drive a young person to drug addiction.

5. Finally, on the intellectual level, examination successes were no less numerous than for those in the control groups. It not only helps to have energy and a clear head, *it helps to be in school.*

The results were so successful that in 1961, only eight years after Dr. Latarjet started his efforts to improve the lot of the French pupil, the experiment was extended to all the regions of France.

We have not been so fortunate here.

A similar program was offered to Abraham Ribicoff, who was then head of HEW, and accepted. Somehow, however, when he resigned from HEW, it was abandoned. The results are what you see. Children are far worse off today, after twenty-six years, than they were when the warning was first sounded.

In France, mornings were devoted to intellectual and artistic training while the afternoons were given over to manual and sporting activities. These were followed by "tea." Tea was a meal, as in England. Some part of the afternoon was set aside for a siesta! Of all things, a siesta! Imagine anyone having the temerity to suggest a midday rest hour for American schools, right in the middle of a school day. Imagine someone being wise enough to recognize that hardworking children might profit from a rest, as they do at camps that are more attached to "rest hour" than to any activity. Almost any other unit can be reslotted, increased, or decreased, but *never* rest hour!

After siesta the youngsters were sent to study hall for supervised study, where, already well exercised and rested, they could then finish their work and go home free to enjoy the evening hours without further responsibilities.

True, the children remained in school longer than did the controls, but the tea, siesta, and sports activities divided the day in such a way as to change the pace and emphasis. The pupils submitted to this unaccustomed rhythm happily and considered themselves privileged, as indeed they were.

Anything can be accomplished if intelligence and goodwill are combined.

The money spent for the increase in physical education brought health and pleasure to the children. It made the teachers' task easier and assured both physical and intellectual successes—and not just for the days when the children were in school. They built a strong health base and they learned habits that would serve them all their lives. France gave them something of value and in time they would contribute to France.

School life now garners six hours of your children's days. The bus steals still more time from their childhood. Only you know how much time they waste on TV and how much they are forced to spend on homework. One can hope that someday there will be someone in America like Dr. Latarjet to help them, but I have seen no sign of that happening.

In September 1985 I was asked to testify before the Senate Subcommittee on the fitness level of American children. I knew, of course, that it was far worse than it had been when your generation was tested, but just to be sure of my facts and figures I asked the graduates of my Myotherapy and fitness school, who have clinics all over America, to go and test as many children as possible before the hearing. It was fall, the first week of school, and about nine hundred children were tested. They *should* have been in pretty fair condition right after vacation. It was, as predicted, far worse. But my findings did not have to stand alone as they did back in the fifties. Another study, released by the United States Department of Health and Human Services and called the Heckler Report, announced that *American youth today carry substantially more body fat than did their counterparts in the 1960s.* They made another statement that was far less factual: *"About half don't receive appropriate physical activity to maintain effectively functioning cardiorespiratory systems."* The next statement gives the lie to the foregoing: *"Twenty-eight percent of them [the tested children] have higher than normal blood pressure. Forty percent have high levels of cholesterol . . . and ninety-eight percent have at least one major risk for developing heart disease."*

Right away you have problems, or rather your children do. If half of America's public school children are getting *the appropriate physical activity to maintain effectively functioning cardiorespiratory systems,* why are so many at risk for developing heart disease? Subtract 50 percent (who in theory are getting exercise) from the 98 percent who obviously are not, and what do you get? I get 48 percent who are *said* to be in good hands, but are not. Now comes problem number one. Who is mistaken? Is it the researcher who proves the children are in terrible shape by medical tests, or the physical education people who claim 50 percent are all right and not to worry?

The second problem is strictly yours: Look at *your* children and find out what is true for *them.* If your child can't pass the K-W test, which is a medically valid test for *minimum* fitness, then he or she is unfit. There may also be other deficiencies, but count on it, *minimum* means *minimum,* and you need not have complicated tests to see that.

The report says that *"The minimum requirement of vigorous activity is generally accepted as 20 minutes at 60 percent of capacity three times a week."* Now, what can you do with that information? First, from checking PE classes from coast to coast we know that three minutes twice a week is all most children get in gym unless they are tall boys. But you should not believe me; you should plan to invest three hours in the present and future health of each child. Go and sit in the gym for three classes. Use a stopwatch to time when your child is moving productively, not merely being in the gym. If you don't have a stopwatch, count seconds (*one*-chim-pan-zee, *two*-chim-pan-zees . . .).

Next, even if your child is getting the "accepted" one hour a week of activity, what is that worth when measured against thirty hours of classes, lunchroom, and another two and one-half or more a week in the school bus? Preschoolers average forty hours a week of TV. What does that young hope of the world of yours watch, and for how long? Now compare your child's activities with yours and then look back on the time your parents spent outdoors in play, walking to and from school and running errands. Next, think of the Vanves experiment and what was accomplished by putting some physical outlets back into the lives of children.

In recent years there has been a great deal of noise about responsibility. Teachers rightfully say they cannot do it all. Parents are within their rights, too, when they say that children are in school more hours than they are awake at home. What is at stake here? It is the child. If both could get together and look at the whole picture, plus the whole child, a great deal could be accomplished. I have found that both parents and teachers are willing to go beyond the edge of duty when they know what direction to take. If you want help from teachers, show them the information on the Vanves experiment (page 53), especially the part where life becomes easier for the teacher when the children are rested and exercised. If you are the teacher, call a meeting with the parents and read them the section on Vanves. You may not be able to change the whole world, but for sure you will be able to change the world for some children. In any case, talk to the children about what you would like to do, test them, and then send a letter home.

ONE TYPE OF LETTER TO PARENTS

On _____, your child was given the Kraus-Weber Test for *Minimum* Strength and Flexibility of key posture muscles. Failure to pass all tests indicates a muscle deficiency that should be corrected at once if the child is to function adequately in daily living.

(Name) _____
passed the test (   )
failed the test (   ).
   The area failed was:
abdominals (   )
hip flexors (   )
back muscles (   )
flexibility (   ).

We request that you oversee the following exercises for ten minutes each evening, whether your child passed or failed. If the child failed any test, extra attention should be given to the failing area.

Abdominals: Have the child lie supine on the floor, knees bent, and hands clasped behind head. Hold the feet down and ask him or her to *roll* to a sitting position slowly. Do ten. If this is impossible, start in the sitting position with hands clasped across the chest and slowly roll down. Do ten. Within a few weeks it will be possible to do roll-ups as well.

Hip Flexors: Have the child lie supine with hands at sides. Bring the knees to a bent position resting above the chest. This ensures that the spine is flat on the floor. Extend legs straight up and return to the rest position. On the second extension lower the feet 6 inches nearer the floor. Watch to see that the spine is still on the floor. At some point the spine will come off the floor. You have then gone too far. Have the child return to the angle of the last successful extension and do ten.

Back Muscles: Lying facedown on the floor with arms stretched ahead, the child should lift the right arm upward and then replace it on the floor. Then lift the left arm and replace. Then both arms at once. Do this series five times. Follow this series by lifting the right leg with the knee held straight. Then the left leg and finally both. Do this series five times.

Flexibility: Stand with feet apart, knees held straight, and hands clasped behind the back. Lean forward from the hips, but keep the head turned upward. Bounce the upper body downward ten times to the center, ten right, and ten left. Follow this by allowing the whole upper body to hang loosely downward toward the floor. Repeat the bounces to center, right, and left.

These exercises are designed to improve the child's strength and flexibility. They will do the same for the parents. By making daily exercise a family activity, much can be done to prevent fatigue, release tension, and improve both performance and appearance.

The Prudden Supplement is not only a valuable tool for use in self-improvement but can also be used for competition, still one of the best motivations for extreme effort. Competition may be held between youngsters of equal abilities who are striving for top honors or between classes, schools, and even towns. This is done by using the point system.

More important than these forms of competition, however, is self-competition. The child who may never be a great athlete can still derive considerable satisfaction as well as a healthy, coordinated body by observing his own steady improvement. This improvement can be put to excellent use with those sports outlined later in the book. Hitherto when letters and trophies were awarded for athletics, the average or below-average student was always ignored.

This led to discouragement and ultimately to a lack of interest in physical activity. Since a high degree of *improvement* can also be determined and rewarded, this need no longer be the case.

Our studies with children show that even eight-year-olds can be made aware of their physical levels and encouraged both to keep records of work and improvement and to do extra work on the side to advance further in the sport of their choice. Each should keep a record of test results, physical measurements (page 37), weight charts (page 37), and the special exercises for individual needs. While it is very possible that a young girl will need abdominal strengthening, strength may be far from her interests, which center more on looking like her best friend who has a "perfect" figure and wears fashionable clothes. The same exercise will contribute to both strength and attractiveness, and the wise teacher will emphasize the latter concern. A boy, on the other hand, may need pectoral stretch for a round-back condition, but be interested only in baseball. The same exercises that stretch the pectorals and strengthen the back will improve his game.

Instructors will find that test results prominently displayed on bulletin boards are prime motivators for improvement. Human beings are so designed that the scrawniest boy could outstrip all contenders if he really set his mind to it. The average youngster does not come within light-years of his potential. It is quite true that the more physically gifted youngsters could put him down, but today they are rarely moved to extend themselves overmuch. In speaking to a group of businessmen at Yale some years ago I asked for a show of hands by varsity athletes in any sport. About 75 percent of the three hundred men present raised their hands. Then I asked how many of them had boys or girls on varsity teams either in high school or in college, and *seven men put their hands up.* Three men had girls who went to dancing school, and two had daughters who were cheerleaders. There were no daughters on varsity teams. Many schools didn't even have varsity teams for girls.

After entering the scores on the record sheet, circle the winning score in each of the five tests.

To find the first-, second-, and third-place winners, set up a scratch sheet. Give the boy with the best score in each test 10 points, the boy placing second, 5, and the third, 3. Add up the number of points each boy has amassed. In the case of a tie, both boys get equal credit.

The second and third testings are entered in the spaces provided in the first box, and new individual scores affixed over the first.

To compare classes for school honors, or schools for town honors, it is only necessary to compare the top scores.

Improvement, a highly important motivator, should be noted and recorded during the second and third testings.

Circle the winning scores as before and box in the scores showing most improvement. Use the same point system, giving 10 points for first place, 5 for second, and 3 for third.

The same system of scoring is used for girls and also when boys and girls are in competition. Each group should be scored separately and later compared.

How Good Are You . . . Really? 59

Class Record of P-S Test for Optimum Performance (Boys)

| Class _____ Sex ____ Date _____ Test Number __1__ |
Name	Chin-ups	Push-ups	Sit-ups	Broad Jumps	Flexibility
Jack D.	1	4	10	60"	T
Tom B.	2	10	7	(79")	+1"
Harry P.	2	12	(15)	74"	(+4")
Dick H.	(4)	8	13	72"	−3"
Jim L.	3	(15)	9	75"	+1"

First Place	Harry P.	29 points
Second Place	Jim L.	25 points
Third Place	Tom B.	23 points

Individual Tests	Top Scorer	Score	Average
Chin-ups	Dick H.	4	2.5
Push-ups	Jim L.	15	9.8
Sit-ups	Harry P.	15	10.8
Broad Jumps	Tom B.	79"(6')	72"(6')
Flexibility Plus	Harry P.	+4"	+1.2"

Scratch Sheet for Optimum Test (Boys)

Jack		Tom		Harry		Dick		Jim	
Chin-ups	5	Chin-ups	3	Chin-ups	10				
Push-ups	10	Push-ups	5	Push-ups	3			Push-ups	5
Sit-ups	10	Sit-ups	5	Sit-ups	5	Sit-ups	3		
Broad Jump	5			Broad Jump	3	Broad Jump	10		
Flexibility	3					Flexibility	10	Flexibility	5
	33		13		21		23		10
	First				Third		Second		

Class Record of P-S Test for Optimum Performance (Boys)

| Class _____ Sex ____ Date _____ Test Number __2__ |
Name	Chin-ups		Push-ups		Sit-ups		Broad Jumps		Flexibility	
Jack D.	1	3	4	[11]	10	[19]	60"	65"	T	+2"
Tom B.	2	3	10	15	7	14	(79")	(79")	+1"	+2"
Harry P.	2	(5)	12	15	(15)	(22)	74"	78"	(+4")	(+5")
Dick H.	(4)	3	8	10	13	19	72"	[78"]	−3"	[+1"]
Jim L.	3	3	(15)	(20)	9	10	75"	77"	+1"	+4"

Scratch Sheet for Winning Scores

Jack		Tom		Harry		Dick		Jim	
		Chin-ups	3	Chin-ups	10	Chin-ups	5		
		Push-ups	5	Push-ups	3			Push-ups	10
Sit-ups	3			Sit-ups	10	Sit-ups	5		
Broad Jump	5			Broad Jump	3	Broad Jump	10		
Flexibility	3					Flexibility	10	Flexibility	5
	33		13		21		23		10
First				Third		Second			

Improvement Scores

——— IMPROVEMENT ———		
First Place	Tom B.	33 points
Second Place	Dick H.	23 points
Third Place	Harry P.	22 points

Individual Tests	Most Improved	Difference
Chin-ups	Harry P.	3
Push-ups	Jack D.	7
Sit-ups	Jack D.	9
Broad Jumps	Dick H.	6″
Flexibility Plus	Dick H.	+4″

ONE TYPE OF PHYSICAL FITNESS REPORT TO PARENTS

A test for optimum physical performance has been given to your child. Below are your child's scores and also the class averages. It is not necessary that one child surpass all others, but it is highly important that every child improve in every area over the course of the year. Emergencies constantly arise in which children (later as adults), are called upon to perform with skill, stamina, and courage. You owe it to your child to see to it that he constantly raises his score.

Average Scores Compared with Individual Scores

Name of Test	September Child's Score	September Class Avg.	December Child's Score	December Class Avg.	May Child's Score	May Class Avg.
Chin-ups	0	2	1	3	3	4
Push-ups	2	7	10	13	15	15
Weighted sit-ups	5	11	17	20	21	20
Broad jump	58"	66"	60"	74"	56"	76"
Flexibility plus	−1"	+1"	touch	+2"	+2"	+2"

Remarks:

The student's arm and shoulder strength shows considerable improvement, but he is still well below the average performance. It is suggested that a chinning bar be installed at home and that he be encouraged to do one chin-up each time he goes through that particular door. (Note: If either chin-ups or push-ups still rate zero, suggest that the student hang from the top of the chin-up and let himself slowly down, taking five seconds for the descent. Use a similar technique with the push-ups.)

Abdominals have improved, as has flexibility, but there has been a loss in leg power, as shown in the broad jump. Daily running over a course previously set up, jumping in place, carrying a heavy pack up and down stairs for ten consecutive minutes daily, would all help in this area. As legs are developed in youth, so do they serve in later years. No one can afford to neglect them.

This student was uninterested in sports before, but is showing considerable interest of late. That is probably because his arm and hand skills have improved and he is making a better record on the field. There has also been an increase in self-confidence and some loss of fatigue.

CHAPTER FIVE
GIRLS AND THEIR MUSCLES

The Age of Aquarius the humanitarian has been ushered in with an avalanche of protest against discrimination. I hope it will eliminate the most international discrimination of all, discrimination against women. It was in 1943—but things haven't changed that much; you get the same reaction today—that I was hurrying along the corridor of the maternity floor looking for someone who could tell me where to find my daughter, who had had a baby only minutes before I got there. "She's still in the delivery room," said the floor nurse, "but she'll be down shortly. Both of them are fine."

I thanked her and was turning toward the typically drab and uncomfortable waiting area to do my thanking for safety of mother and child to whatever celestial overseer takes care of these things, when I was detained. "Aren't you interested in what you got?" the nurse said in a rather disapproving tone. It was hot and I was tired, but I stifled my first urge to say that I presumed it was a baby and evinced the expected interest in the sex of my first grandchild. "Why, it's a *boy!*" she said with a china smile that stretched halfway around her head. I flunked again. I was just so glad that a baby had arrived safely and that my own child was all right that I couldn't get out more than, "Really, imagine that!"—and then I began to seethe.

That's where it all starts, in the womb. I had been as guilty as the next one. I'd called my first baby Peter from the time I found out that it was on its way, and that's how I came to have a little girl named Petie. Then there was David, who turned out to be Suzy. It hadn't begun there either: my father had given me boxing gloves for my eighth birthday, and every letter from him began "Dear Pal . . ."

I wonder what it is we've all got against girls. It certainly shows up in physical education and sports in general. There are all sorts of clubs for little boys—Little League, Cookie League, and Biddy Basketball, to name a few—but little girls aren't even recognized as human. I can still remember sitting next to a small girl in the lobby of one of our university's physical education buildings. I was there to make a speech; she was there to get a swimming lesson. She was a good swimmer, she said; the whole team of ten-year-olds were good swimmers, but they never got a chance to prove it—there was no competition for the girls, only for the boys. I thought of the fabulous ice skaters, the beautiful young Olympic swimmers, divers, skiers, and of late, gymnasts, and ground my teeth. Of course the day would come when little girls could compete, but it wouldn't happen for that particular child.

That's been the whole trouble. Things change so fast for the bad and so slowly for the better. Way back in 1930 when we still had competition for girls (a lot of us still played boys' rules in basketball, and hockey was grueling enough to get you to spit blood when the weather got cold enough), a lady (it *had* to be a lady) wrote a paper claiming that girls were delicate and that any overexertion such as running or jumping would scramble their reproductive organs.

More boy babies than girl babies are born, but more girls make it to home plate.

More girl babies survive the first year of life, while children are still making up their minds if they want to stay.

Today in America the average woman can look forward to eight years of widowhood if she is as old as her husband. A pretty lonely prospect. Delicate indeed! Let's see what the tests said.

Little boys aged six enter first grade with a physical failure rate of 62.3 percent, but little girls of that age come in with 44.7 percent. The girl children from "advantaged" families didn't do quite that well, however. They had a 53.3 percent failure when they were six. I can remember when I had an institute at White Plains, New York. Many of the children were brought there by chauffeurs, who *carried* them in and placed them on the gym floors for an hour of conditioning. At the end they were *carried* out again. I never felt we had much of a chance in that one hour a week.

By the age of nine, in spite of the activity groups available for boys, they still had a failure rate of 58.6 percent. The girls who had no help at all were still ahead with 50 percent. In the private schools, where they had a little more action, girls were down to 27.9 percent.

By the time the ripe old age of twelve was reached, the boys' failure rate had reached 68 percent. The girls were still ahead with 59 percent. In the private schools, where they had to be given equal time in the gym with the boys by right of equal tuition, the boys had 42.8 percent failure. The little girls, who were quite definitely in that interesting period when reproductive organs, scrambled or not, were developing, had a failure rate of 22.8 percent. In Europe the same age girl, with presumably the same type of organs, had a failure rate of 4.6 percent. Isn't that sad!

No, there's nothing the matter with little girls except adult confusion. You ask your daughter who gets the gym after school. It has to be the boys' basketball team. Who gets the field? The boys' football team. If there are two gyms, a new one and an old one, who gets the new one? The answer is almost always the same. It shouldn't be an unequal arrangement even if the boys do have to fight the wars. The girls still have the babies, and whatever the girl's physical experience has been is bound to reflect on the children. The tomboy with plenty of exercise makes the best mother. She will not overprotect, and she will encourage action. The children of skiers will ski. If mother is a tennis player, they will play tennis; if she skates, they will skate. If she sits in front of the TV, more than likely that's where you'll find the kids from three to nine and all day Saturday and Sunday.

At this moment a word to both mothers and teachers: If you are slim and attractive, if you take exercise seriously and if you wear attractive, suitable outfits for your work, girls will want to be like you. If you are out of shape and you say to the kids that you know you are out of shape, they will say to themselves, "That's a fact." Then if you say that you intend to get into shape with your classes and that you expect them to go right along with you, ten to one they will give you a chance to prove it. You can always feel at least a little superiority, since you have this book. That gives you quite an edge. *But*, if you are overweight, if you dress in street clothes for class (or wear a housedress for your mother-daughter session at home), and if you give them the do-as-I-say-but-not-as-I-do routine, you're dead—and so are their chances of ever becoming what they could become—healthy, strong, attractive, and tireless.

It's up to you. They are there and they are waiting. They are waiting for you.

CHAPTER SIX
THE FIRST STEP—WARM-UPS

The teaching of exercise, whether to your own children or to the children of others, is an art. However, it is an art that can be learned—even on the job. One of the reasons exercise was given up back in the 1930s was because it was taught so poorly. Also, one must remember that exercises suitable for another generation, or even for another nationality, need not be right for today or for Americans. Today's children need a challenge because both challenge and change are all around them. At the same time many are far weaker and have less determination than the boys and girls of a few generations ago. Repetition isn't the answer—they find it dull and also uncomfortable. Further, they can see no reason for "punishing" themselves and are rarely possessed of the self-discipline that would make it possible even if they were convinced it was a good thing. But exercise is essential to life, and the secret lies in making it exciting and fun. The needed ingredient is music, the *right* music, and that changes every few years. Certain qualities remain constant, however; music that has a quick, light beat or a steady, throbbing rhythm is always in.

GENERAL DIRECTIONS FOR GETTING STARTED—HOME

Let's say that you have discovered that your children are out of shape and it looks as though nothing short of an atomic bomb would move the school to give more hours to physical activities or improve the content of the existing program. The fastest way to influence change is to do it yourself. The earlier you start, the less opposition you will get. Invite several little friends to join the class and begin with the costume.

Exercise clothes must fit close to the body, but when you are just starting out, you may not want to invest much money, nor will you want the parents of your children's friends to do so. What's inexpensive and what works? Require each child to bring a pair of white underpants and dye them navy blue. Half your problem is solved. Every child has a white T-shirt, but what would make it into an "exercise shirt?" Go to a millinery shop and buy one of those little decorative shields that can be sewn onto the left side of the front of the shirt where older kid's shirts have pockets. Now you have a costume and the little group will look like a real "class."

What about foot covering? Ballet dancers have ballet slippers. Baseball players have baseball shoes. What is your class going to wear? If the floor is safe, they are going to wear nothing on their feet at all. Feet are being rediscovered even as I write. For years they have been stuffed into sneakers, which turn a foot of any age into a hoof. Shoes, no matter the form, limit action and prevent the foot muscles from developing properly.

Today people have no trouble finding very attractive exercise clothes if they want to make the investment. For yourself, make the investment. You want to look good and feel good about yourself. You also want to set both the stage and the tone. If you wear a leotard and tights, be sure there are no feet on the tights; they are dangerous and can slip. A broken leg is very discouraging.

Where should you have your class? I started mine in my living room, but I found it too "familiar" to my own two children. I was on the Girl Scout Council, and they allowed me to start a class in the Scout House. In return I was to take on all comers. No problem, I thought. I started with ten, and within six weeks there were seventy-five children taking "conditioning" classes at the Harrison Girl Scout House. Over half of them were *boys!* No one seemed to mind, and we almost doubled every year, bringing in older and older groups until I finally had every age. That's what can happen, but you can control it by renting some time in a dance studio, a church, a service club, or a community center.

Suppose you want to get started in a school. The same costume works very well for starters, and it doesn't tie you to anything. No one has made an investment. If you are the teacher, you won't have to face parents who either don't want to pay for "gym" clothes or can't. Every kid has white underpants and a

The First Step—Warm-Ups

white T-shirt. Navy dye is cheap, and you might even be able to get the Home Ec. Department to do the dyeing. In the parochial schools where I set up such programs, there were no locker rooms. As in England, the children came to school wearing their "gym" clothes under their regular clothes. The advantage provided by uniform dress is uniformity and anonymity. When a group performs the same movement in the same outfits, the group takes on form. Line can be seen and appreciated. Children enjoy art and they like to make it themselves. They love to be part of something bigger than themselves and they love to do that to music.

So, with a good record player, some exciting records, and a group of little people who are ready for anything, you will be on your way, whether in the Scout House, the Woman's Club, the Boy's Club, the church basement, or your own living room. If you are in school, you *may* get the all-purpose room, but then again you may have to settle for much less. Settle (at first). You will be able to change things in time—and the children will help you.

EXERCISE FORMAT

No matter where you hold your class, no matter the age of your students or their sexes, no matter their condition or ability, the overall format should be the same. If you have a format right from the start, you will never wonder what to teach, what you could do next, what you omitted that should have been included, or even if you are doing the right thing. You will be, and both your body and those of the children will thrive.

Begin by forgetting. Forget the misinformation foisted on the public in the seventies and especially the eighties. Forget "Go for the burn," and "No pain . . . no gain." Forget the pictures of people hopping up and down, clapping their hands and shouting "Whhh-eeee!" Forget the straining weight lifters, the miserable-looking joggers, forget the whole caravan as they stagger down the road to the past. What you will teach your little charges will be fun, exciting, and safe. You will hurt no one—not even yourself.

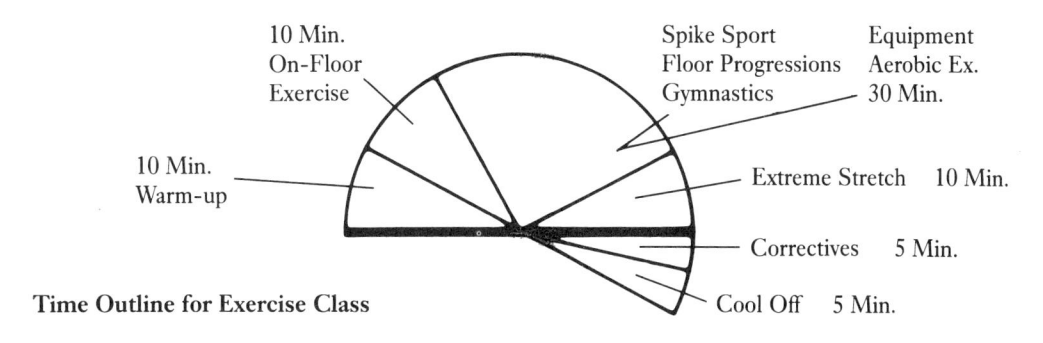

10 Min. On-Floor Exercise

Spike Sport Floor Progressions Gymnastics

Equipment Aerobic Ex. 30 Min.

10 Min. Warm-up

Extreme Stretch 10 Min.

Correctives 5 Min.

Cool Off 5 Min.

Time Outline for Exercise Class

WARM-UPS

Put your group, large or small, into a circle. Why? Because you can see every last one of them, and they can see you. *You* are going to be the one they look at. There will be no "back-of-the-class shenanigans" because there is no back of the class. While they are in that circle, you are in control.

Warm-ups are very special exercises and they come first, before anything else. They have a very special part to play in the success of your class—and your own safety. A warm muscle is 20 percent more efficient than a cold muscle and, incidentally, 20 percent safer. If you warm up in the locker room before addressing the ball on the first tee, there is a 20 percent better chance of getting off a good shot. Warming up before going onto the ice to try for an Olympic medal gives you a 20 percent better chance than you would have had going out cold. Why?

Cold muscles are tense and inelastic. They do not respond to orders the way warm, elastic muscles respond. If you have had a hard day emotionally, your muscles will be especially tight. If you overstretch one of them, it doesn't give, it tears. It doesn't tear the whole way and wave like a flag in the breeze, but a few fibers here and there do tear, and that is a wound. What do wounds do?

Wounds heal and they leave scar tissue behind. If there is a big wound, there is a big scar. If the wound is a microinjury, it will heal, leaving a microscar. One of those might not be capable of doing much of anything to cause you distress, but bunches of them certainly will. Most athletic careers are lost to bunches of microscars that finally gang up on their host.

Right now you are probably wondering what scars have to do with anything. You have dozens, so what?! When you get to the chapter on myotherapy and pain, you will learn about trigger points. They cause the pain most people suffer when they throw muscles into spasm. You need not be a world-class athlete to attract the trigger points that cause sidelining. You could easily have back pain, headaches, knee pain, wrist or shoulder pain, and it would have the same cause—trigger points. We all have them, they have a penchant for scar tissue. That's a good reason for not hurting yourself when you know full well how to avoid it. In exercise and sports, you avoid injuries by starting with warm-ups.

Warm-up exercises are designed to get the heart beating faster so that larger amounts of warm, oxygenated blood flows faster to the extremities you expect to use in the activity. You do *not* warm up by running around the track, doing jumping jacks in place, or hopping up and down as in "aerobic dance." If there is a tight muscle anywhere in your body, those activities will cause that muscle to tighten and even to cramp. Warm-up exercises are done from a standing, spread-leg position and involve arm swings, waist twists, hip and shoulder rotations, half and full knee-bends, toe rises, ceiling reaches, overhead reaches, crawl strokes, backstrokes, breaststrokes—anything that will not strain muscles but will get the heart beating and raise a sweat. When there is a light film of sweat just under your nose, you can feel that (a) you are warm enough for the next step; and (b) you are *safe* enough to go on with the program, whether it be exercise or a game . . . or the run down the ski trail. Your muscles are ready.

Stretch is another confusing word to many people. When jogging was the thing to do, one could see joggers walk out of their homes and over to the nearest tree. There they would stretch their calf muscles as they leaned into it. Or they would put a leg up on the nearest fence and stretch hamstrings and back muscles. Every time they did that, they hurt themselves a little. In time, that damage, plus running on cement, drove 50 percent of the serious runners off the roads and thousands of amateurs as well. You stretch lightly when you are warm . . . and seriously when you are sweating bullets. Serious stretch is done last, according to the class outline. That's when well-used muscles are soft as butter.

Repetitions confuse people too. In the olden days when most of our "calisthenics" were copied from German gymnastics, we played the same dangerous game we have just relinquished: "Go for the burn." In essence what that means is that you do repetitions of the same exercise until the muscles are so full of waste products that they are burning with pain. The muscle is saying, "Stop! You are hurting me." But alas, we have never been taught to listen to our bodies—just to our teachers. The German teachers felt that the last ten arm circles (which you should never do anyway) after you felt as though the arm would fall off, were the only ones with value. That is nonsense of course and contributed to the average American's dislike for calisthenics. Those calisthenics died due to disinterest and were resurrected by movie stars in the late seventies and early eighties. After hordes of people were injured, the idea went into limbo again.

If you were one of those who followed that line of action, you may have begun to hurt. Don't worry, it's not age that is descending on you, it's muscle spasm. Check with the chapter on Myotherapy and get rid of the pain. Then adopt a different way of exercising and you will have all the advantages and none of the disadvantages of the recent exercise formats.

When leading your class, keep the repetitions to between fifteen and twenty seconds and then get on to another exercise, one that works a different part of the body. In my summer workshops we work *physically* five hours a day, and the people can range from six to eighty. They neither tire nor hurt. They don't stop either. The trick lies in resting one set of muscles while using another.

Stiffness happens all the time. All it means is that you haven't used that set of muscles recently. When I rode in roundups, we each had three horses in the remuda. If I stuck to those three horses, I was never stiff at night, no matter how many hours I rode; my muscles were used to their gaits and had learned to accommodate to them. *But,* if I rode a borrowed horse, even for an hour, I crawled into my bedroll stiff as a board. The next day was worse and the third day worst of all. That applies to overdoing in exercise too. The day you do it is okay, but you pay the next day. On the third you may think you've done yourself in. Not so; the next day you'll be better. But you can avoid two miserable days by changing your exercise every fifteen to twenty seconds. You can return to that exercise a little later, say after exercises that worked other parts of the body while you rested the parts you used first. You can rotate that way for hours, just as you can alternate running with walking for a long time. What you must not do—ever—is "Go for the burn."

WARM-UP EXERCISES

You are now ready to start, and you can make a good start even if you only have three children. I started with ten, and as the numbers grew, so grew my ability to handle both the increased numbers and the need for more complicated exercise. Not only that, I discovered how different children are, one from another. There are the physically adept and ready for anything. There are others who have never had a chance to develop agility and coordination. Some have the endurance of ninety-year-olds in nursing homes. There are the shy and the bold. There are children who have already developed eye-body coordination from playing games like "Follow the Leader" or copying their parents who are involved in sports. How do you work with such a mix? With music and fun.

Put your any-size group into a circle. All eyes will be on you, not on each other. That takes care of peer pressure. The peers are too busy trying to do what you are doing.

---

8. THE SWIM

• *Start with the feet well apart and the knees stiff.*

• *Bend forward from the hips and use the "dog paddle" straight ahead for eight counts, then eight right, then eight left. Finish with eight to the center.*

(Note: Check to see that the children's backs are flat; there is no bounce in the torso; and the arms reach as far forward and to the sides as possible.)

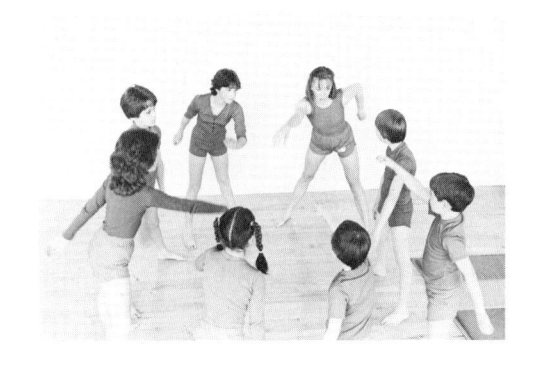

9. WAIST TWIST, UP

All sports demand separation between the upper and lower parts of the torso. A good-looking body demands the same. All sports that rotate the body—tennis, golf, skiing, for example—require strong, well-developed muscles at the waist.

• *Start with the feet apart and the legs straight.*
• *Bend both elbows and bring the fists in front of the chest. Twist the upper body to the right, leading with the right elbow.*
• *Swing immediately as far to the left as possible, leading with the left elbow.*
• *Count eight twists with the right arm only and proceed to the next exercise.*

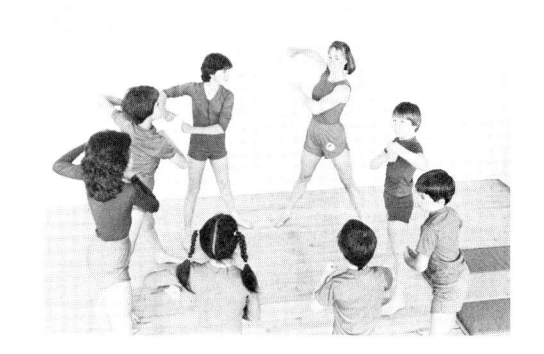

10. WAIST TWIST, DOWN

This exercise also works the waist, but in addition puts some pressure on the back muscles and stretches the hamstrings.

• *Bend forward from the hips, keeping the back parallel with the floor. Continue the arm and waist twists, except that the hands seem to punch a punching bag on a short pole.*
• *Do eight, counting the right arm only.*
• *Alternate twice with exercise 9.*

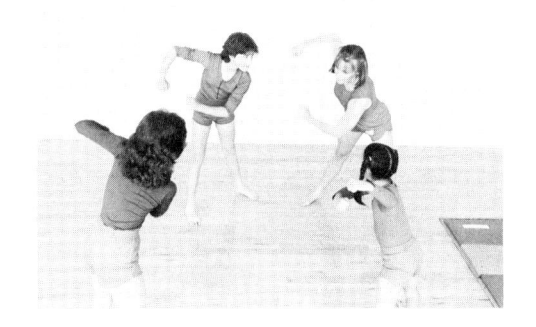

11. OVERHEAD REACH

This exercise relaxes the shoulders and strengthens the sides of the torso. It is especially helpful for any parent or teacher who uses either a typewriter or a computer. Dentists, surgeons, and artists, too, will benefit, as will people who use hands and arms in their profession. *All* these exercises are good for children.

- *Stand with the feet apart and the right arm thrust straight up into the air. The left hand is pressed against the left thigh.*
- *Bend the upper body to the left and slide the left hand down toward the knee. This will bring the right arm across to the left.*
- *Take time to stretch each child's arm so that he or she is aware of the direction. For most children, once would be enough.*
- *Have the children draw their hands in to cover their right ears. Thrust out and pull back to cover four times. Then lean to the right and repeat with the left arm.*
- *Alternate four times.*

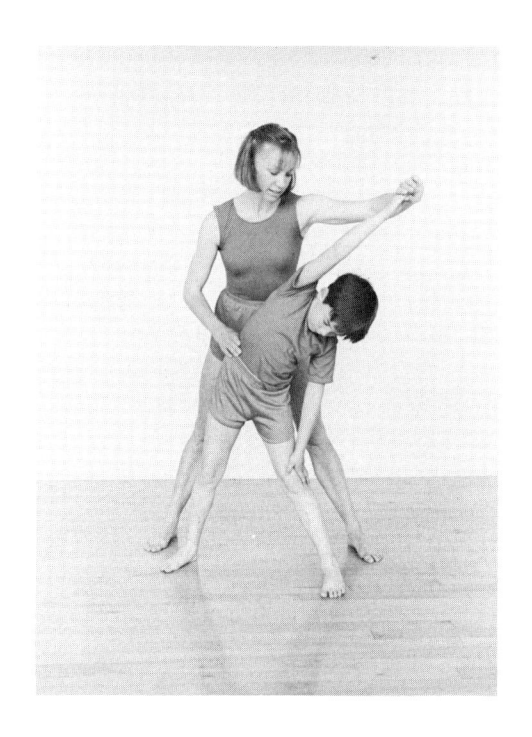

> Note: You used your arms first, torso muscles second, and then back to a combination of arms and torso, but differently. Now it is time to change the area of action.

12. KNEE BENDS

When children are young, the knees bend easily; constant practice is responsible for the facility they possess. It is important that they retain this ability and that it continue to be easy. As with every other joint in the body it is essential that knees be put through the full range of motion each day. While children are little, they spend a lot of time scrambling around on the floor, and knee action is not a problem. As they grow older, the opportunities diminish. This is especially true of children who live without the benefit of stairs. However, if you are forewarned, you will be forearmed. If your child or class is stairless, see page 148. In addition, take every chance you can to get down on the floor yourself. Your legs are just as important as the child's.

Something else: In America we have very little real information about exercise; we flow with the fads. In the 1930s, most houses had stairs and no one thought anything of climbing them. In the 1950s, we began to build split-level houses and "one level" was a selling point. Girls were not supposed to develop muscles, and the school bus arrived. In the 1960s, one of those PE folk who said jumping would loosen a uterus said also that deep knee-bends would cause meniscus injuries. You may still be harboring those bits of misinformation. Get rid of them.

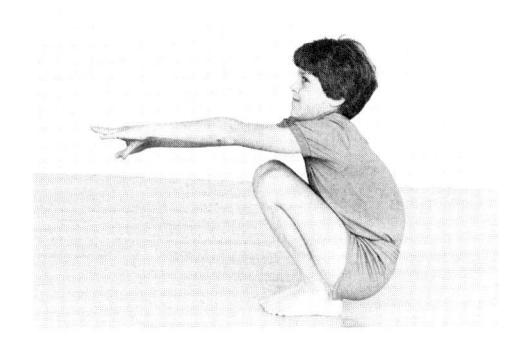

• *With the feet together and the heels flat on the floor (you may have difficulty, but most of the children won't), go down into a full knee-bend with arms outstretched in front. Make the descent as well as the ascent as slow and controlled as possible. If you or the children have trouble keeping your balance or pressing the heels to the floor, hold a couple of weight bags in your hands. Do exercise xx to stretch the heel cords.*
• *Do four knee-bends, dropping your arms to your sides as you rise. Extend them as you sink.*

Now that you have exercised the legs, change the working area back to the torso.

The shoulders are the killing field in the American body. Most of what we do involves them and often at stressful times. Writing, playing an instrument, driving, even watching TV involves shoulders. When we are under stress (which includes watching the exciting TV show) the shoulder muscles tighten. Most headaches emanate from the shoulders, no matter what those headaches are called. The more often you tie the following exercises in with classroom work or household chores, the better for you. The earlier you can make them part of a child's day (or evening), the better for the child.

13. SHOULDER SHRUG SERIES

• *Pull the shoulders up to cover the ears. Hold for a count of three.*
• *Press the shoulders down hard and make a long neck. Hold for three.*
• *Round the shoulders by dropping the head and turning both hands back to back.*
• *Press the shoulders and arms back as you lift both chest and head. Hold for three. Repeat this series often throughout the day. It is best to tie this one into things that happen regularly—change of classes, recess, before starting a new activity—if you are the teacher. If you are the parent, look at your own schedule. What do you do every day? What do you do at regular intervals?*

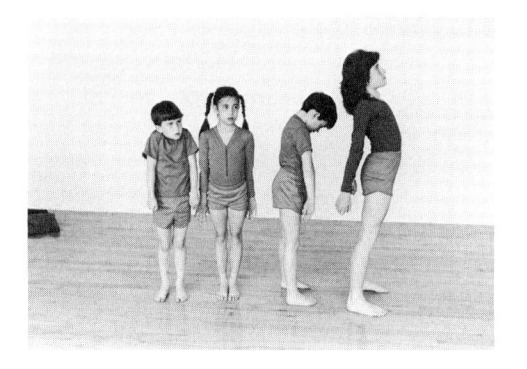

The next exercise comes in two parts. No one thought anything about it when these children's grandparents were in school, because those children had good legs. This is no longer true for many children. While deep knee-bends are more or less safe, since one leg serves to splint the other, one-legged knee-bends take practice, even the supported or partial kind.

14. HALF KNEE BENDS, SIDE

• *Stand with the legs well apart and bend the right slightly. It should just cover the toes. Look down and make doubly sure that the foot is entirely covered by the knee and that no toes are sticking out to* either *side. This patterns the leg correctly and prevents augmenting any already acquired bad habit of pronation.*

The First Step—Warm-Ups

• *Straighten the leg and tighten the entire leg from hip to ankle.*
• *On the next count, bend the other knee, again being careful to cover all the toes.*
• *Alternate sides counting to eight with the right leg only.*

Keep in mind that while American legs are underworked, American shoulders are overworked in sports, hobbies, and most of all in our occupations. Occupations include *every* occupation ever undertaken, and that means starting with "student."

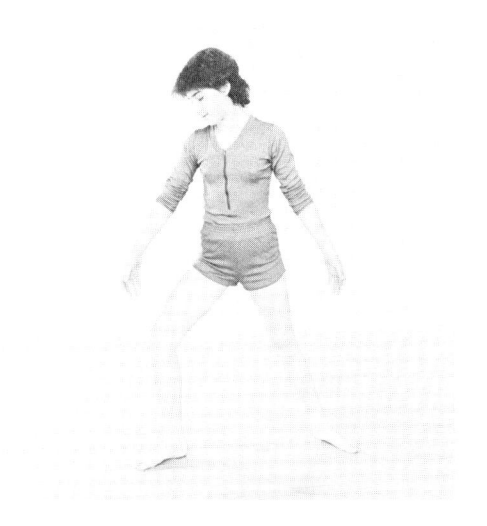

15. SHOULDER ROTATIONS, SIDE

• *Reach the right arm out to the side at shoulder level. Rotate the arm counterclockwise until the thumb points straight up toward the ceiling.*
• *Keeping the arm at shoulder level, rotate the arm clockwise until the thumb points straight backward.*
• *Do four shoulder rotations to each side and then add the next exercise.*

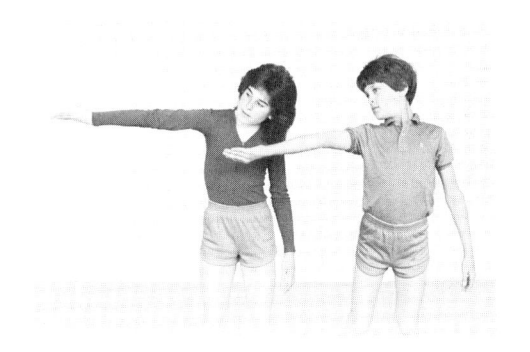

16. SHOULDER ROTATIONS, FRONT

• *Repeat the shoulder rotations, but with the arms reaching forward. Alternate, four to a side.*

• *Four shoulder rotations with each arm in both directions make up one set. Do two sets as warm-up, then do two sets several times a day, especially after writing tasks. Combine them with exercises 18 and 21 to prevent (or correct) round back.*

The next exercise releases the stress of sitting. Ask yourself, what do American children do most of the time!!! It works well between classes and even between activities within the class period. It should be made compulsory during *all* television commercials.

17. HIP ROTATIONS

• *Stand on the left leg and turn the right foot outward as far as possible.*
• *Then turn the right foot inward as far as possible. Alternate directions four times, counting only the outward rotations.*
• *Do the same with the left foot. Those make up one set. Do four sets. Be sure that everyone works as hard as possible: This one is easy to fake.*

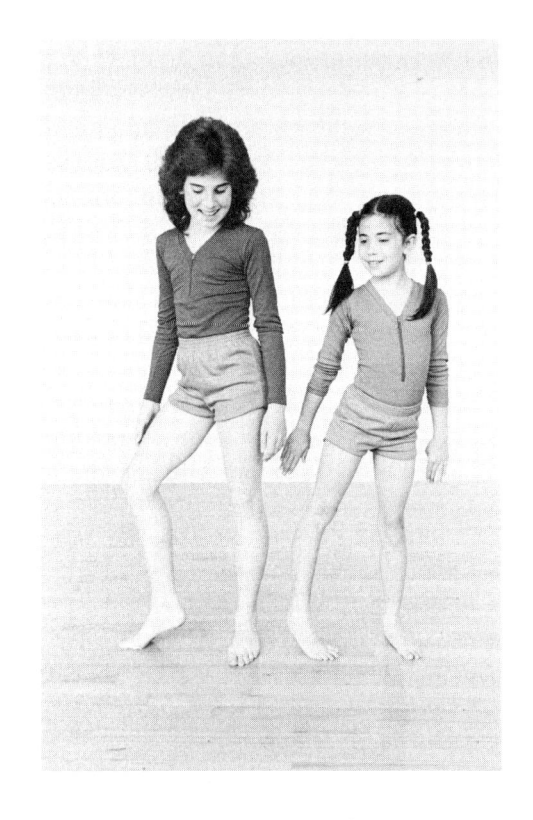

The next exercise should wear the American flag. American children do two things to cause round shoulders: They sit crouched or slumped, and they stand with their hands crossed over their chests. These postures are a sure sign of tension and uncertainty when it doesn't express lack of self-esteem and actual fear. Children sit or stand this way when they feel inadequate. The habit can be bred out of them with exercise, an understanding of what they reveal when they stand that way, and reminders. It should be understood (but maybe you, too, need reminders) that kids follow examples. Whose example are they following? Recently I heard a man, much beloved by his children, tell his daughter to stop folding her arms across her chest. Ten minutes later I watched him hide behind his. He was under considerable business stress—and there was the sign. If arms feel heavy, clasp your hands *behind* your back. It gets your chest up and out. It puts up a front. *Front* says courage, control, and "I'm just fine thank you." Other people accept that message just as they see and record signs of inadequacy. The treatment accorded to adequate and inadequate people is distinctly different. In addition, "front" is a little like the whistling by the little boy in *The King and I*. He whistled when he was afraid and pretty soon he became as "brave" as he made believe he was.

18. BACK STROKE

• *Stand with the feet apart for balance. Place the back of the right hand on the right cheek.*

• *Press the right elbow back as far as possible* without turning the body. *When you first teach this exercise, or try it yourself,* hold that elbow press-back *for a second or two.*

• *Then,* slowly *circle the lower arm back and around without letting the elbow come forward. One try will assure you that something is definitely stretching.*

• *Alternate the backstroke with each arm four times, counting only those done with the right arm.* Slowly *work up to sixteen.*

The next exercise is essential for proficiency in any sport and in the prevention of adult back pain. We are finding that back pain is attacking younger and younger people. It is rife in high schools and even in junior high. Why? It is a condition resulting from sedentary living.

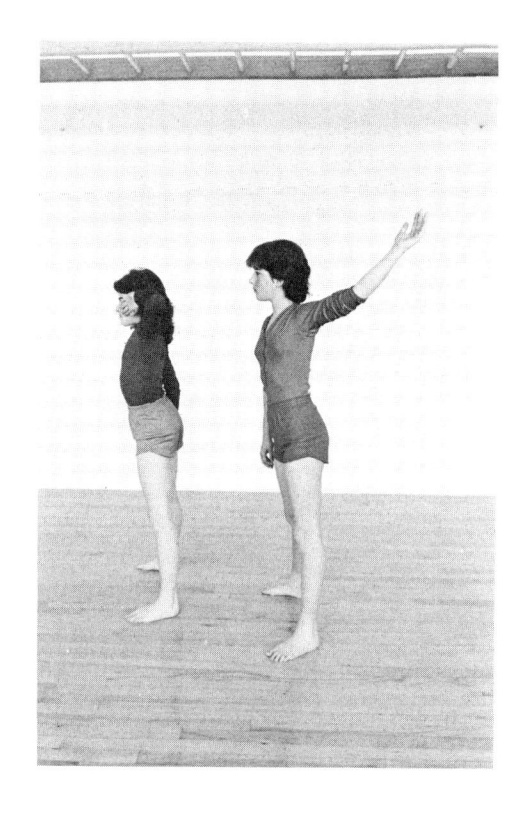

19. PELVIC TILT, STANDING

- *Stand with the feet apart and the knees slightly bent.*
- *Thrust the seat out and back, arching the back at the waist.*
- *Then, without straightening the knees, thrust the pelvis forward to make a straight line down the body from chest to knees.*
- *Do eight pelvic tilts standing.*

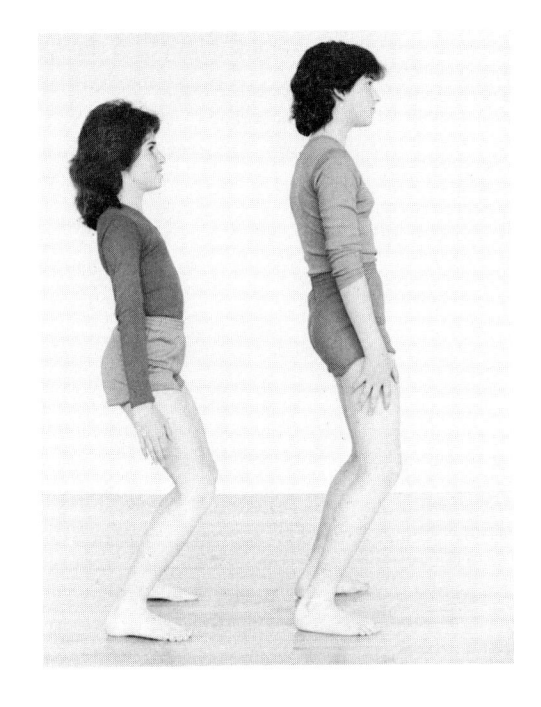

20. PELVIC TILT TO TOES

- *Bring the feet together. Thrust the seat forward as you bend the knees slightly and rise to the toes. The head will remain at the same level.*
- *Start with four and work up to eight.*

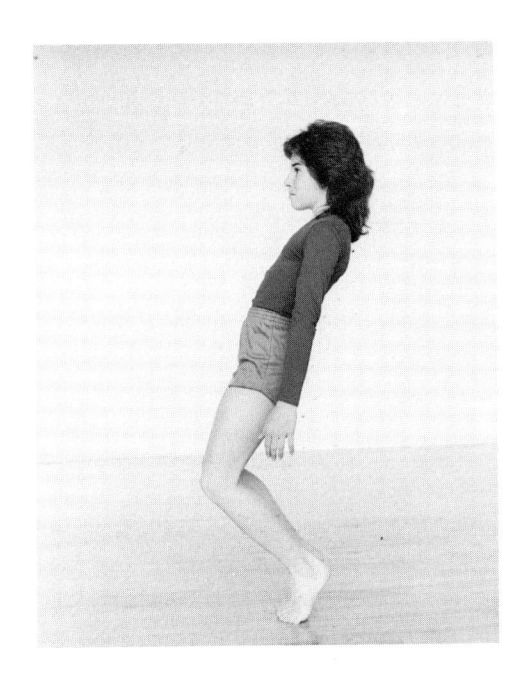

21. SNAP AND STRETCH

This is the second exercise that should be considered *must-do-daily* exercises.

- *Stand with the feet well apart and bring bent elbows to shoulder level, hands touching in front.*
- *Snap the bent elbows back on the count of "one."*
- *Bring the hands back to the touch position on the word "and."*
- *Fling both arms wide on the count of "two."*
- *Return to the hand-touch position on the word "and."*
- *Do eight snap-and-stretch exercises.* Don't let the arms drop below shoulder level.

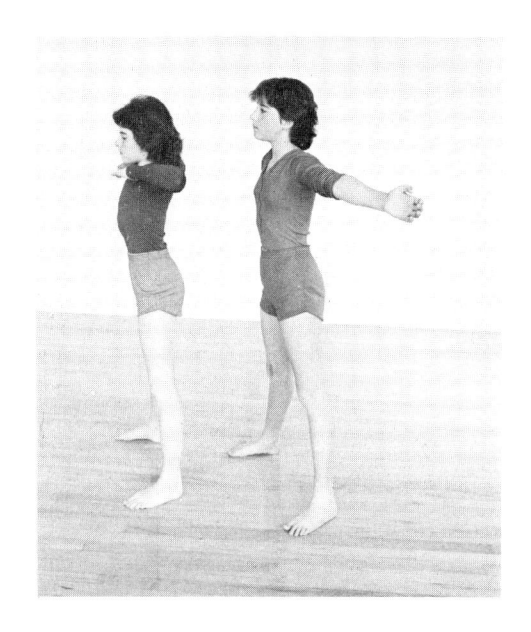

Most of the children's bodies and your own will now be warm enough to go after those forever-shortened back and hamstring muscles. Keep in mind that three things shorten those muscles:

- *Disuse, which happens whenever we sit, is the worst*
- *Overuse, which happens when children have to lift heavy loads (we have found this only with farm kids)*
- *Tension*

Everyone is subjected to tension, but some either feel it more than others or lack outlets that can dissipate it. You can do this exercise vigorously—as after-warm-ups—or gently, more as a push to full ROM (range of motion) several times during the day.

22. FLEXIBILITY BOUNCE

• Stand with the feet well apart, the knees held straight, and the hands clasped behind the back.

• Lean forward from the hips, keeping the head up and the back as level as possible.

• Bounce the upper body downward eight times while keeping the head up. The stretch will be felt behind the knees.

• Next, allow the whole upper body to droop downward, completely relaxed. Do another eight bounces in this position.

• Stand straight and then bend the body to the right, still with the legs apart and straight and the hands behind the back.

• Repeat the head-up bounces and the bounces in the drooped position, eight each.

• Do the same to the left. Finish with eight each, up and down, in the forward position. This makes up a set. As soon as possible, extend the exercise to two sets, but do one set (with light bounces) often throughout the day.

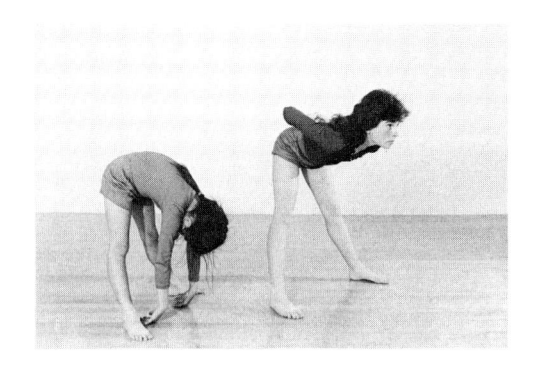

CHAPTER SEVEN
STANDING EXERCISES

As long as you have your class, however large or small, *in a circle,* you are in control, so use the circle as long as possible. *Every* child can see you, and they don't have to worry about their own performances—*they become you.* If the music is good, you should become the music. Don't think about it, it will happen. In the circle you can also see each person. One of the main "tricks" to being a good teacher *is* seeing *everyone.* Seeing, absorbing, and retaining. These are the keys to learning, with one addition—doing. Exercise is certainly doing.

You are probably one of the people Barbra Streisand sings about: people who need people who are the luckiest people in the world. If you *need* people and manage to *be with* people and bring to those people something they need and want, you have it made. Of course everyone *needs* exercise. Use your talent to make it such fun that they begin to *want* it. Then *they* will have it made.

One of the first things any teacher should know is the children's names. If there are ten little kids and two of them are yours, no problem. The first day you will know that the redhead's name is Scott. The child who fell and skinned her knee is Pam. The child whose mother was late coming to get her is called Joanie and is always on the verge of tears. When the mother is late the third time, you will know why Joanie is insecure, and rather than express irritation, you will be extra kind to Joanie. I used to wonder what those children went home to. Now, many years after I was where you are, I know. My fuse is short with parents, but I try not to ever have a short one with the children. Fairness and expectation are good watchwords. If you expect great things of children, you get great things. If you are fair, you will be respected. If you are respected, you *may* garner some love, but don't go into teaching for that reason or you'll be disappointed. I have found that making lives a *little* better and the world a *little* better is reward enough. What you will have is laughter and fun. That is guaranteed. In a world where "youth" is paramount, laughter and fun are the magic that buys it.

So, now you are all warmed up and ready for the next step—standing exercises. You are still in your controlled circle and still standing. All you need to do is change the record or the tape.

Feet are top-order in importance. Most people count the baby's toes and after finding there are ten, forget the feet altogether. Shoe manufacturers are quick to provide hard-soled shoes for new little feet, which should be allowed to develop without such bracing. One of the reasons we *never* wear shoes in an exercise class is the need for foot development. It's true, there usually are ten toes, and every single one of them is fully equipped with muscles and tendons, blood and nerves, flesh, skin and bones. Every one has a circulatory system that depends upon cramp-free legs to funnel nutrition to it and to carry away its waste products. Understand that—*every single toe*. When the foot is unshod, all of it gets a chance to work and develop. But when you put a shoe on that foot, it becomes a hoof. Only part of it can work *and never to full range of motion.*

If you or your spouse has a long second toe (see page 435), your child probably has the same anomaly. In that case both of you, or all three, should go shoeless as much as possible. If you are a teacher, take the time when you test to check all your little people for the long second toe. On page 436 you will find out how to test.

23. MOUSETRAP, HOT PENNIES

• *Stand with the feet close together, the knees straight.*

• *Roll onto the outsides of both feet so that the space between the feet could hold a small mouse. Be sure that both the toes touch and both the heels; otherwise the mouse could get out.*

• *Now flatten both feet, trapping the mouse inside. Do four.*

• *Begin again with feet flat and parallel*

Standing Exercises 83

as before. Pretend there are ten hot pennies on the floor just under your toes.

• *Lift up the toes to cool them. Lower them again. Do four.*

After you are sure the mousetraps are neat and closed at each end and the toes lifted high off the hot pennies, alternate the two, eight times.

Many older people who wear shoes all the time and never exercise their feet other than through walking (if that!!), cannot lift onto their toes and have no right-angle break between toes and foot.

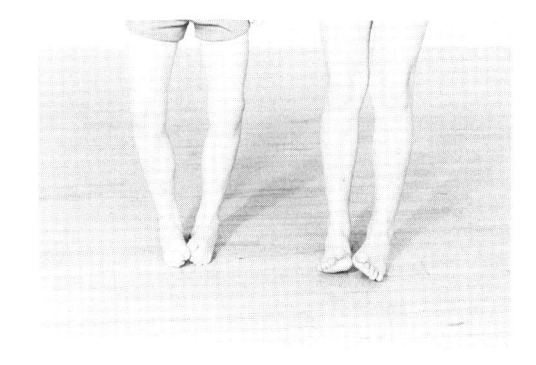

Check your own. Children still can, and that *must* be maintained.

24. TOE RISES, SINGLE

• *Stand on both feet and then press one foot forward as you bend your knee. Check for a good forward position of the instep.*

• *Replace the heel on the floor and press the other instep forward as you lift the heel and bend the knee.*

• *Alternate for sixteen.*

Toe rises are essential for foot strength, balance, and control. The children with the long second toes will have trouble with balance at first (see why on page 435). There are two tricks that help with balance: Make the whole lower body into a pole by tightening hips, thighs, knees, calves, and ankles. The second trick is concentration. Look at an unmoving spot on the wall.

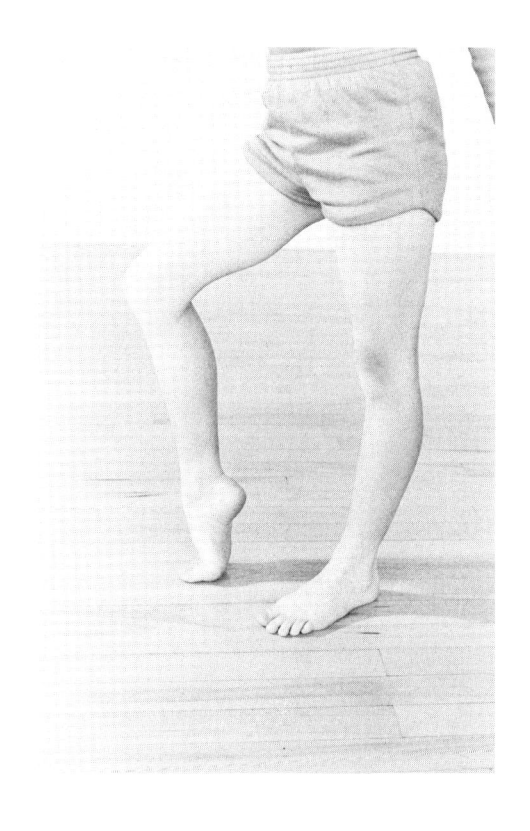

25. TOE RISES

• *With the feet together, rise as high on the toes as possible. Lower to rest on the floor. Do eight.*

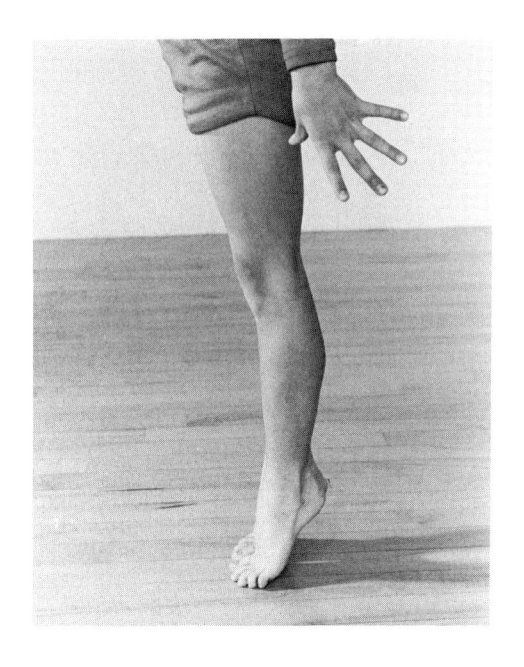

26. THE ELEVATOR

This exercise is a form of toe rise that calls for good control. Start with an elevator that goes up four floors and *slowly* proceed to eight. Say to the children the following:

• *"This time we are going to go up in an elevator. Go up off the floor just a little, which we'll call the first floor."*

• *"Now go up another little bit to the next floor. Stay a minute to let some people off."*

• *"Ready, up to the third floor. Hold it for passengers."*

• *"Right to the top. Hold."*

• *"Now we go down in four counts, one to a floor."* Repeat four times.

27. EDGING

• *Stand with the feet together and bend both knees just a little.*

• *Roll over onto the right edges of both feet. (Check to see that the feet actually roll over.)*

• *Now roll to the other side.*

Standing Exercises

- *Keeping the knees bent, arms away from the body, and head level, shift from side to side sixteen times.*

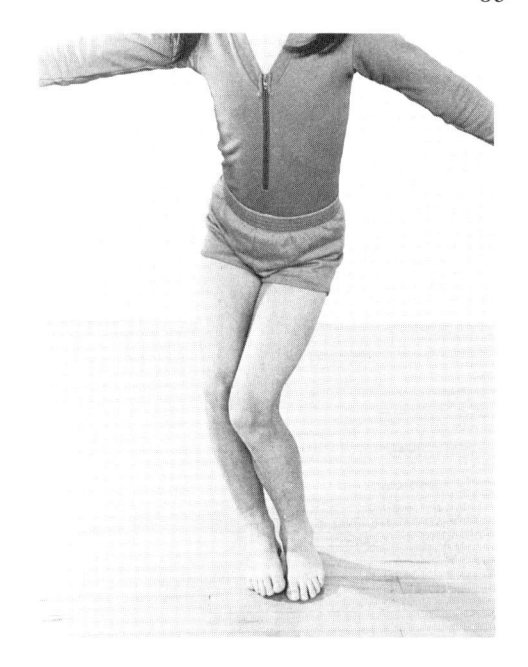

Go through the foot series twice at each class, not necessarily in succession. The children will soon be good at it and will be better prepared for the floor progressions (starting on page 107). When both are a part of their everyday routine, they will begin to do well at sports.

---

28. HAND WALK-OUT

- *Stand with the feet well apart. (The farther apart the legs, the easier the exercise.)*
- *Lean forward from the hips and, keeping the feet anchored, walk the hands out until the body is at full stretch.*
- *Walk out to each of four counts. Come back, however, in two and use counts "three" and "four" for standing erect. Start with four and work up to eight. Keep the knees straight.*

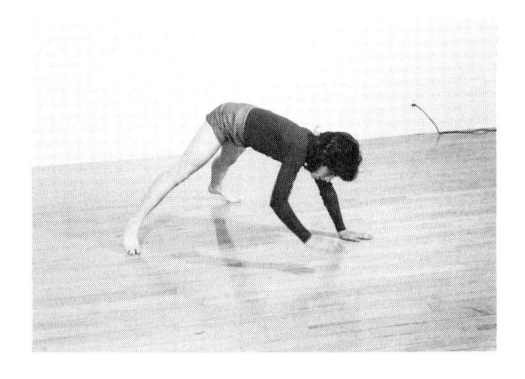

The next two exercises belong in the standing series, but the preparation is in the kneeling section. Pass over these until you have prepared with the easier exercises.

29. THREAD NEEDLE, STANDING

• *Stand on all fours, legs wide and straight.*
• *With the weight on the right hand, bring the left arm under the body.*

• *Swing the left arm up toward the ceiling, following it with your eyes. Do four with the left arm and then four with the right.*

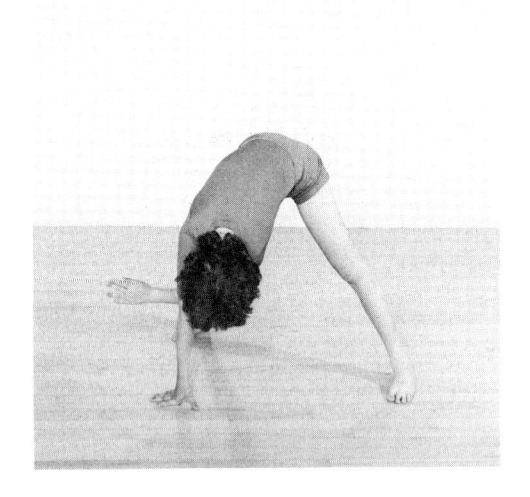

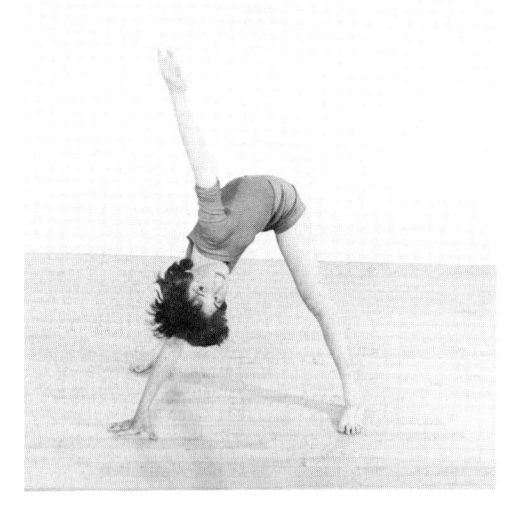

30. FORWARD FALL, STANDING

• *Stand with the legs spread wide. (The wider the spread, the easier the exercise.)*
• *Bring the hands to a point just in front of the shoulders.*
• *Lean way forward from the hips while keeping the legs absolutely straight. Reach for the floor with both hands.*
• *Fall forward and catch the body on the outstretched hands.*

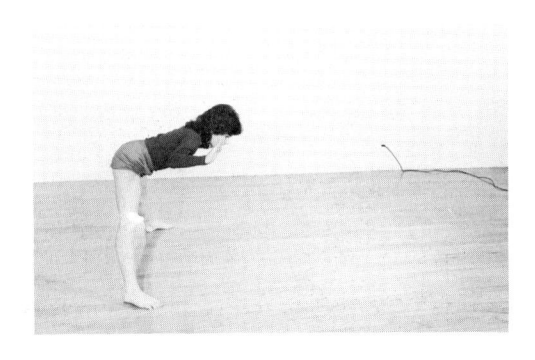

Standing Exercises

• *Arch the body down as you bring the head up.*
• *Bounce down gently four times and return to the standing position, using two-hand steps as you did in exercise 28.*

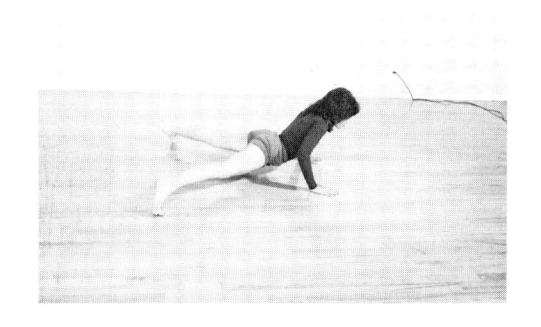

The next series of exercises is a lot of fun, but calls for extra work and control by the teacher, since you are about to lose that valuable teaching aid, the circle.

Pair up the children as close to size as possible and explain that pushing is an exercise of *balance* as well as *strength*. This might be a good time to remind them that bigger kids don't pick on little kids, because that's cowardice.

31. SHOULDER PUSH

• *Stand shoulder to shoulder with the outsides of the feet pressed against each other. Do* not *link arms.*
• *Both children bend the elbows pressed against their partners.*
• *Each then grasps the partner's upper arms with the free hand. (This prevents breaking away and falling due to momentum).*
• *Each presses as hard against the other as possible. Most of the time the push won't go anywhere.*

Hold for ten counts.

• *Do three holds for ten counts and then reverse the feet and repeat, using the opposite sides.*

Most of the time the children will hang there in a kind of dynamic balance.

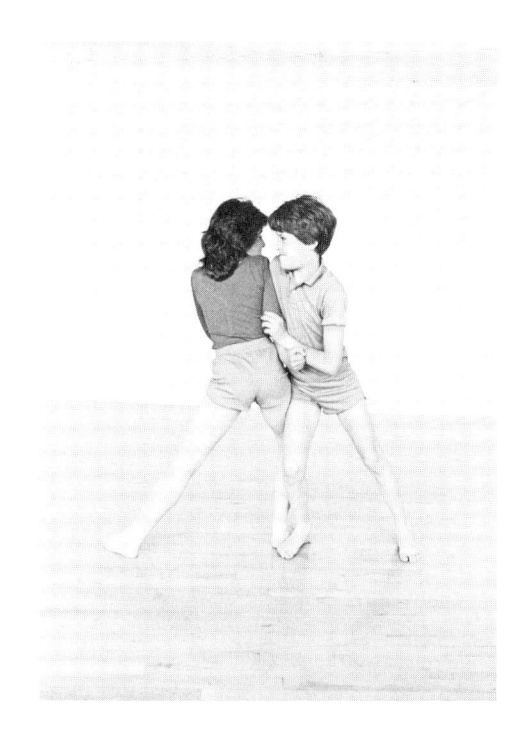

Sometimes (and watch for it) there is a stronger child who finds he can push his partner over. The easiest way to handle that is to pair him or her with a stronger partner. *You* may have to be that partner. Explain at the outset that the idea is to hang there, each pushing as hard as possible, but *not* to "win." Show how even the strongest could be pushed over by you, but you are trying to find that balance point where you both meet.

32. RAM PUSH

• *The partners face each other and place their hands on each other's shoulders. At a given signal they start to push against each other, trying again to reach the balance point. Hold for ten and release. Do three.*
• *Change the foot positions and push again for three sets of ten.*

The minute adjustments each child must make to the other's pressures are like scales for the pianist: One cannot begin either too soon. The next exercise will prove how much they have learned about balancing two bodies against each other. *Explain* that we all have a mechanism for controlling our muscles and that it must be developed *before* we try to become dancers, athletes, or indeed do anything physical.

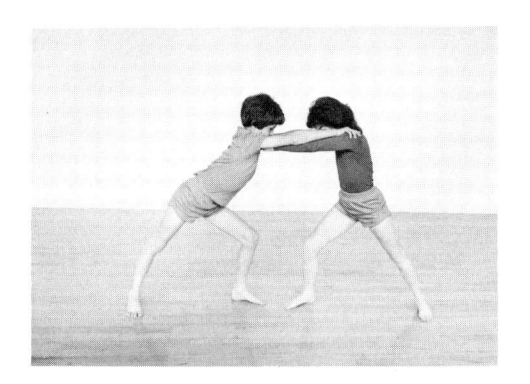

33. ONE-FOOT BALANCED STAND

• *Stand again with the right feet pressed against each other.*
• *Have the children grasp each other's wrists.*
• *Lean back and try to establish a balance point where each child will be able to lift the free foot and stay suspended. Try three times with each foot for a count of ten.*

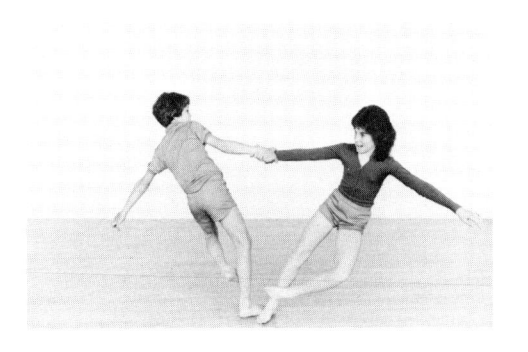

MUSIC

When you do *any* exercise that requires control of this kind, use slow, fluid, steady music. Muscles react to music. This is especially important if you work with children who have spasmed muscles, as children with cerebral palsy do. The *muscles* will respond to passive exercises at first. Later the response will carry over into the child's efforts to move to music.

CHAPTER EIGHT
KNEELING, SITTING, AND LYING EXERCISES

There are as many different ways to exercise as there are muscles, multiplied by the qualities of those muscles. The exercises that strengthen are the opposite from those that stretch. Those two qualities taken together, in the proper timing and intensity, give us coordination. No muscle can work to its full potential without *both* qualities. Imagine how frustrated I was when a fine, courageous, Olympic skier came to me just before the FIS and said he'd like some extra training. In those days the skiers' training consisted only of skiing—no exercise, no running, no apparatus, and no weights. I tested his flexibility and found that his *vorlage* (ability to bend the ankle forward, which depends on hamstring stretch) was nil. It was too late. That should have been spotted and remedied when he was a child and had his first pair of skis.

KNEELING EXERCISES

Back to the circle! The kneeling exercises bring your flock, however large or small, back under your complete control—all the better for their time away.

Kneeling, Sitting, and Lying Exercises

34. ANGRY CAT, OLD HORSE

• *Start on hands and knees. Press the back up like an angry, spitting, hissing cat. (Sometimes children like to provide their own sound effects.) Be sure the head is down and arms held straight.*

• *Drop the back into a sag to look like a tired old horse with a swayback. Do eight.*

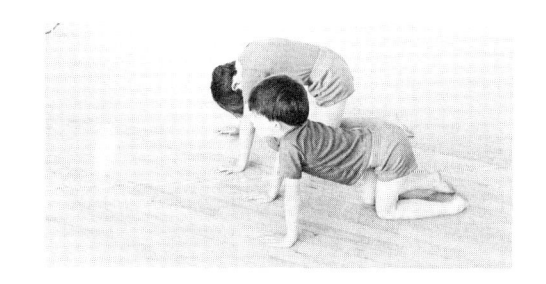

35. KNEE-TO-NOSE KICK

This exercise tightens up the seat, and the seat is a very telling feature. Wobbly rear ends are unattractive. They also shout of a lack of self-discipline. You will never see one on a dancer or athlete.

• *Still on hands and knees, bring one knee as close to the nose as possible.*

• *Next, stretch the leg backward and up as high as possible. Do eight with each leg to make up a set.*

• *Do three sets.*

You have just worked the back, abdominals, and legs. Rest them as you stretch the chest and arms and build strength in the upper back and arms.

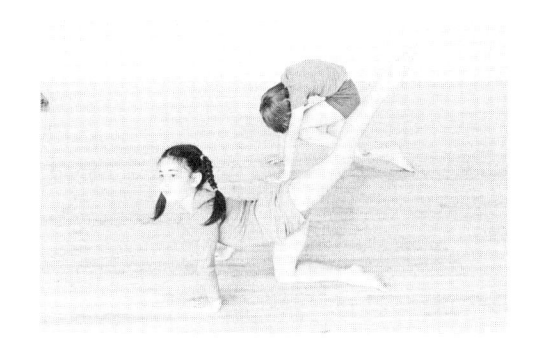

36. THREAD NEEDLE, KNEELING

• *Start on all fours with knees a little apart for balance.*

• *Thrust the right arm under the chest and out the other side between the left arm and the knee.*

• *Next, thrust the same arm back out and straight up toward the ceiling. Follow the hand with the eyes.*

• *Do eight with each arm.*

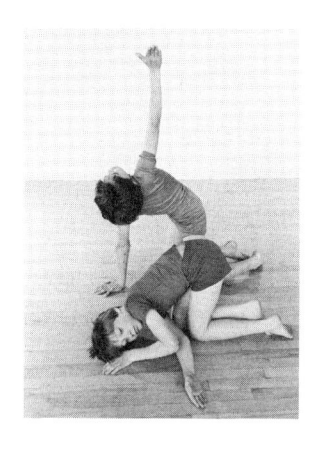

37. SWING AROUND

The next exercise gets the seat and legs again, and the waist.

• *Still on all fours, swing one leg forward to a point ahead of the hands.*
• *Then swing the same leg back around over the kneeling leg. Turn to look over your shoulder far enough so that you can see the crossed-over foot. Do four to the side.*

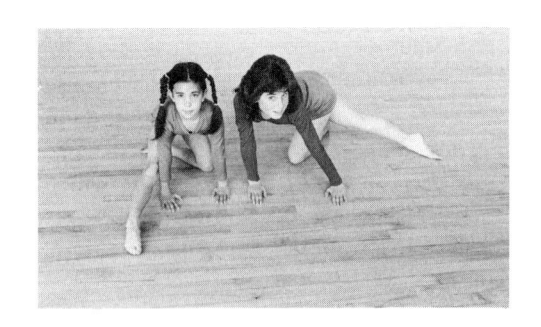

38. PELVIC TILT, KNEELING

The Pelvic Tilt, whether prone (as in the limbering series), standing, sitting, or kneeling, is of prime importance. It flattens the abdominals, tightens the seat, and strengthens the pelvic floor. You as the teacher should make a habit of doing many pelvic tilts every day.

• *Start kneeling with the knees slightly apart. Sit on your heels.*
• *Rise from your heels as little as possible as you press the pelvis forward to make a straight line from chin to knee.*
• *Then arch the back as you tilt the pelvis back.*

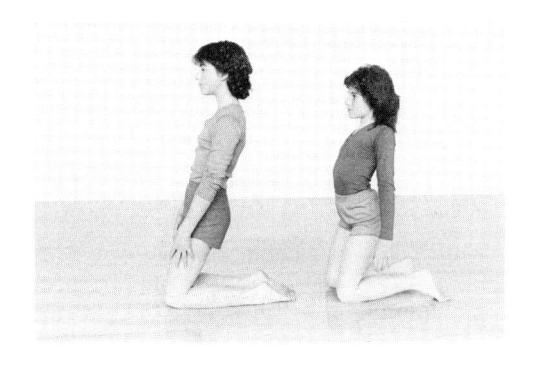

• *Try to keep the head level as you work the pelvis between chin and knees. Stay low. Do four.*

39. THE HYDRANT

The name of this exercise always starts the class giggling, no age limit! It is a hard exercise, so begin with only a few.

• *Start in the hands-and-knees position.*
• *Bring the bent knee out to the side, trying to make it level and even with the back.*

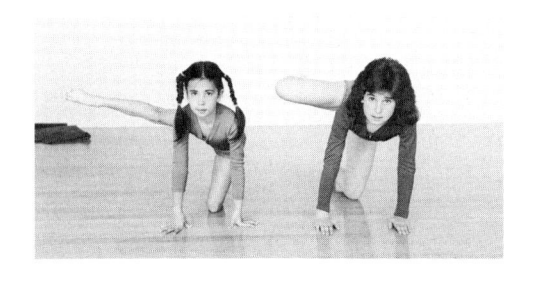

Kneeling, Sitting, and Lying Exercises

• *Holding that lifted position, extend the leg fully to the side.*
• *Retract the leg and place the knee on the floor. Do four.*

• *Repeat to the other side. As strength improves, add four to each side. Still later, add a third set of four to a side.*

40. FORWARD FALL, KNEELING

The next exercise calls for arm strength and also for courage. Remember, little people do not have far to fall, but still it's scary. To take the fear out of it, just wave good-bye with both hands as you fall. They will follow. Later, when they are sure of themselves, try for a straight body with no bend in the hips.

• *Kneeling in the circle, bring both hands to shoulder level so that the children know where they belong.*
• *Next, wave good-bye across the circle as you fall forward to catch yourself on outstretched arms. Do four, always waving good-bye.*

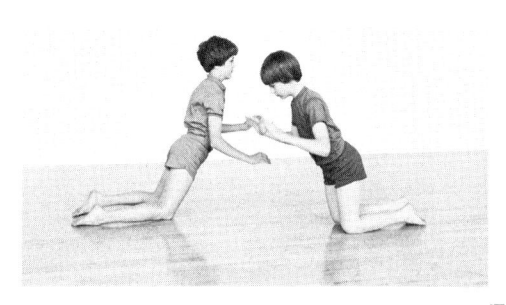

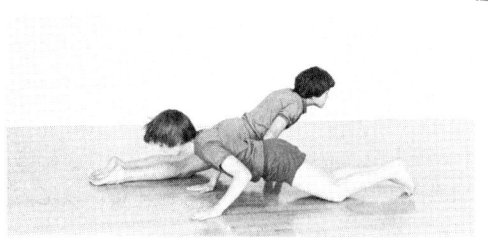

41. PEANUT PUSH

This exercise really has three parts. Start doing the first and second positions *long* before adding the third, the Peanut Push with the chin. Once you can do that push with ease, use the catback return.

• *Start with the kneelback, the seat on the heels, and the arms stretched out in front. Press way down to stretch the arms and chest.*
• *Rock forward onto the hands as you arch the back and bring the head up. This is the practice exercise.*
• *When you feel that that part is easy, start as in position one with your chin almost on the floor.*

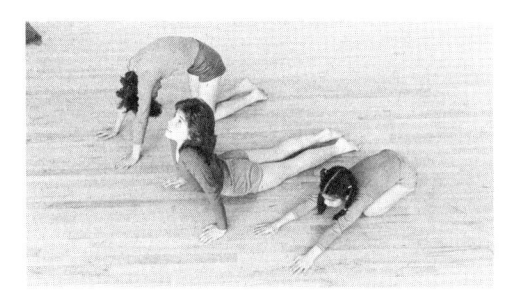

• *Stay low and pretend to push a peanut across the floor as you move the upper body out of the arched-up position. Do* not *push upward until you are at full stretch.*
• *From that position, push the back up into the angry-cat position and press back to the heel-sitting start. Do four.*

SITTING AND LYING EXERCISES

The number of possible exercises multiplies again when you consider how many levels are involved. So far we have had standing, and kneeling; sitting and the very lowest level, lying, are next. Lying down exercises are done either, prone (facedown) or supine (faceup) or on one side.

42. THE LIMBERING SERIES

These are the very *best* exercises for people with aching backs. Even children get back pain, especially when they are ill, have a high fever, or have to stay in bed for any length of time. That's one of the reasons people get back rubs. These exercises are far better than massage—and you can do them for yourself.

42A. SUPINE, KNEE TO NOSE

* *Lie supine with the knees bent and the feet slightly apart.*
* *Bring the left knee as close to the nose as possible as you lift the head to meet it.*
* *Lie back down* and then *extend the leg straight out.*
* *Return the extended leg to the starting position and do the same with the right leg. Alternate for eight.*
* *When you have completed the exercise, drop your knees to the right and roll onto your right side.*

Children, who rarely have stiff necks, don't seem to mind how their heads rest, but you and your friends will. Curl your right arm up under your head to be comfortable.

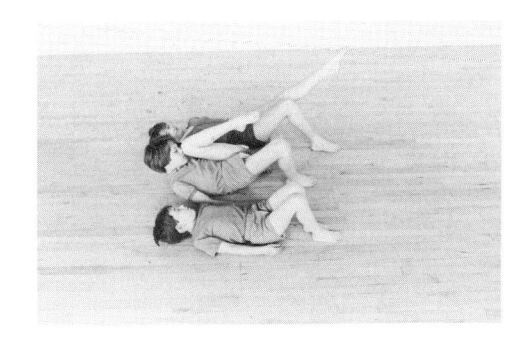

Kneeling, Sitting, and Lying Exercises　　　　　　　　　　　　　　　　　　　　95

42B. RIGHT SIDE-LYING STRETCH

• *Bend the left (or upper) leg and bring it as close to the chest as possible. Help with one or both hands if necessary (usually not for children, but all too often for grown-ups).*

• *Extend the leg straight down, about eight inches above the resting leg.*

• *Lower and* relax *for a count of three. Repeat four times and then roll over to the prone position.*

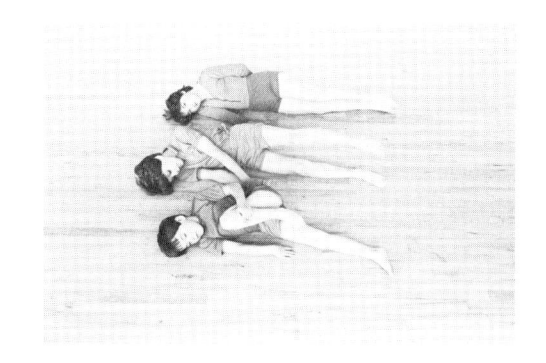

42C. PRONE GLUTEUS SET

Actually this is the easiest position in which to do a Pelvic Tilt, and it is one of the best exercises for an aching back. (The Side-Lying Stretch, above, is *unquestionably* the best; see the chapter on Myotherapy.)

• *Rest your head on your arms and relax while rolling your heels outward. This relaxes the buttocks.*

• *Roll the heels in to touch each other and tighten the seat muscles as much as possible. Pinch the buttock muscles together. Hold for a slow count of four.*

• *Roll the heels out and relax for a count of three.*

• *Roll the heels in and tighten the buttocks as before . . . and then pull in the abdominals as you hold for a count of four.*

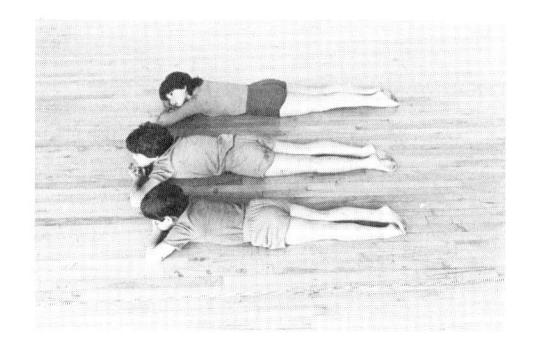

• *Roll the heels out again and relax for three. Do four of the buttock-abdominal tightening and relaxing.*

42D. LEFT SIDE-LYING STRETCH

• *Roll the body onto the left side and repeat the Side-Lying Stretch (exercise 42B) with the other leg.*

• *Roll onto your back.*

42E. PELVIC TILT, SUPINE

- *Rest your head on your hands and bend both knees.*
- *Arch the back as much as possible. There should be an arch that a small mouse could hide under.*
- *Press the spine down to flatten the mouse and at the same time tilt the pelvis up. The abdominals disappear from view. Hold this position for a slow count of four. Relax.*
- *Arch, flatten, and hold; relax. Do four.*

If you will make this series of exercises a daily routine for every child in your care, your whole family, and for any friends who are dear to you, you will be able to get rid of backaches and, more important, prevent them in the future.

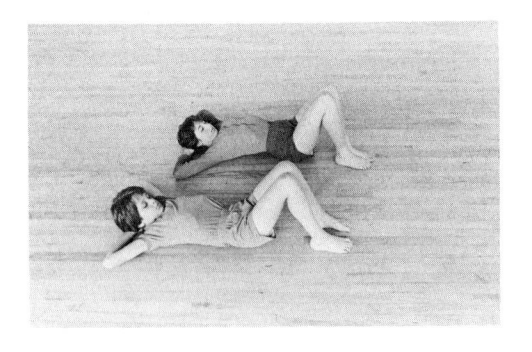

CHAPTER NINE
FLEXIBILITY EXERCISES

Flexibility is every bit as important as strength; without it no child can attain full potential. The important thing to remember about it is that flexibility exercises come *after* the body is thoroughly warmed, even hot and dripping with sweat. Then the muscles are elastic and soft as butter.

Before we start, let me again ask you to forget any injunctions you have heard against "bouncing" to achieve stretch. That type of stretch is called *ballistic stretch* and has served dancers and gymnasts well for centuries. That is why *all* of them are flexible. As I said before, the latest "discovery" is called *static stretch*. America is full of "latest discoveries," such as push-ups from the knees for girls, no chin-ups for girls, no jumping for girls, no deep knee-bends for any of the children ... and now "static stretch." In a static stretch you hold a stretch at its ultimate for forty to sixty seconds. To see the difference in results, visit a dance studio using ballistic stretch and then a gym where the coach uses static stretch. The children of that group will have no flexibility. The dancers could spread their legs east and west. Warning: If the teacher of the dancers has adopted static stretch, look out. *Some people will follow anything.* Some of those teachers who used static stretch and noticed the poor results have resorted to ballistic stretch, but they call it *pulsing.* In this book (and all my books) we use ballistic stretch. Why? Because it works, *and none of our students has been injured by it in forty years.*

43. STRETCH SIT-UP

- *Sit with straight legs close together.*
- *Round your back as you lean forward toward the toes. Keep your head down.*
- *Keeping the head down, roll slowly back, trying to touch each button of the spine to the floor.*
- *Point the toes. That stretches the anterior tibialis muscles in the lower legs. They make a great difference when it comes to running.*
- *When you are flat, stretch both arms above your head and then* swing *up to the sitting position. The momentum of the swing prevents any overwork for the psoas. Do four.*

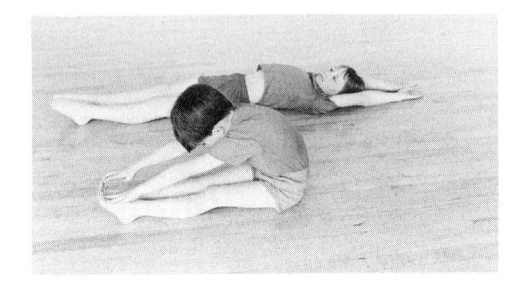

Children are *so* smart, and we ask *so* little of them. Sometimes it's because *we* don't know enough. Teach them about those muscles that are so important to them. *Anterior* means in front. *Tibialis* is the muscle running along the *tibia,* the large bone in the lower leg. The *fibula* is the little bone on the outside. Get a colorful anatomy book and teach them about their bodies so that they will understand and care about them.

---

44. SPREAD-LEG SIDE-DROP

This exercise works a number of areas: It stretches the chest (which helps the round-backed); it works the waistline and abdominals (useful for the kids who still have straight-up-and-down figures and, at twelve, don't like it at all). The forward reach stretches the back and hamstring muscles.

Flexibility Exercises

- *Sit on the floor with the legs spread wide.*
- *Drop the upper body to one side as you twist the waist in that direction as far as you can manage.*
- *Land on both hands and bring the chest and one ear to the floor.*
- *Sit up and lean forward to touch the toes as you swing around to repeat the drop to the other side. Alternate for eight.*

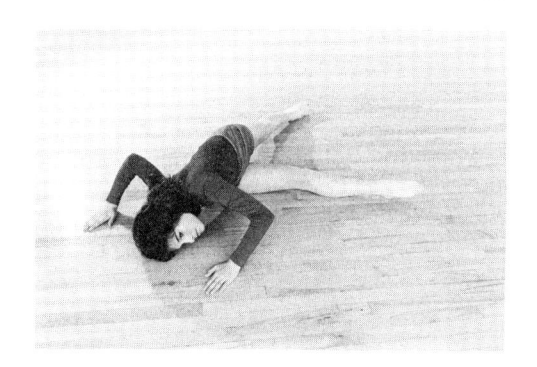

When people are lying on one side and are asked to "roll over onto the other side," they go through a whole series of unnecessary movements. In most cases they move over onto their backs, lift their hips, and set them down on the other side. There is a simpler way. Just curl up, on whatever side you are on, and roll over with hands and legs out of the way. When the roll is terminated, stretch out on the other side.

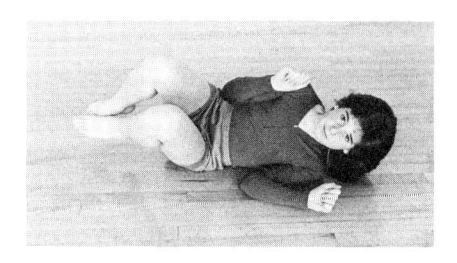

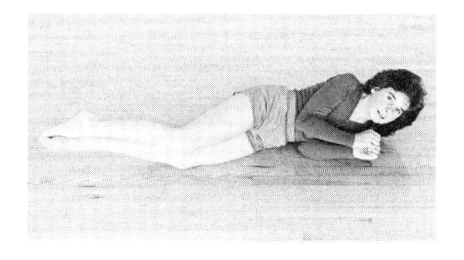

45. SIDE LEG LIFT

- *Lie on the right side, resting on the right elbow with the left hand on the floor in front of you.*
- *Lie with your weight on the side of the pelvis and lift the top leg. If you are on the pelvic bone and not back on the hip, you will not be able to lift the leg very high, which is correct. Do eight to a side.*

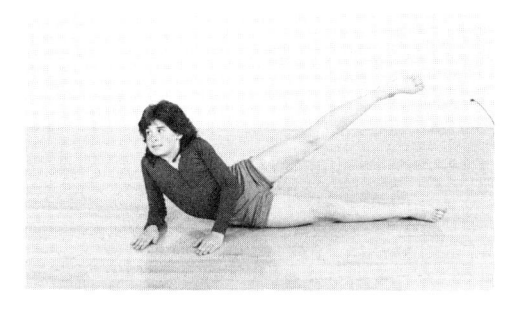

46. CURL ... EXTEND ... CURL

• *Start on the right side, curled into the fetal position.*
• *Extend the body on its side to the fully stretched position.*
• *Roll in the extended position to the other side and then curl up tight again.*
• *Extend again and roll.*
• *Curl again into the fetal position as at the start. That makes one set. Do four sets.*

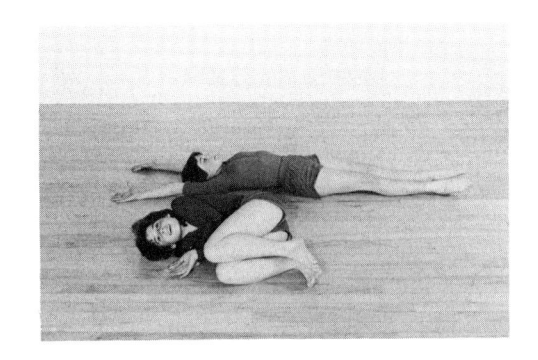

47. SIDE KNEE BEND, EXTENDED

• *Start on the side with the body extended, both hands on the floor in front of the chest. Point the toes. Rest on elbow.*
• *Lean back very slightly to take the weight onto the hip, and bring the bent knee in back of the shoulder.*
• *Keeping the knee as close to the shoulder as possible, extend the leg straight up.*
• *Return to the bent-knee position.*
• *Extend the leg to rest just above the other leg. Do four and then* roll *to the other side and repeat with the other leg. Do four.*

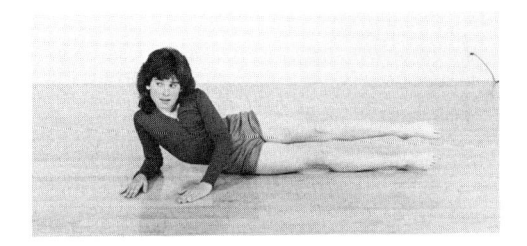

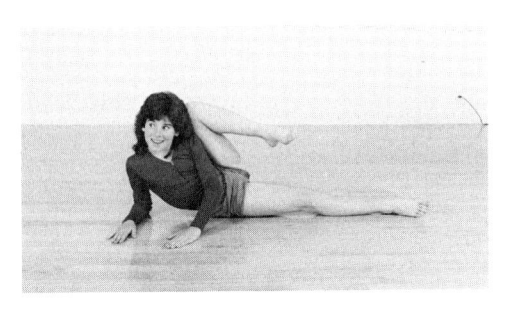

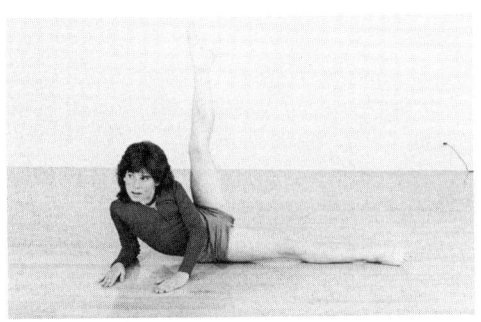

Flexibility Exercises

48. SUPINE KNEE-TO-NOSE KICK

• *Lie supine, resting on the elbows, legs together and extended, with the toes pointed.*
• *Bring the left knee to the nose.*
• *Keeping it as close to the nose as possible, extend the leg straight up.*
• *Return the bent knee to its knee-to-nose position.*
• *Extend the leg to the starting rest position. Alternate for eight.*

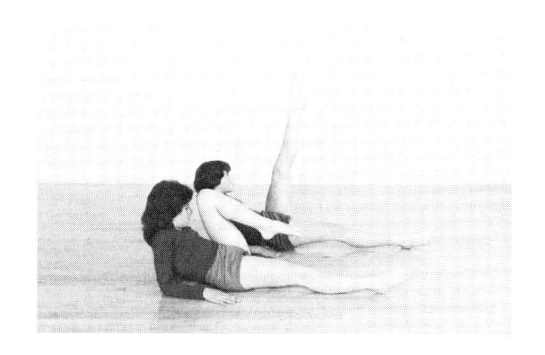

49. FORWARD-BACKWARD LEG SWINGS

• *Lie on one side, both hands on the floor in front. Rest on one elbow.*
• *Swing the top leg first forward and then back eight times. Be sure that the legs are held straight and the toes are pointed.*

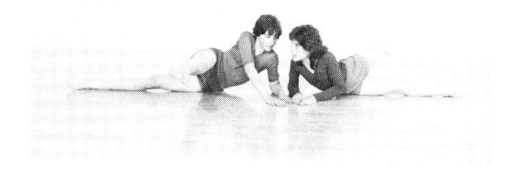

50. THE FLAGPOLE

• *Lie supine with the body stretched long and the arms stretched on the floor above the head.*
• *Raise one leg straight overhead.*
• *At first, "walk" up that leg hand over hand until the ankle is reached.*
• *Roll back down with the hands free. Leave the leg aloft.*
• *Do four climbs with each leg.*
• *As soon as the abdominals are strong enough, swing both hands from the floor above the head and reach for the ankle with no intermittent steps. Do four on each side.*

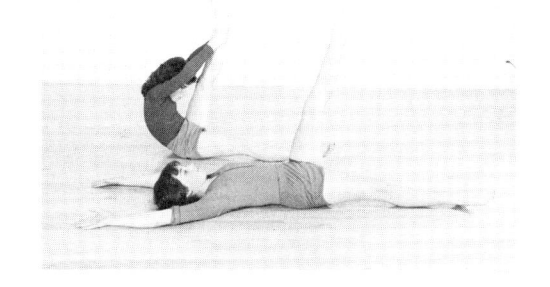

51. HAND-HELD LEG STRETCH

• Lie on the right side, resting on the right elbow.
• Take the instep of the left foot in the left hand. Be sure the extended leg is straight and the toes are pointed.
• Stay on the side and do not tip back onto the hip.
• Keeping a tight hold on the instep, extend the leg overhead. Be sure that the knee does not bend.
• Return to the bent-knee position. Do four extensions with each leg.

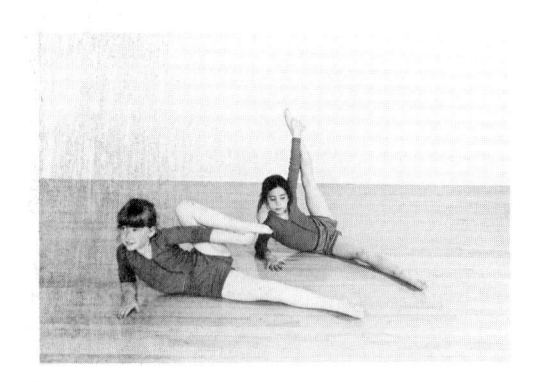

52. LEG SPREAD, HEAD DOWN

• Spread both legs, grasping the insteps with both hands.
• Pull the head down in short, easy bounces. The aim is to touch the floor, but take your time.

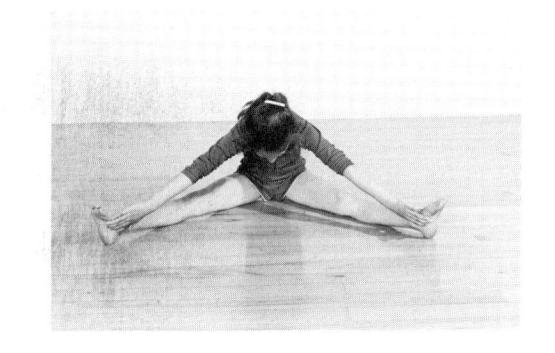

53. LOWER-BACK STRETCH

• Sit with the feet drawn up to the crotch and sole to sole.
• Grasp both ankles and pull your head down to touch the toes in eight easy bounces.
• Sit up to rest and then repeat. Do three.

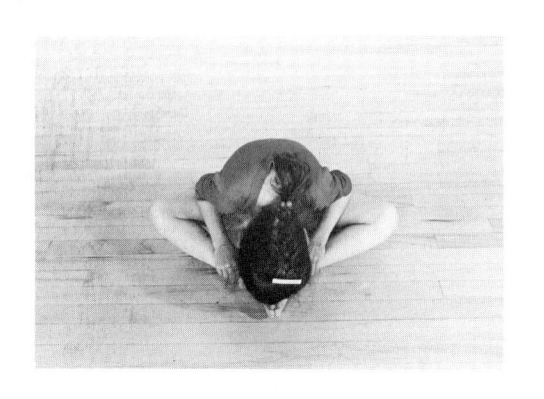

Flexibility Exercises

54. CROTCH STRETCH

- *Sit with the knees bent, feet sole to sole and drawn up to the crotch.*
- *Grasp the ankles in the hands as you press down with elbows on knees. The aim is to press them flat on the floor. This one is easy for kids, almost impossible for grown-ups.*

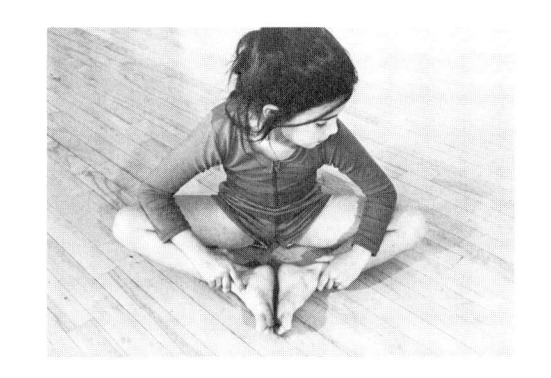

55. LEG SPREAD, EAR TO KNEE

- *Grasp the right ankle with the right hand and pull the right ear down to touch the knee in eight easy bounces. Do the same to the other side to make up a set. Do four sets.*

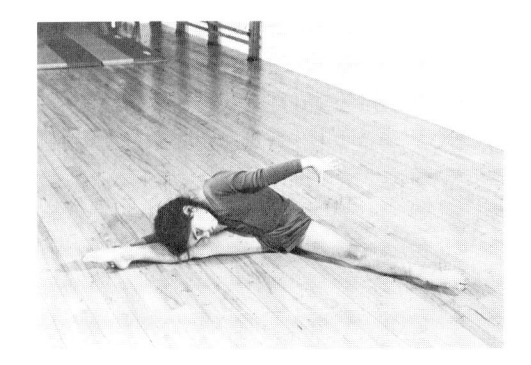

56. LEG SPREAD, HELD ALOFT

- *Start with the ankles held in both hands, knees out to the side and feet off the floor.*
- *Extend straight legs out and up. Try to hold for five seconds. (If you roll back, duck your head.)*
- *Do three, trying to keep the back straight.*

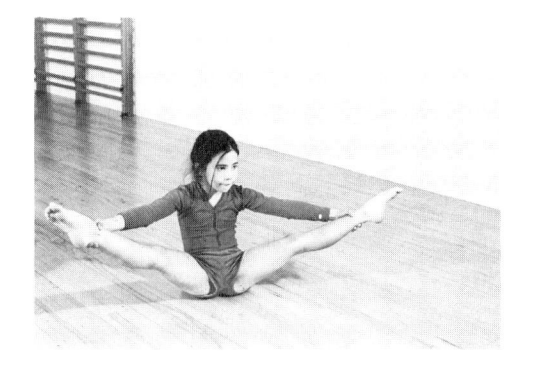

57. KNEE TO SHOULDER, ASSISTED

• *This calls for passive stretch in which the teacher does all the work and the child tries to relax.*
• *Press the bent knee into the shoulder for eight presses on each leg to make up a set.*
• *Do four sets.*

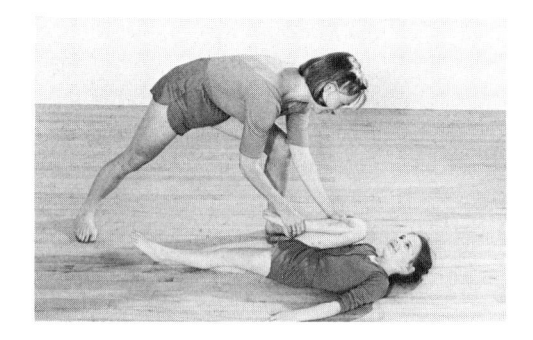

58. STRAIGHT-LEG STRETCH, ASSISTED

• *The child lies supine with both legs straight.*
• *He or she raises one leg straight up while keeping the other flat on the floor.*
• *The teacher presses the leg back toward the child's head.*
• *Use eight presses on each leg for a set. Do three sets.*

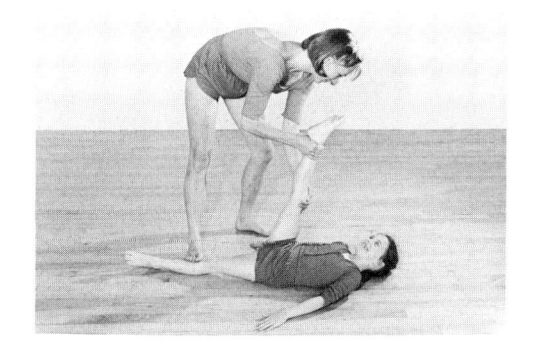

59. KNEE TO ARMPIT, ASSISTED

• *Bend the knee outward and up into the armpit in eight presses. Use eight presses on each leg for a set.*
• *Do three sets.*

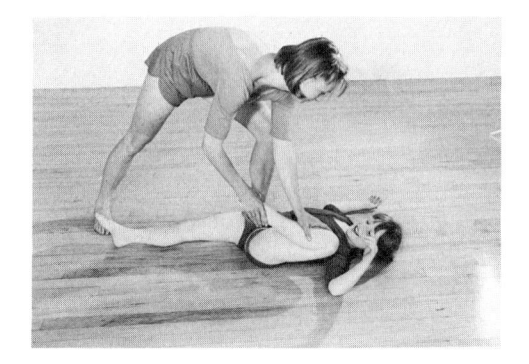

Flexibility Exercises

60. PRONE BACK BEND, ASSISTED

• *The child lies prone and presses the upper body up onto straight arms.*
• *The legs are then bent and the head bent back.*
• *The teacher tries to make head and feet meet with eight easy presses.*
• *Rest a few seconds and try again. Do three.*

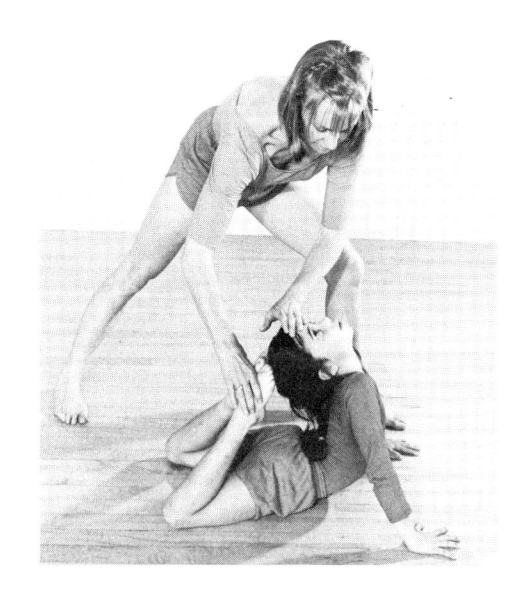

61. PRONE BACK BEND

• *Immediately after doing the assisted back bend (exercise 60), the child should try to do the exercise alone.*

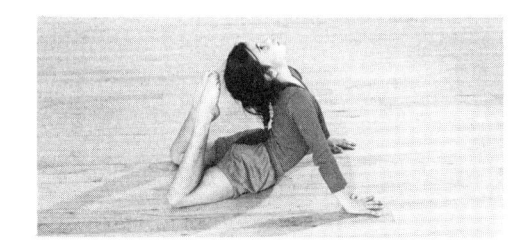

62. HAMSTRINGS AND GROIN STRETCH

• *Stand with the feet well apart and lean forward from the hips.*
• *Hand-walk forward until the body is at full stretch and resting on the hands. Keep the head up.*
• *With feet facing forward and the knees straight, press the weight back until the heels touch. Drop your head down between your shoulders. Rock backward and forward eight times. Hand-walk to the standing position.*

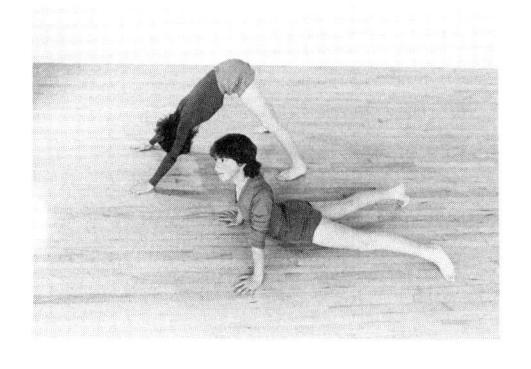

63. FLEXIBILITY BOUNCE

- Stand with feet widespread, hands clasped behind the back.
- Bend forward from the hips, keeping the head up and the back flat.
- Bounce the upper body downward in eight bounces.
- Drop the upper body downward, completely relaxed, for eight bounces.
- Repeat the same exercise, first to the left and then to the right.
- Repeat this exercise often throughout the day.

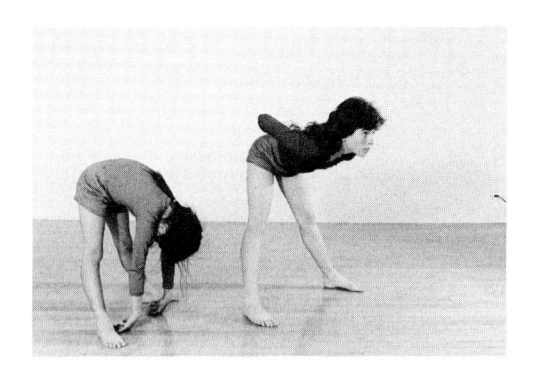

CHAPTER TEN
ACROSS-THE-FLOOR
PROGRESSIONS

Now we begin to get into the "candy" of exercise—movement across the floor. This is the part *everybody* loves, and it is also the easiest part of the exercise class if you play it right.

For the first progressions use a brisk rhythm. Every rhythm you provide will pay vast dividends to your little students. Not one of them will ever cripple himself or herself with the statement "I just don't have any rhythm." That's information the subconscious doesn't need. It isn't true in the first place; everyone has rhythm. What else keeps hearts beating? The people who say they don't, just never had a chance to listen to music and move to that music.

If you are exercising in your living room, move all the furniture back and start in one corner. Corner to corner, diagonally, will give a longer stretch for movement. When the children finish in the far corner, teach them to stroll back around the edge of the room to the starting corner. If they are working in pairs, teach them to split at the end and each stroll back on a different side. This turns your floor progressions into a form of interval training in which the body works hard for a given time and then rests on the way back. This may not be apparent when they are doing walks, but they will appreciate it when they are leapfrogging across.

If you have a very large group in a big room, divide them into four smaller groups, one to a corner. The group you lead is called number one no matter which group you lead during the entire series. You should skip from group to group for two reasons: Followers do better when they are right behind the leader, and you want to be able to see everyone at some time. Right from the start watch for the superior student so that you can fashion a "leader group." They can be given extra training and become your assistants. If you will take the time, they can be better assistants than any comparable group of adults, since they have no bad habits to unlearn. For example, every dancer is scarred by his or her first teachers. Habits are learned early. What you will be teaching is *basic movement*, movement without frills or fancy furbelows, just the real thing.

When your group starts across the floor, that alerts the youngster leading the group *to your right* that her turn is next. As soon as your group is out of the way, group number two starts across as your group gets in behind the next group waiting to go across. That frees you to watch everyone else from the center of the room. When the third group has reached the corner you started from, and the fourth is halfway across, you return to your group to lead the next movement. Later, when you decide it's time to lead group number two (the one that was on your right when you started), everyone will know his position has changed. Your *new* group has become number 1, and the one on your right, number 2, and so on.

WALKING

Walking is considered to be an easy exercise requiring little skill. If you watch the children one by one, you will see every example of terrible posture you have ever heard about. Shoulders round, heads poke forward, hips swing, and feet turn in or out. What you might miss when they are standing still you will see as soon as they walk.

64. THE WALK

Walks are done to brisk, jaunty music. Try to give your little people the idea that they should walk as though they were starting off down the road headed for someplace they want very much to be.

Across-the-Floor Progressions

- *Walk with head up, chest out, and arms relaxed.*
- *The most important part is to stay with the beat.*

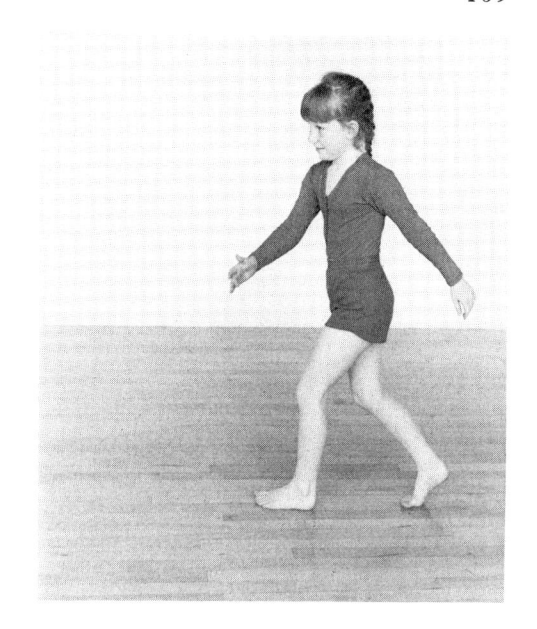

65. TURNED-IN WALK

If you have the idea that this should be easy for everyone, look how difficult this little boy is making it. If he and others like him are allowed to complicate simple movements, they will never be able to learn the difficult ones that go with games. Note the tightened pelvis, arched back, tilted head, and turned-in hands that are getting the same message directed toward his feet. Then watch for them in the children you are teaching.

- *Turn your toes in as far as possible and walk across the room.*

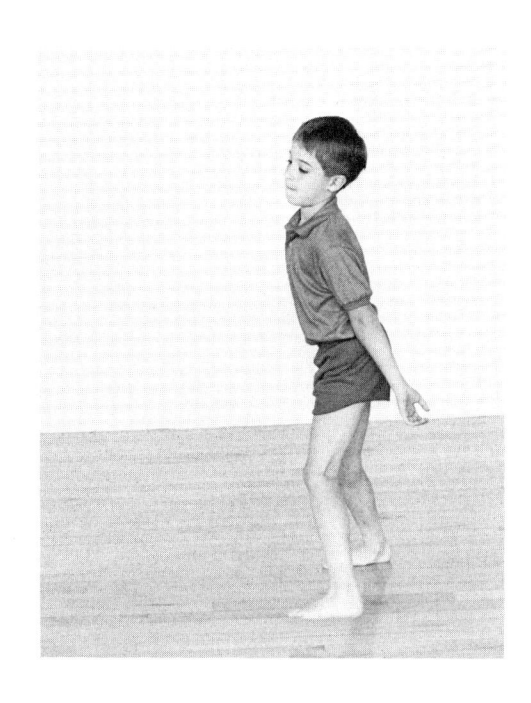

66. TURNED-OUT WALK

By this time the children think you look wonderfully silly and they love it. You have scotched the fear that they will look, and then feel, awkward. They now know they can do what you want and also that you don't mind looking silly.

The boy in the picture is a very happy little fellow. His kind are apt to be somewhat obstreperous at first. If there are two of them, they will surely find each other and often be convulsed with giggles. This is a challenge worth the effort. These become the loved and the followed ones. You will be able to get them under control with lavish (*when earned*) praise.

• Start by turning your feet out and bending your knees. Be sure to tuck your seat under. This exercise shows up the swaybacks.

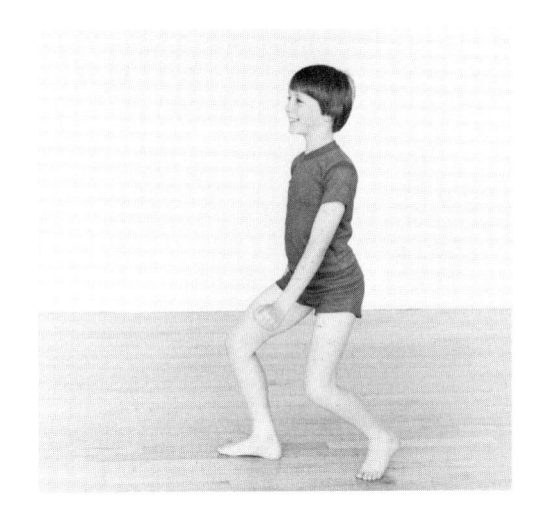

• Walk with nice big even steps. Remember, seat tucked under.

67. TOE BOUNCES

The child in this picture could be described as a fairy or a tiny sprite. Toe Bounces were just made for her. She will do them extremely well and must be complimented. Never take it for granted that a child who does well doesn't need praise, affection, and notice. Often that's the one who is most neglected at home.

Every child will do something well at one time or another. It is almost more important to watch for that one time than to watch for things needing correction.

• Walk across the floor high on the toes. Bounce a little at the height of the step.

• Be sure to keep the head up and arms relaxed. Make a lot over the bounce; it will later lead to skips.

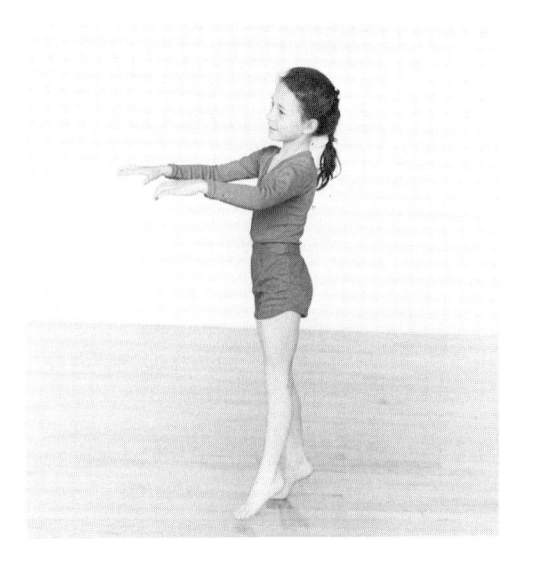

Across-the-Floor Progressions

68. KNEE LIFTS

This exercise strengthens the *quadriceps*. Those are the thigh muscles that are responsible for good performance in games. Pointing out what muscles work for what gives people a reason to exercise. Keep in mind that what is learned young sticks. (The better the vocabulary, for example, the more interest in reading.)

• *March across the room to the beat.*
• *Lift the knees high with each step, chest out, and head up. Relax your shoulders.*

69. HIP TWISTS

This is a combination exercise. The steps are taken on the toes with the already-learned bounce, but with each step forward, the toes are pointed *inward* in order to bring the hip around. Don't worry about the arms at the start. Later, note that they work in opposition to the legs. The further the reach across the body, the better the twist—and the results.

• *Pretend there is a line drawn on the floor all the way across the room.*
• *Step on that line with every step you take on your toes. At the same time, turn your toes in and add the bounce you just learned.*

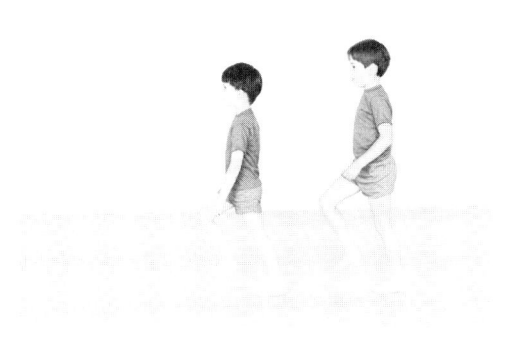

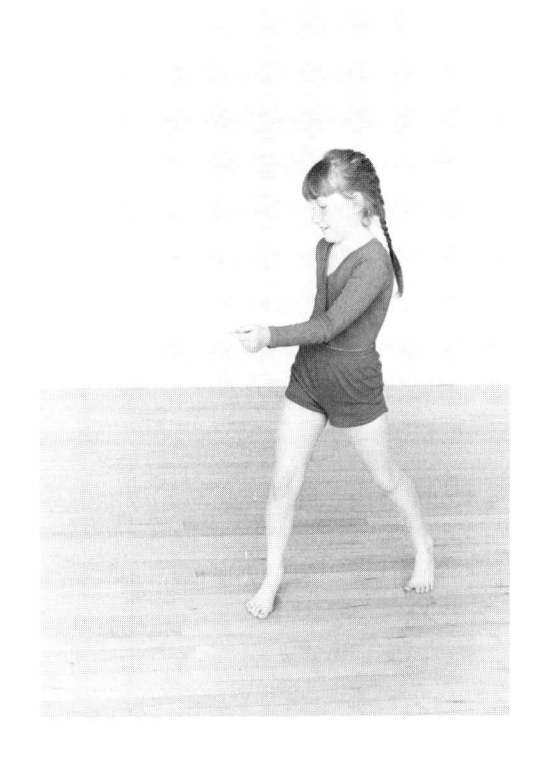

> Important Note: There is no need to give the children detailed instructions. Just DO it. It's "Follow the Leader" at its best.

70. DOG RUN

Children love the floor, and grown-ups should use it for more than walking. The Japanese, who use the floor for living, maintain good leg muscles throughout their lives. We complain of "rusty knees" early on. We should learn how people acquire the assets we lack. For example, the Austrians, who also have good legs, walk a lot, as do the Swiss and the Italians.

• *Get down on all fours and (paying attention to the beat of the music)* with the hands, *run across the floor.*

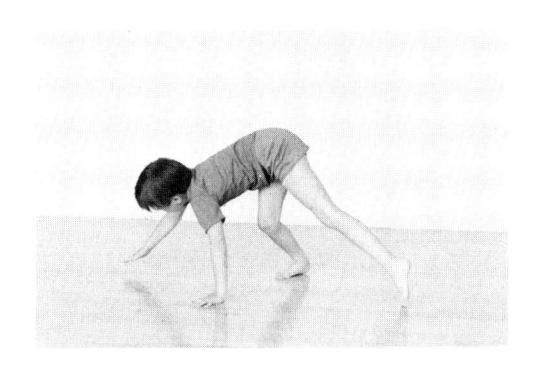

• *Let the feet follow along. In time, they, too, will follow the beat.*

71. ROW A BOAT

This exercise works the *abdominals* and arm muscles. It stretches the chest muscles, called the *pectorals*. In addition it stretches the lower back, that area most at risk when it comes to teenage and adult pain.

• *Sit on the floor with your back facing the other corner of the room.*
• *Keeping the legs straight and together* with toes pointed, lean back as far as possible, placing your hands at the end of the reach.

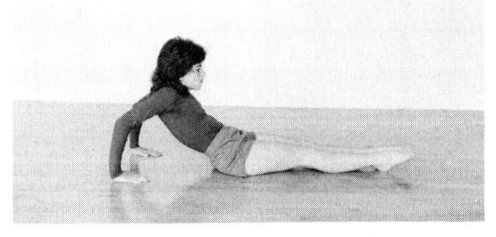

Across-the-Floor Progressions

• *Press down on your hands and push your seat back between them as far as you can before your hands leave the floor near your ankles. Progress in this way across the floor.*

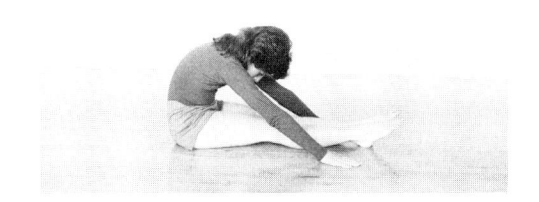

72. SEALING

Most American children do not climb trees or have access to other kinds of arm-, hand-, and chest-muscle-building activities. Part of the reason is a lack of safe outdoor places to play; more important is the lack of leadership and role models. This is a tragedy of major proportions. Most people want their sojourn on earth to mean something. If you can give even a few children a chance to build good bodies, you have done something of incalculable value.

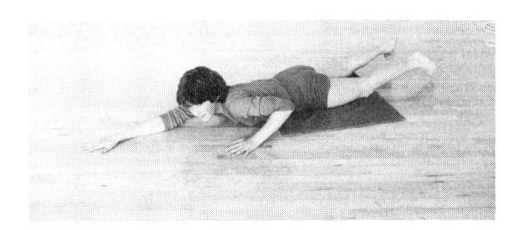

• *Lie prone on the floor, facing the opposite corner.*
• *Using just your lower arms, drag your body across the floor.*

73. DOUBLE-LEG JUMPS

If the children's feet, legs, and lower back muscles are strong, this is easy. If they aren't, they will try to perform with substitutions. The easiest to spot will be the one-two beat. Instead of jumping both feet at the same time, one follows the other, with the strongest leg taking off first. Another way to go is the "hitch," in which the upper body bobs back and forth.

• *Take a wide stance with bent knees and hands on knees.*
• *Try to jump primarily from the feet.*
• *Do the double jumps across the floor.*

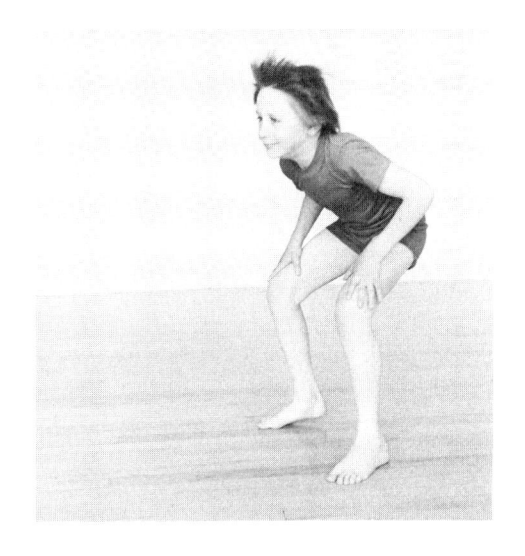

74. CRAB WALK

• *Stand sideways to the corners and get down on all fours.*
• *Move sideways across the floor, trying to keep the beat. It doesn't matter whether the feet keep time or not; that will come. The hands are the beat keepers. Encourage a wide reach.*

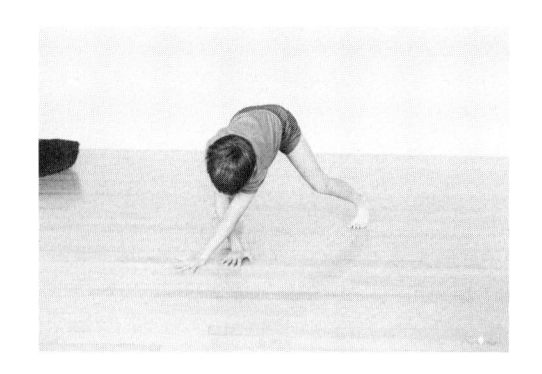

75. FOUR-FOOT BACKWARD WALK

• *Sit down with your back facing the corner you are to head for.*
• *Place the hands and feet on the floor and bend both knees.*
• *Lift your seat from the floor and proceed backward on hands and feet.*

76. HORSE KICK

This exercise works many parts of the body, probably *all* the parts. Children love it. Don't be overly particular about the beat here; just let them get across.

• *Go across the floor, kicking your feet up behind you as high as you feel you can control.*
• *Watch out for the horse ahead of you. Don't get too close.*

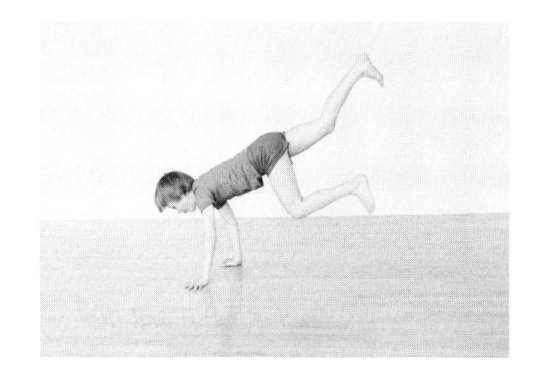

77. WALK HANDS, BOUNCE FEET

The next exercise looks very hard and is quite impressive, but isn't so bad. It's really a combination of the hands in the Horse Kick (exercise 76) and the legs in the Double Leg Jump (exercise 73).

• *Start by doing about twenty double-leg jumps in place. Everybody together.*
• *Next, get down on all fours and march your hands to the same beat.*
• *Now, walk your hands and jump your feet at the same time across the floor.*

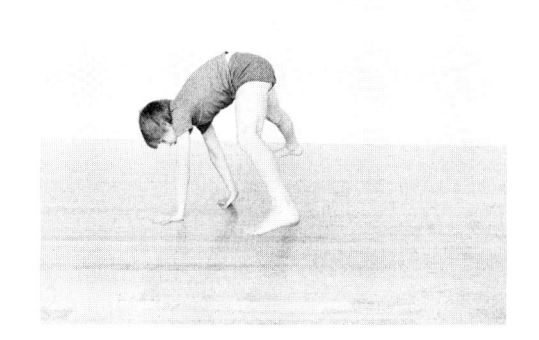

78. WOLF IN THE GARDEN

This exercise strengthens the anterior tibialis and is the exercise that helps the most when feet are flat or not very strong. Before we can do the exercise as we see it here, we must play a stationary game.

• *Pair your charges and have one sit on the floor with legs close together.*
• *That partner's toes become the garden gate as they are turned inward to touch and hold.*
• *The other partner's fist is the wolf. He places his fist between the ankles of "The garden" and tries to break out.*
• *The garden gate holds tight, keeping the toes together.*
• *The pull is for five counts and then release. Do three of these.*

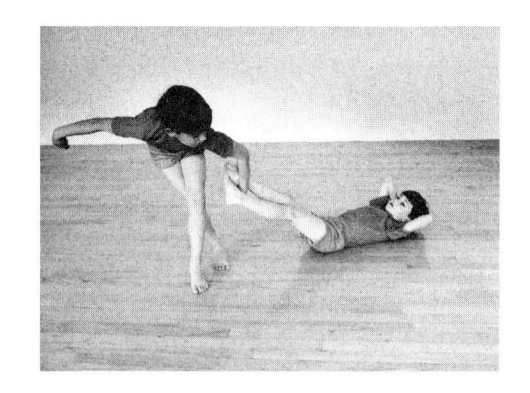

• *Now you are ready to go across the floor, the wolf pulling the garden gate after him. The wolf puts his fist inside the garden gate's ankles and starts to pull him across the floor.*
• *Only the wolf has to worry about walking to the beat; the garden gate just goes along for the ride.*

79. FROG HOP

• *Place your hands on the floor well ahead of your feet.*
• *Jump both feet forward to rest* outside *of your hands and as much ahead of them as you can manage.*
• *Try to hop to the beat.*

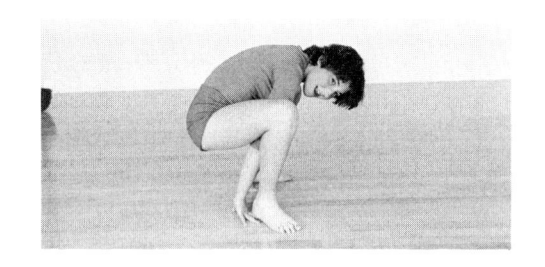

80. APART-TOGETHER JUMP

• *Jump your feet apart on one beat and together on the next beat.*

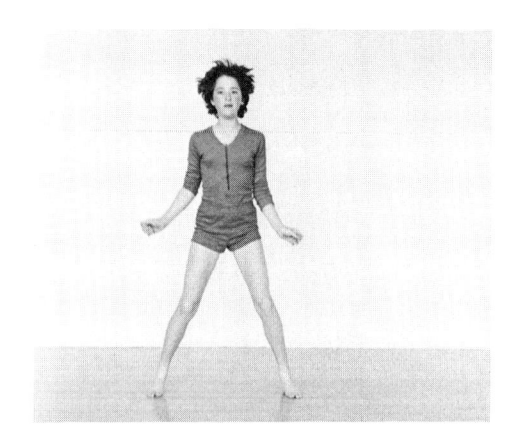

Keep in mind that the slower the beat, the higher you must jump, so try out your music *before* the class.

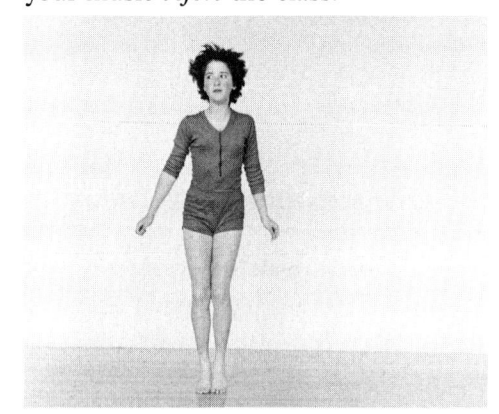

81. SIDE-TO-SIDE JUMP

• *Keeping your legs together, jump both feet from side to side. Stay with the beat.*

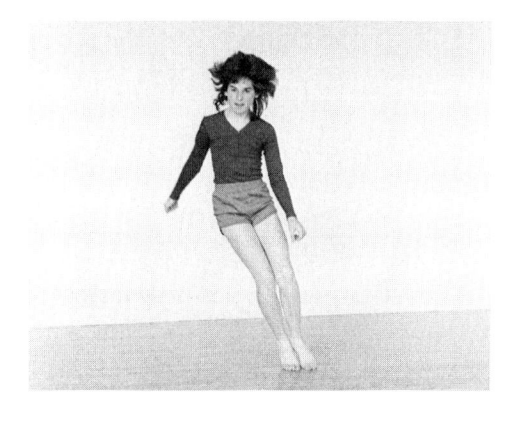

82. SKIPS

Skipping is something that every child *used* to learn on the way to school, but no longer. There isn't much constructive action going on in the school buses.

• *Begin with lots of practice with exercise 67, Toe Bounces. This will provide the needed strength to* both *legs.*
• *Start with forward skips. Don't explain skips, just* show *them.*
• *Skip backward, watching to see that the heels touch the floor.*
• *Skip sideways. Remember to lead with* both *sides.*

Now we begin to add small equipment. We have already used a wand in the lifts. A wand is usually 36 inches long. The expensive way is to go to the hardware store and buy dowels 36-inch-long and ½-inch thick. The cheaper way is to have everyone bring in an old mop handle or broomstick. Cut those to the 36-inch length. *Paint your equipment.* Kids like bright colors, and so will you. Don't use a mix of leftovers; get bright new red, white, blue, and yellow enamels. If you are going to do this, make it enjoyable.

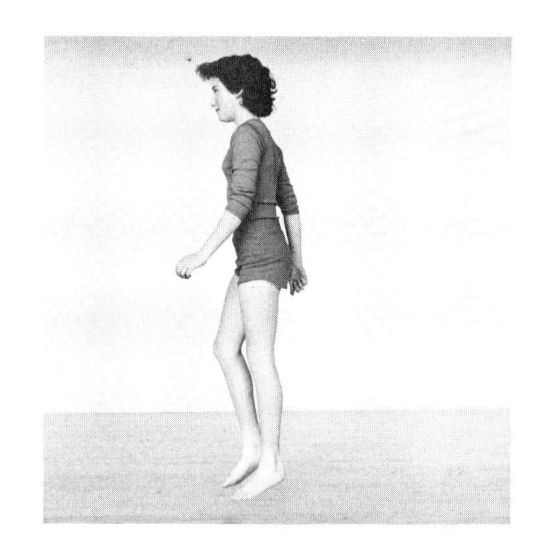

83. DOUBLES RUNS

• *Partners hold onto the same dowel and run across the floor to the beat.* Now you find out how much harder it is to work with someone else than alone. The teacher's job becomes harder, too; you now have personalities to deal with. You will find that "best friends" may want to be partners. Nothing against that, unless they are both poorly coordinated. If they are, they can't help each other. Sometimes the pair will be perfectly matched; they will be "dancing" and loving it. Taking on a clumsy little friend will *not*

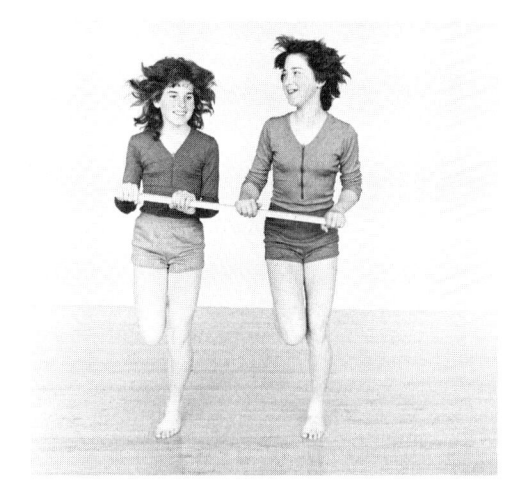

be in their cards, they think. You must think both ways. Let them have several satisfying turns across the floor and then split them to become "teachers." Ask for their help with the others. It won't be too long before that help won't be needed anymore.

84. DOUBLES RUNS, BACKWARD

• *Partners, holding the same wand, run backward to the beat.*
• *Pay lots of attention to heels; they must come down to touch the floor on each step. This stretches the gastrocnemius muscles in the calves. Strong, flexible calves make the difference in all sports and in both gymnastics and dance.*

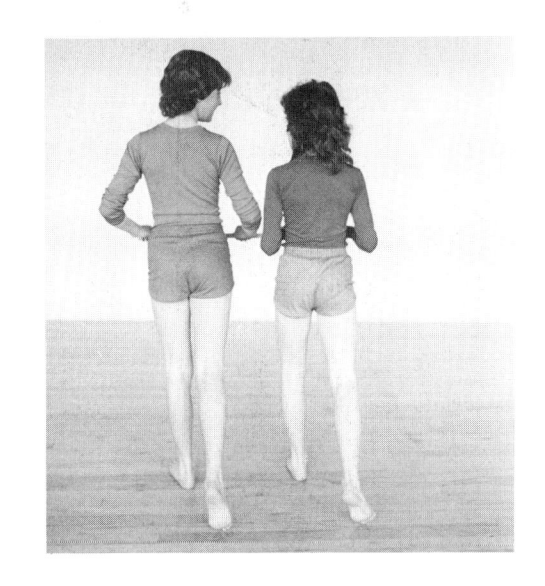

85. DOUBLES CROSSOVER

The crossover exercises, in which one foot is required to cross over the other and then cross back, are *supposed* to be impossible for handicapped people. Should you be working with handicapped children, know from the start that most of the "supposed to's" are actually cop-outs used by people who don't know how to get the required results. It's all in how you teach, the music you choose—and how much you want success for your pupils.

• *Stand on the right foot and cross the left*

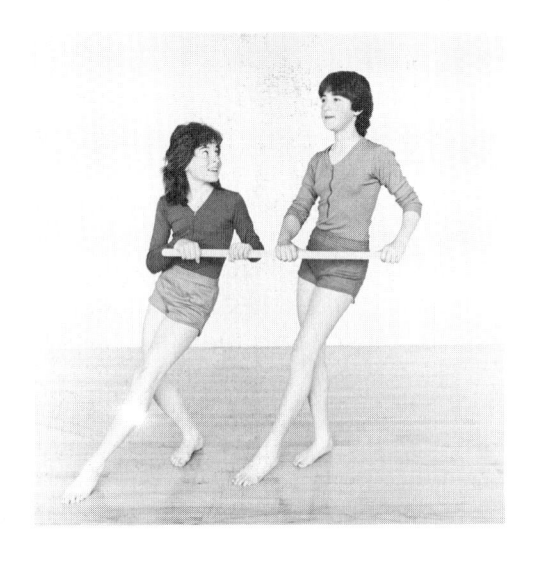

foot over the right to touch the floor on the outside of it.

• *Return to the start, and this time stand on the left foot.*

• *Cross the right foot over and return it to the standing position. Alternate for several counts while standing in one place.*

• *When the rhythm and movement are going nicely, you* start moving, just a couple of inches forward and back, *and they'll have it. Cross the floor in pairs holding onto wands.*

Of all the steps my adult students find hard, this simple crossover move is the worst; that's because they have never been taught to *look . . . see . . . report back to the brain.* Imagine what they have missed all their lives!

86. JUMP ROPE

Jump ropes were the special prerogative of little girls and boxers until the 1930s. At that time a misguided person in physical education sounded an alarm: *If girls jump up and down, their reproductive organs will get scrambled.* It was bad enough that a professional person could be so silly, but far worse was to come. Thousands of others followed like sheep. Americans do that—often. Jumping of any kind was denied to girls. We lost the fun of playing boys' rules in basketball, lost the chance to compete in anything. We lost a lot. Now, of course, we have disproved all of it, but several generations of girls were disenfranchised. Now we are again allowed to run and jump, but only a few actually *do* it. The permission is there, but the leadership is missing. Not for your group!

When you buy jump ropes, get sash cord. It's heavier and better than the lightweight, colorful ropes offered in toy stores.

• *Stand on two feet with the rope resting on the floor just behind your heels.*

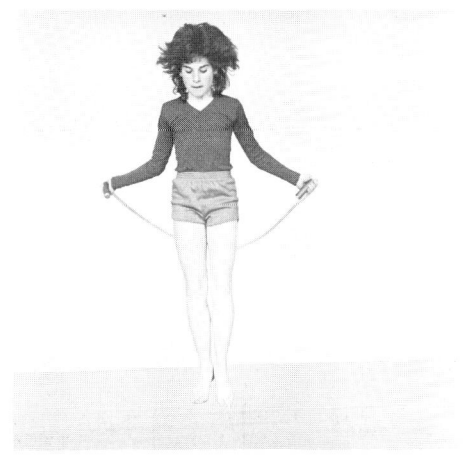

• *Swing the rope over your head to a point just in front of your feet, and* when it has stopped, *jump both feet over it. Repeat that a number of times and then try to jump over it without waiting for it to stop. Try that a few times.*

• *Soon the children will be able to coordinate the rope with the jump.*

• *The next move is to jump over the rope as it passes under your feet and take another jump while the rope is passing over your head. If you can do it, they will get it. If you can't do it, find a friend who can and have him or her visit your class one day.*

87. JUMP ROPE, RUNNING

This was the rope trick that made running to school fun.

• *There isn't any way to explain this except to say, "Run, and turn the rope over your head fast enough to go under each foot as you go."*

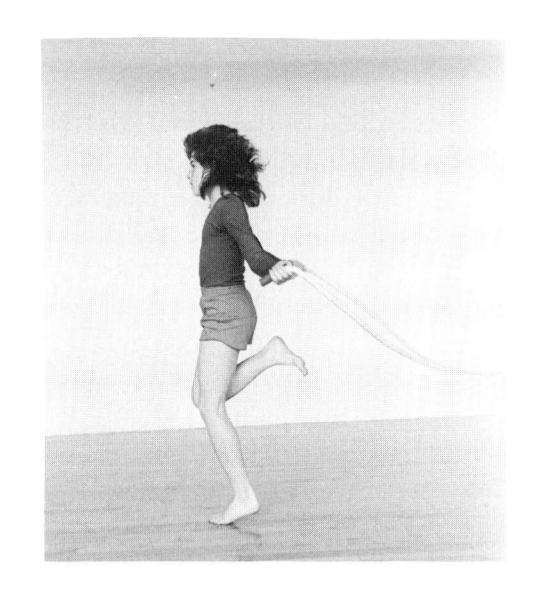

88. JUMP ROPE, BENT KNEES

• *After you can jump rope standing straight, start to do it with slightly* bent knees. *Try to get lower and lower.*

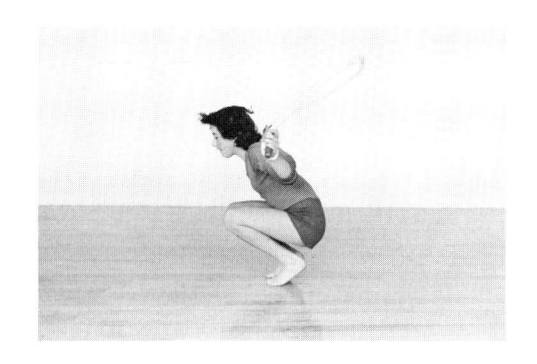

CHAPTER ELEVEN
THE RUSSIAN SERIES

There was once a time, long ago, when things Russian were accepted in this country. People wore Russian boots. (Russians were the only people that we knew of who wore boots.) Then there were Russian blouses. They were of silk and usually had expensive fur trimming at the neck in a high collar. The fur also ran down the left side of the front and as trimming around the bottom. The fur was usually karakul. Then the blouse was belted or sashed, and people who wore them felt very romantic and just a little bit far-out. We called that look *bohemian*.

In addition, there were words like *dasha* and *troika*. We didn't know about the awful trials the new regime was visiting on the Russian people, so dance teachers didn't feel nervous about teaching Russian folk dance to their pupils. There were also Russian ballet schools; many people felt that they were the best by far, and they were right. What these Russian teachers taught was the same thing taught to them when they were starting out back home in Mother Russia. It required strong bodies, but back then, we had them too. The ballet schools didn't ruin children forever, because their little bodies were strong enough. Today is another story. Ballet *can* and *does* hurt children. Before you turn your child over to something as demanding as ballet, be sure he or she can do most of the exercises in this book.

The following exercises are not easy. They are not even medium hard. They are *very* hard, and the children who do them must *want* to do them and be willing to work hard. To say they are exciting and fun is an understatement. To say they take good legs and make them far better is the absolute truth. Once mastered, they provide strength, rhythm, challenge, and satisfaction. These are special exercises, to be done later, when the children are much stronger. Even then teach them one at a time.

89. TWO-ARM AND ONE-ARM FLOOR PROGRESSION

We can continue our floor progressions with two from the Russian Series.

• *Begin in a deep squat; place* both *hands on the floor in front of and a little to the right of the right knee.*
• *Jump your body forward ahead of your hands, still in the squat.*
• *Bring both hands forward and a little to the left of the left knee and jump forward ahead of your hands again.*
• *Proceed across the room, taking the weight first on one side and then on the other.*
• *Be sure the music is right, neither too slow nor too fast. A lot of Russian and Hungarian folk music can be found in public libraries, just waiting to be taped.*
• *Once you can do the two-arm progression, try the harder, one-arm floor progression. Start in the deep squat and place the right hand on the floor a little to the right and as far ahead of the right knee as possible.*
• *Spring forward, kicking the leg high as you rotate around the arm.*
• *Do the same with the left and alternate across the floor.*

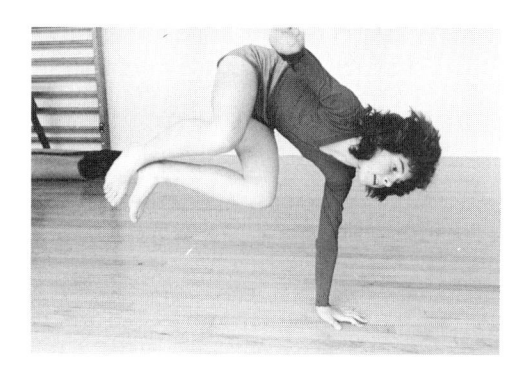

90. CHANGE-LEVEL SIDE EXTENSIONS

Russians, Austrians, Swiss, Italians, and many other nations have far fewer knee injuries than we do. One of the reasons is walking. For the people of those countries, walking is a way of life, and in all but Italy, physical education is considered an important part of the school curriculum for *all* the children. While

The Russian Series

Italy had the best results when I tested Italian, Austrian, and Swiss children, they had the poorest economy and no money left over for gyms. What they did have was a hilly country and the need to get around on their own legs. We are an affluent nation and have no such need. For that we pay a price in leg and foot injuries. *Your children need not pay that price.*

• *Start standing straight with arms at your sides.*

• *On the first count or beat, jump down into a deep knee-bend, elbows at shoulder level and bent, hands touching. Hold flattened hands at chest level with fingers touching.*

• *On the second count or beat, jump up with both legs spread wide and feet flat on the floor. Fling the arms wide and a little above shoulder level.*

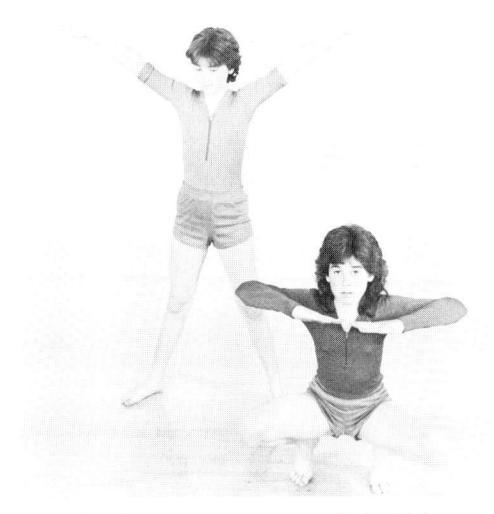

• *At the start you may do* half knee-bends *to learn the beat and the form of the exercise. As legs improve, go deeper and deeper.*

• *Still later, after lots of practice you can jump up to take the weight onto one foot as the other is lifted into a side kick.*

91. LATERAL KNEE BEND AND SHIFT

Before you can do this exercise properly, you will need some preparation. The preparation should be done weeks before asking the children to do the finished step.

This is done in place.

• *Start standing with legs spread wide, arms at sides.*

• *Drop down into a deep knee-bend on the right side with arms outflung for balance.*

• *Return to the standing position with arms down.*

• *Tighten every muscle you can find, starting with the legs and moving up through the tightened pelvic and abdominal muscles. Hold that. Explain to the children that they are doing an* isometric contraction *and tell them exactly what it is.*

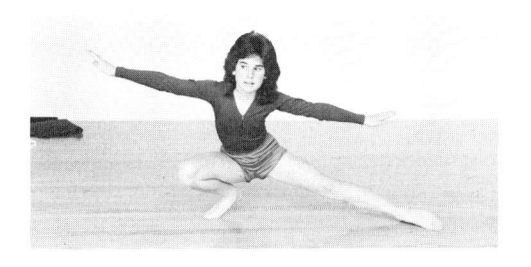

• *Repeat this exercise to the left. Alternate for eight.*

ISOMETRIC CONTRACTION

Simply put, in an isometric contraction the muscle contracts but no movement ensues. When I was a kid, girls did it when they pressed their hands together in a prayerful position chanting

I must
I must
Develop
My bust

Actually the muscle contractions, done over a long period of time, will develop bulk in muscle, but this exercise fell out of favor when it was discovered to be a less-than-perfect (or even very good) way to develop muscle. One of the reasons was that when enough contraction is put to the muscle to really develop it, the oxygen supply is cut off. *Isotonic Exercise* (in which the contraction causes movement, as in weight lifting) got far better results than *isometric*, and the gains lasted longer, even when those using it were forced for one reason or another to stop exercising for a period of time.

Why is it important that you know this and that the children know this? It is very important as a safety measure. The so-called "fitness boom" that took place in the seventies and led to innumerable injuries, *could* have been a good thing. It hasn't been. People became aware that they ought to be fit, but they had no idea how to go about it, because since 1930 physical education had been treated as "play." Games were substituted for *education.* That left at least three generations open to the leadership of people who knew very little about the human body and nothing whatever about exercise. You and the children need to know all about both. They (and you) need the protection of knowledge against the so-called fitness experts, who are any and everything but. Don't be deceived by titles. The Ph.D's are just as guilty as the cheerleaders who became exercise teachers. Was it their fault? No, it was the colleges that "educated" them, and it is still going on today, full force. The responsibility for most football injuries lies at the doors of trainers and coaches who were mistrained in school. Dance injuries are usually caused by teachers who were untrained where muscles are concerned. *You must stand between injuries and your family, your students, and yourself,* and the first weapon is common sense. The second is knowledge. Read the chapter entitled "Sports in America" in my book *Myotherapy: Bonnie Prudden's Complete Guide to Pain-Free Living.* The facts are there in detail.

92. SIDE-EXTENSION THRUST

Way back in the chapter on warm-ups you began preparing for this exercise. If you have spent some time on the foregoing exercise, Lateral Knee-bend and Shift, you are ready for this one.

- *Drop down into the deep knee-bend with knees turned out.*
- *Place your hands on the floor in front of you for support. Later you will not need them there.*
- *Holding the squat on the left leg, thrust the right leg straight out to the side.*
- *Hop your seat up a little way into the air, which will unweight the left leg.*
- *At the same second, retract the right leg and thrust the left out to the left side.*
- *Repeat slowly several times.* Do not try for the finished position immediately. Give yourself practice and patterning.
- *When you are ready, carry bent arms in front of the chest.*

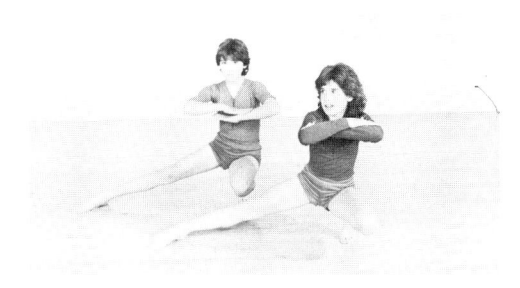

PATTERNING: WHAT IS IT?

This is another thing you need to know. When you *pattern* a body into a series of movements, slowly and close to perfectly, for some time—and then let what you have taught "cook"—an interesting thing happens: You can do that series of movements perfectly, much faster, and with strength and flexibility, *even after* a "vacation" from doing them!

If you have a child taking piano lessons and you can convince that child to learn a new piece by playing it so slowly that he or she can count to three between each chord, and play it that way without a hitch for two weeks, you have a surprise coming. Take the piece away and hide it for three months; when you take it out again, the child will be able to play it without a pause almost up to speed. Your tennis lessons "cook" over the winter and your ski lessons over the summer. Watch how much better your class performs after vacation.

ABDOMINAL AND GROIN STRENGTHENING

The next exercises require strong abdominal and groin muscles if the children are not to be frustrated and either perform poorly or hurt themselves. If every coach had that attitude, athletic injuries would be cut in half. And if you allow a child of yours to go out for a sport without the backup of a good body, you will be as much at fault as the coach. Keep this in mind, *sports in America do not build good bodies, they use the good bodies that come to school already fashioned.* The children are usually safe until junior high school, which is the first time many of them ever see the inside of a gym. Junior high is no-man's-land where physical education is concerned. It is where proficiency is demanded of children who cannot pass even the minimum test. Those who don't have it, and know they don't have it, retire to the sidelines and accept the *fact* that they are "klutzes." This prevents any real development. Perhaps they don't know it and are game to try anything. They will try—and fail. That opens up two possibilities—an injured ego or an injured body. Often both go together. Don't think that just because the youngster doesn't talk about the misery of "gym,"

nothing is happening. It may well be. A sure sign is the request for a note excusing the child from gym on any pretext. Sometimes it isn't really pretext but a combination; she really does have menstrual cramps, but well exercised, happy-with-gym-classes girls are rarely bothered by cramps. If they are, get rid of them with help from the Myotherapy section (chapter 34). A boy may have an asthma attack in gym, but if he does, he is not being taught correctly or the right thing. Check, too, with the Myotherapy chapter for how to alleviate asthma. Go and sit in those classes—and do it often so that the teacher can't put on a "show" for you and then go back to business as usual when you aren't there. *Know what you are looking at.* I started exercise classes for my two children after watching one gym class. That's how I got into this in the first place. I wasn't sure of myself either, but I learned, and half the time it was the children who taught me.

93. TRIPLE BIKE

• *Lie supine and rest back on your elbows. Use the well-known bicycle motion with your legs about six inches straight out in front of you. Count eight on the right leg only.*
• *Leave your elbows tight to the floor and roll over onto the left hip; repeat the biking motion for eight. Do the same on the right hip.*
• *Start back in the center and lift both legs and arms off the floor and do eight more. That makes one set. Do three sets.*

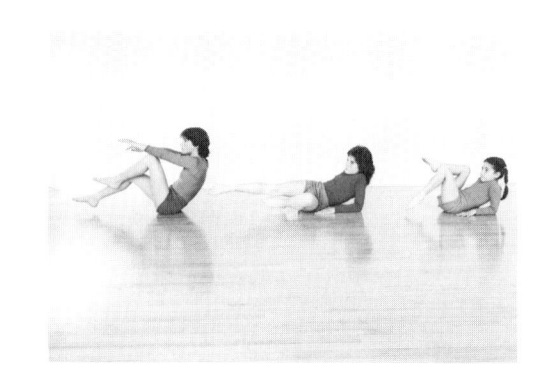

The Russian Series

94. TWO-LEGGED SIDE THRUSTS

• Start again in a deep squat and place the left hand on the floor on the left. Be sure the weight is evenly distributed between that hand and the pulled-in feet.
• Jump the legs to the outthrust position with legs apart, the left well out in front and the right leg back.
• Retract to the squat, but leave the left hand on the floor. Do four on each side. Do some other exercise not requiring the arms for a minute or two, and then add the next exercise.

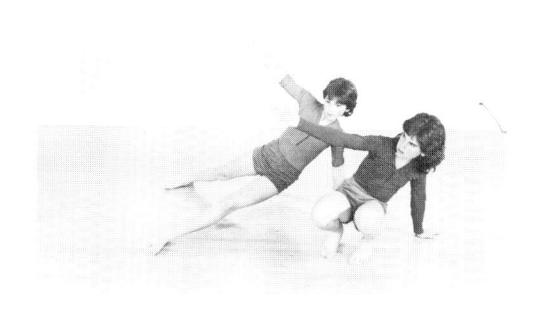

95. HUB OF THE WHEEL

• Start as for the Side Thrusts (exercise 94) and repeat the thrust and retract. As you repeat the four and add four more to make eight thrusts and retracts, turn in a circle to make a wheel with leg spokes. Do the exercise with legs to both sides.

96. ALTERNATING FORWARD THRUSTS

• Start in a deep squat and thrust the right leg out in front.
• Retract that leg and thrust the left leg forward. Retract. Do several this way until the pattern is set and the muscles know what is expected of them.
• Now add the little jump as you thrust first one leg out and then the other without any stop in between. Do eight and then have everyone walk in circles, first one way and then the other, to unkink the leg muscles.

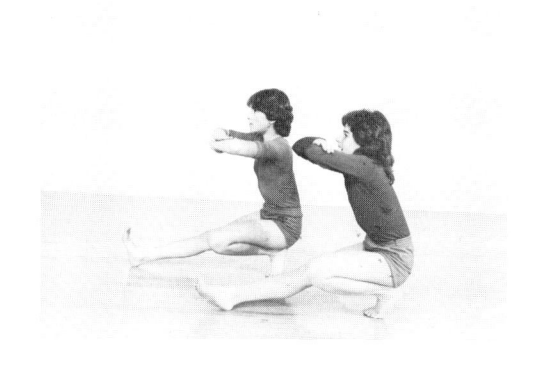

CHAPTER TWELVE
TUMBLING

Tumbling is valuable on many levels, and the first that comes to mind is coordination. The little body that develops coordination can perform well in almost any sport. Coupled with rhythm, coordination is the ticket into any physical activity and provides the assurance of success.

Tumbling develops *proprioception*, the ability to know where the body is in space. This prevents many accidents and lessens the possibility of serious injury should an accident occur. On two occasions, the ability to instinctively do a shoulder roll saved my life. Not long ago the ability to instinctively do a racing dive onto a floor prevented what might have been multiple fractures, because the impact of a spinning fall was spread evenly from chest to thighs, and the only result was skinned elbows. At the moment of crisis, there is rarely time to think about what should be done. Long practice as a child is the best guarantee of doing the right thing *without* having to think.

Tumbling also develops courage and self-assurance. Those are two qualities that, like a good self-image, feed over into all the other facets of living.

Tumbling

Tumbling *uses* the strength, flexibility, coordination, and judgment we have been developing with the exercises. It prepares for gymnastics, and gymnastics is the natural arena for small, wiry children. It prevents awkwardness for those children who will be tall. Lastly, it's great fun.

Tumbling *should* begin when the child starts to crawl. In my book *How to Keep Your Child Fit from Birth to Six*, I show how a baby can be helped into an elbow stand and then a handstand *before* it can crawl. Why do that? It's fun. The baby *feels* a new feeling and *sees* a new view, or the same view from a different aspect. That alone is good training. But suppose those important years were not used to build the little body? You miss your best chance. You can't start any sooner, and since the sooner the better, sooner is now.

97. SOMERSAULTS

All tumbling stunts are a matter of patterning, and that depends at first on an adult. You are very much there at the beginning, but the sooner you can turn your duet into a solo, the better for everyone.

• *Have the child start on a rug or a mat, kneeling down and placing the hands flat, fingers pointing forward and toes curled for takeoff.*

• *The* spotter *(you) places firm hands on either side of the bony pelvis. This gives you complete control. As the child pushes off with both feet,* guide the stunt straight forward. *If the tumbler straightens the back, there will be a breathtaking landing on a flat back. You want a very round back, so press down on the pelvis; that pressure will keep the starting round-backed position.*

• *As the seat and legs go over, use your hands on the sides of the thighs to continue the straight direction. It usually takes about twelve guided somersaults before a child is ready to solo. Make much of the first solo.*

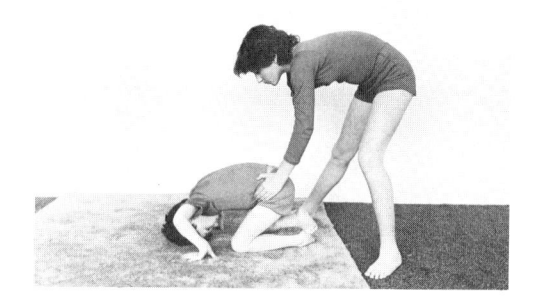

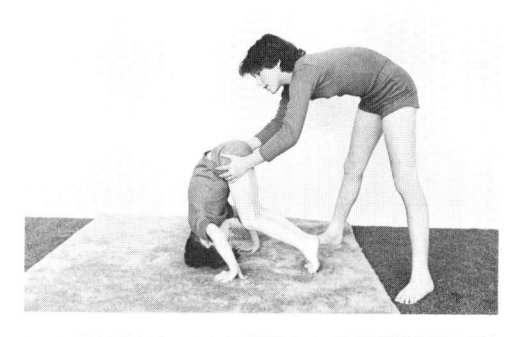

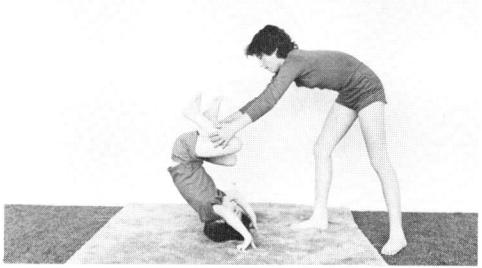

98. SOLO SOMERSAULT

- *The preparation for the solo is the same. Place the hands with fingers pointing forward. Curl the toes and push off.*
- *Now we begin to look for form. The move is done in a slow, controlled manner. The use of slow, fluid music is very helpful, as it is with all slow movements and those requiring balance.*
- *The body stays curled, the legs together and the toes pointed, until the sitting position is attained.*

There are many variations on this stunt once it is done well.

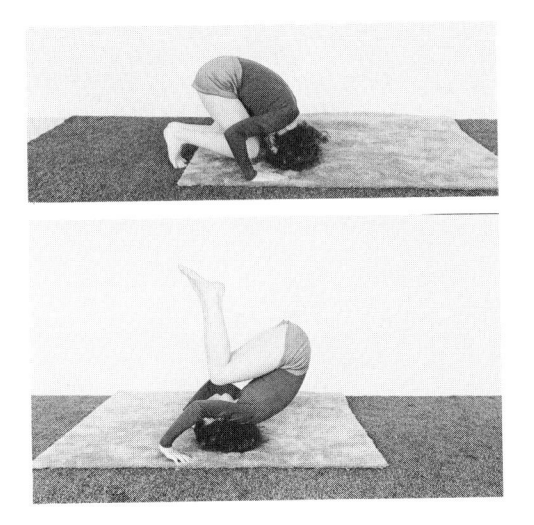

99. SOMERSAULT OVER, STOP

- *In this stunt you do the same as above except that you bring the feet in close to the body and end in a squat, ready for the next somersault.*

The foregoing exercises should ultimately be done to a slow 4/4 beat. *Over . . . hold . . . three, four. Over . . . hold, three, four,* and so on. When the rhythm is established, pairs can work down the mat side by side. If your class is large, always allow a full count of four in between starting pairs. Some children have been scared away from doing somersaults—or embarrassed out of doing them. They may have had that straight-back fall, which hurt. They may have been shamed by others. The cause isn't important, but getting around it is. Many children can't turn over forward, so we go in by the back door.

100. BACKWARD SHOULDER ROLL

- *Have the child lie on his back and bring both knees toward the face.*
- *Help him to lift the hips and support them at the waist. At that point, tell him to hold his nose with his knees. That will be cause for giggles. (Giggles are very useful when someone is frightened. How can holding the nose hurt!?)*

Tumbling

• *Next, place his knees on the floor next to his right ear and tell him to* look at his knees. *This will turn his head in the right direction and a strained neck can be avoided. Then, controlling the body by holding the sides of the pelvis, press him over onto his knees. Big surprise! It was so easy.*

• *Do the same to the other side. Don't allow the children to be just one-sided. An accident requiring instinctive response doesn't always choose the good side.*

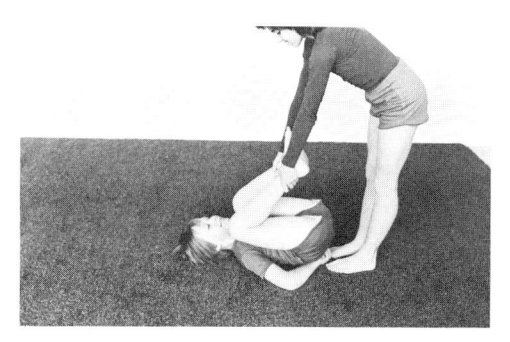

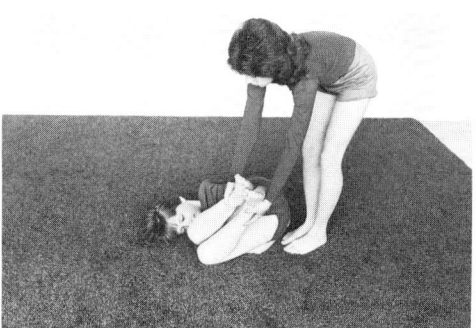

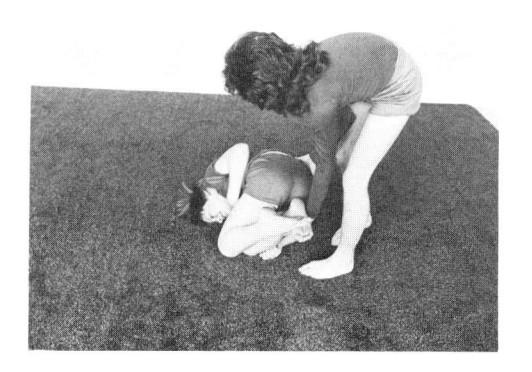

101. FORWARD SHOULDER ROLL

This is another injury preventer. You have seen football players take terrible spills and, by doing a shoulder roll, roll right away from trouble with no jarring impact. That goes for almost any forward fall. If you can curl and roll, you rarely fracture.

- *Kneel on the right knee.*
- *Bring the left knee out to the side in the bent-knee position.*
- *Place the foot in the turned-out position about three inches to the rear of the right knee. This will assure a straight roll rather than one off the mat.*
- *Place the left hand on the floor with the fingers turned inward.*
- *Now, holding that position, try to put your right shoulder and right ear on the mat.*
- *The spotter grasps the tumbler under the left thigh and, for small children, the right shoulder (for bigger ones, the right side of the pelvis).*
- *As the child pushes off, the spotter spins him as if he were a wheel. Do these rolls to both sides.*

Start as early as you can to develop responsible spotters. Give equal time to teaching both stunts and spotting, and note which children can be depended on. Go after the others, too; they need the practice even more than the naturally responsible ones do. Praise for good spotting is the best aid.

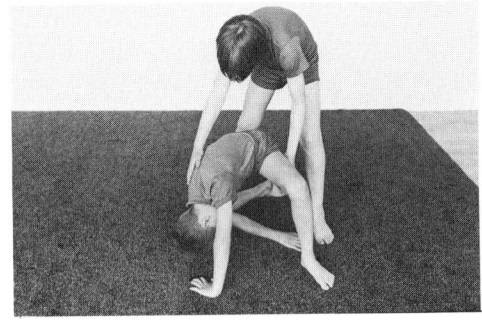

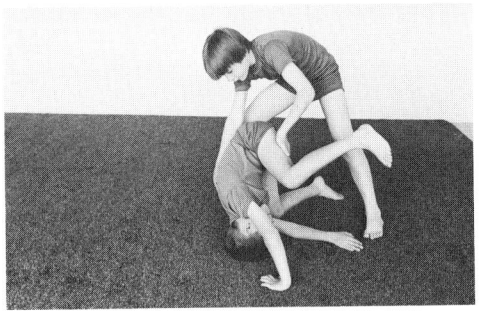

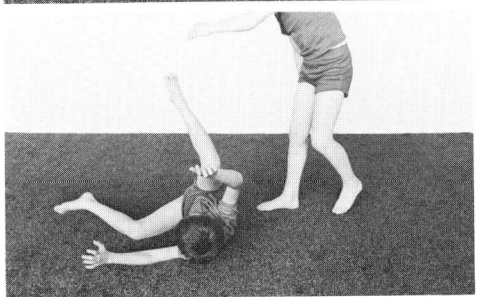

102. SPREAD-LEG SOMERSAULT

This stunt calls for arm strength and good abdominal muscles as well as a flexible back.

- *Start with a very wide stance, hands flat on the floor.*
- *Lower the head very slowly toward the floor, trying to place it as close to the feet as possible. Tuck the chin on the chest.*

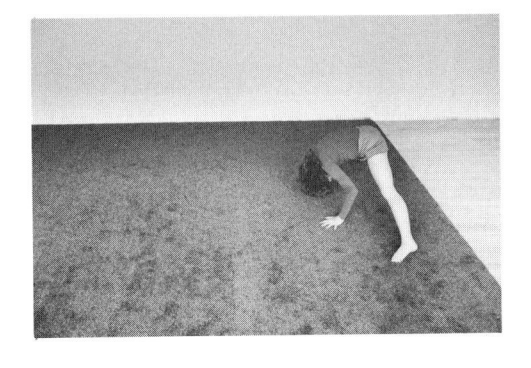

Tumbling

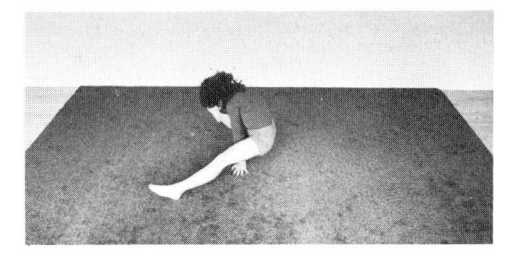

• *Push off* hard *and think "sit UP" as you go over.*
• *Quickly bring the hands around so that they face backward just under the thighs.*
• *Use the momentum of the turn, the down pressure of both legs, and the up pres-*

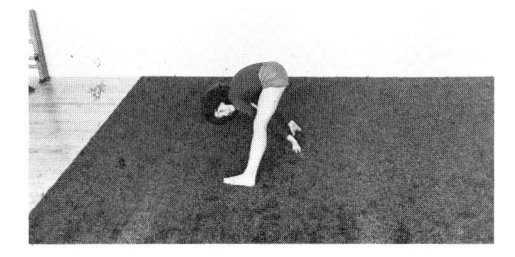

sure *of both hands to lift your seat off the mat. Tuck the head and go again.*
• *Don't hesitate. Place your head on the mat as close as possible and repeat. Once learned, this is good for four or five somersaults down the mat.*

103. TAILOR'S SOMERSAULT

This is a fairly easy progressing somersault. Most children sit cross-legged without even thinking about it.
• *Once they can do solo somersaults, ask* them *to do them ending in a cross-legged position; then push off and do another and another. The tighter the ball they make of themselves, the easier.*

104. REVERSE TAILOR'S SOMERSAULT

• *Do two tailor's somersaults. After the second, stand up with the legs still crossed.*
• *Untangle your legs by turning around to face the way you just came.*
• *Do one tailor's somersault back toward the starting spot and end cross-legged.*
• *Stand, turn, and do two tailor's somersaults forward again.*

• *Progress, two forward and one back, to the end of the mat.*
• *Don't send a second tumbler or pair of tumblers after the first until they have completed* two *forward-backward somersaults. As they start their third set of forwards, send in the next pair.*

105. SHOULDER STAND

• *Press the body up straight to stand on the shoulders.*

• *Support the stand with hands at the waist. Try to make the bodies stand straight.*

• *When you have that under control, start at the top of the lift and bring straight spread legs down, an inch at a time. This will force a balance act in which the legs work against the rest of the body. The object is to control the descent so that two people can work together to form designs.*

• *Keeping the hands at the waist, curl up like the girl on the left. Lower legs should be vertical and toes pointed.*

• *Next, extend both legs over the head to touch the floor as you lay both arms flat on the floor.*

• *Curl, and return to the sitting position.*

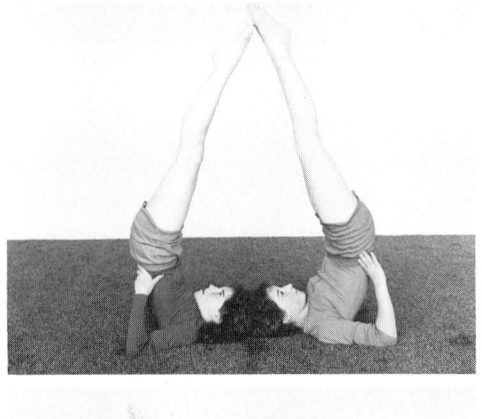

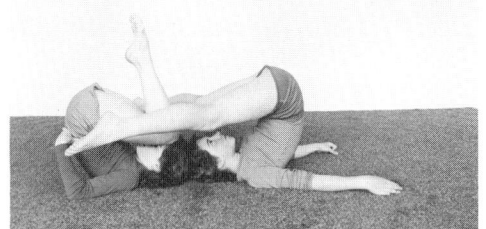

106. HEADSTAND

When you do headstands, be sure that the child's neck matches the body. If the child is overweight, that neck may not be able to support the heavy body. Fat is not to be ignored. The sooner it is gotten off, the happier and healthier the child will be.

• *The spotter and the tumbler kneel, facing each other.*

• *The tumbler places her head on the floor and her hands back toward her feet, but with fingers pointing forward. The bent arms make ideal platforms to kneel on. The head and hands form a tripod.*

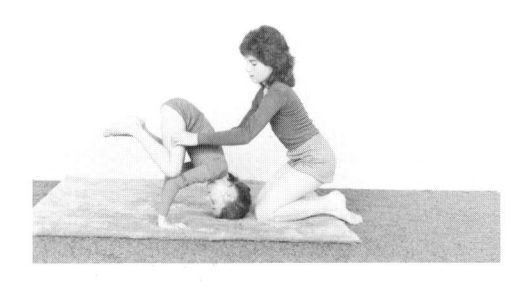

Tumbling

- *The spotter controls at the thighs or pelvis.*
- *When balance can be maintained kneeling on the elbows, the legs are slowly raised.*
- *From the straight-upward position the legs and body curl back down to the knees-on-elbows position.*
- *The spotter keeps control until the tumbler is sure of her ability to go up and down from the knee-elbow-kneel.*

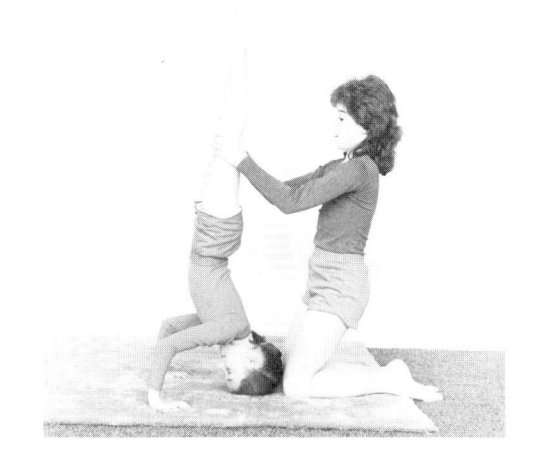

107. SOLO HEADSTAND

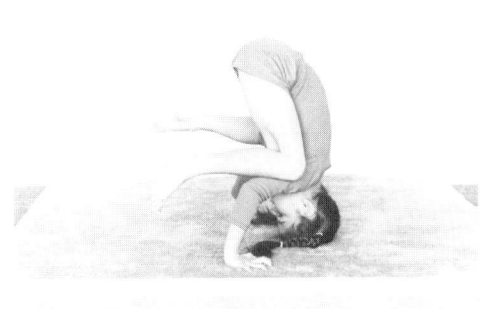

- *As back, abdominal, and leg strength improve, the tumbler takes control.*
- *Start in the kneeling position and proceed to the knees-to-elbows-stand.*
- *From there, raise both legs straight up.*
- *The descent is made possible by practice with the shoulder stands. Keep the legs straight and lower them slowly as the back leans further back as balance.*

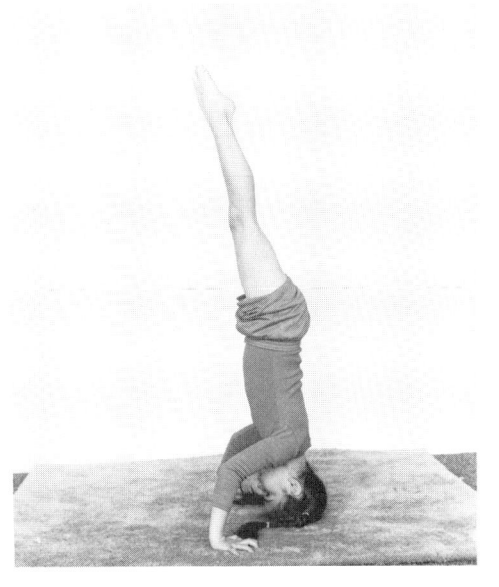

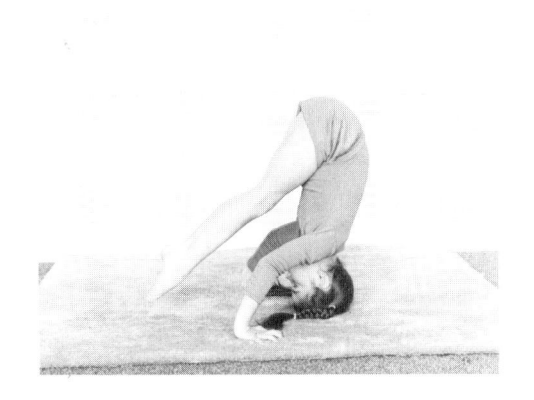

108. HANDSTAND

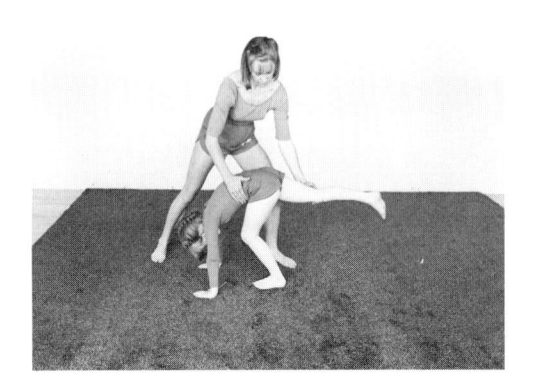

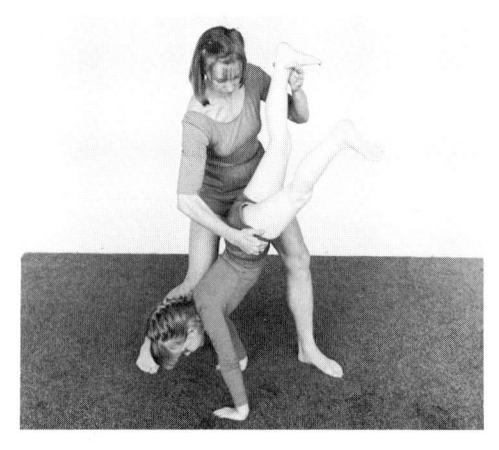

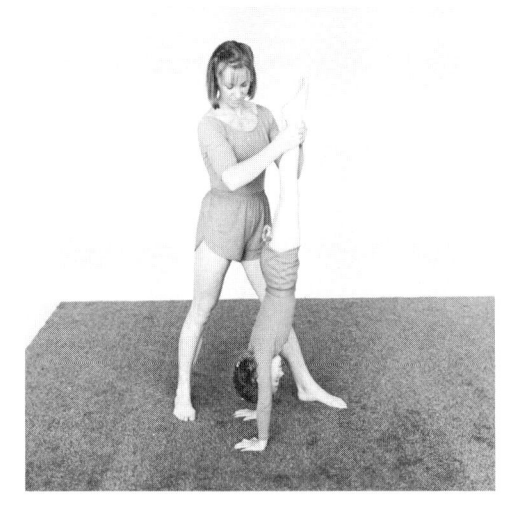

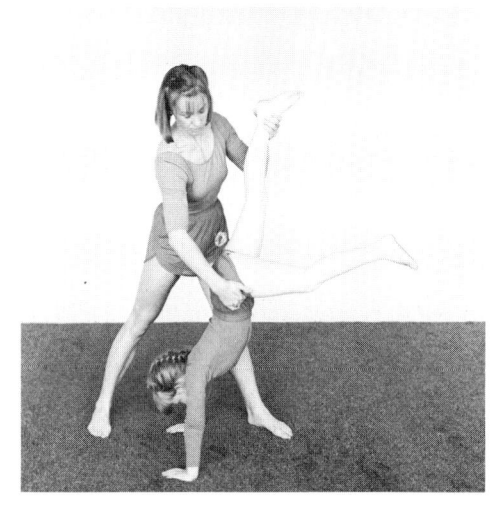

- The tumbler places both hands on the floor and looks at a spot between her hands. (It helps to put a small object there so that there is something definite to see.) That focus will keep the head up, and that head position will ultimately control the stunt.
- The tumbler lifts the leg nearest the spotter and at first, taking it in hand furthest *from* the tumbler, the spotter lifts the little person into the air. The other hand reaches across to grasp the bony pelvis. (This assures everyone that the acrobat cannot fall on her head.)
- The spotter then straightens the tumbler's legs and tells her to tighten her seat and point her toes. Those two actions serve to stabilize the body into a pole rather than uncontrolled segments.
- The return is very important. The child is held at the pelvis and told to put one foot down under her nose.
- When the foot touches down, the spotter pushes back on both sides of the pelvis and the child will stand up. The patterning has begun.
- Keep the handstand legs under control for at least twelve tries, and the pattern is set.

Tumbling 137

> If a child has trouble with tumbling, notice what parts of her body are weak and use the equipment (pages 145–227) to strengthen them.

109. KICK-UP HANDSTAND

Try to free the tumblers from your care as soon as you can. If they can tumble on their own, they will—constantly. Constant practice makes for perfect performance. Children *feel* like turning cartwheels, somersaulting down a hill, rolling, spinning, falling, climbing. The better their coordination, the more fun they will have and the more options they will have when it comes to exercise in the future.

• *The spotter stands a little to the side as the tumbler raises both hands, advances one foot, and picks out the place she intends to kick off from.*

• *While it is no longer necessary to catch the pelvis, the spotter is nonetheless ready for anything. With practice she can hold her hand up and the tumbler will be able to put her heel into it.*

• *The spotter lets go as soon as the balance point is reached and the tumbler makes the straight-leg descent, bringing one foot under the nose. Use both legs alternately for kick-up so that both sides will be evenly developed.*

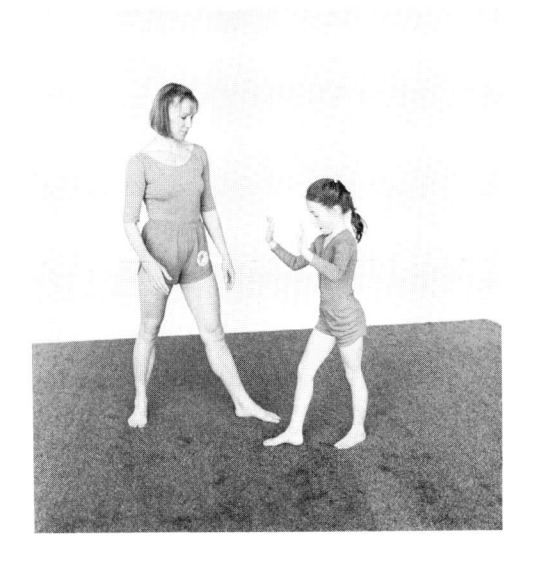

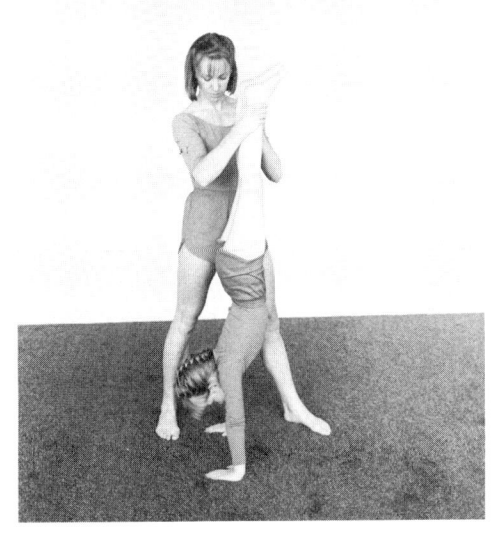

110. WALL HANDSTAND

• *Handstands can be done against a wall, thus freeing the spotter to work with other children.*

• *The tumbler faces a wall and picks out a spot for her hands that seems right. If it is too close, she will come back down at once; if too far away, she will have to really reach with her legs. The first three tries should be spotted. After that each tumbler learns the right distance.*

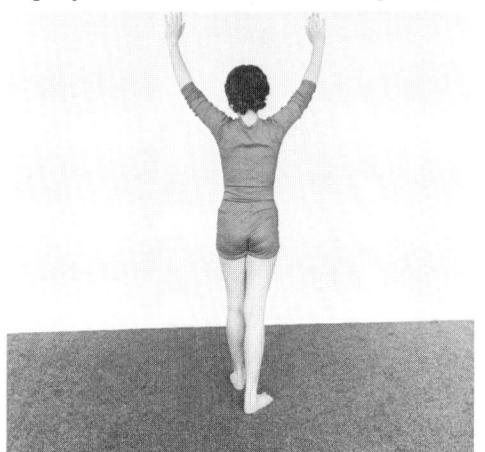

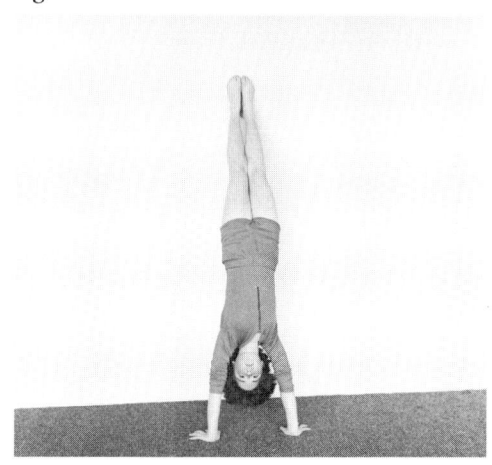

111. BACK BEND

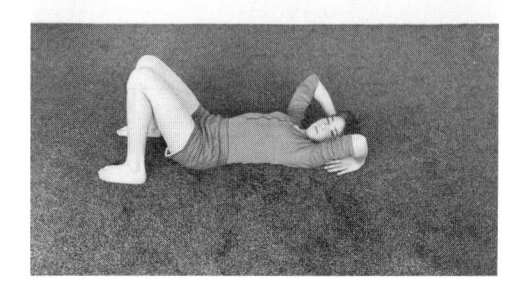

One stunt leads to another, and while all exercises prepare the body, there are specific exercises that help with specific stunts. The *assisted Prone Back Bend #61* gets the back ready for this exercise and also for the Walkover (exercise 112).

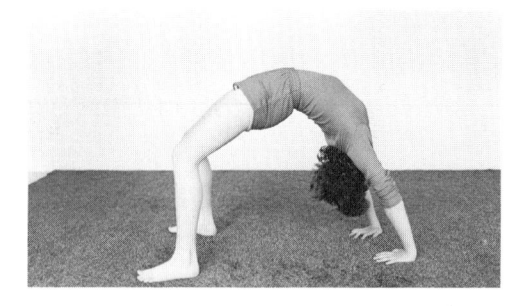

• *Lie supine with the feet apart and the knees bent, bringing the heels as close to the seat as possible.*

• *Place the thumbs in both ears with the hands sticking out like large ears.*

• *Bend the hands back, slipping the fin-*

Tumbling

gers out of the ears and near to the shoulders.
• *Press the body up into an arch and tip the head back.*
• *Lower and repeat five or six times.*
• *Once this becomes easy and the arch is really high, the spotter grasps the pelvis and rocks the child's weight onto her hands, back to her feet, again to the arms; as the weight heads for the feet the second time, the spotter pulls her to her feet.*
• *Practice this until the tumbler can do it herself.*

112. WALKOVER

If the spotter is big and the tumbler is small, the first Walkovers can be done over the knee of the spotter.

• *The spotter kneels on one knee as the tumbler prepares for a handstand.*
• *When the apex is reached, the spotter lowers the child into an arch over her knee.*
• *The spotter then presses down on the thighs and lifts the upper back; the tumbler stands up. Soon she will be able to combine the Handstand (exercise 108), the Back Bend (exercise 111), and the Walkover (exercise 112).*

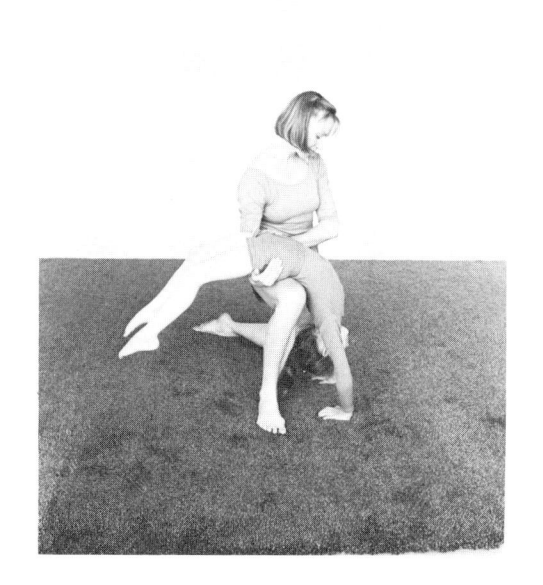

113. CARTWHEEL

Cartwheels begin as "gnome jumps." Gnomes are very short and they like it that way because they can get into and under things big people can't get into or under.

• *Pretend that you have drawn a magic line across the floor. It's a magic line for squatty little gnomes only. Squat down on the line with your left foot toward the other end of the line on the other side of the room.*

• *Look straight ahead and pretend there is a large king gnome sitting straight ahead of you. You* must *keep your eyes on that king gnome. That's the rule. There's only one safe time when you can look away and that's when you put your hands on the line facing* away *from the king.*

• *Place both hands on the line with the fingers pointing* away *from him. You are quite safe now, but you want to get to the other side of the line. How to do it?*

• *Take your weight on your hands and jump your feet right around your hands to land on the line facing the king. Safe again.*

• *Jump-around-turn, one at a time, all the way to the end.*

• *When the tumblers can do nice turns, they can forget the king and having to look at him and only being safe while turning.*

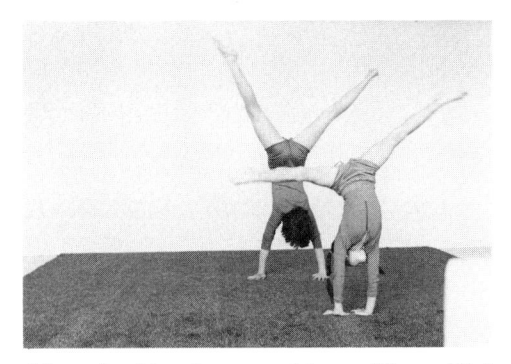

Now the idea is to combine a Horse Kick (exercise 76) with both feet in the air as you turn.

• *Pretty soon the horse kick turns will get higher and higher; a cartwheel is very near.*

• *Straighten out the horse's legs as you jump and keep the legs wide apart. That will make them land one at a time. The wider, the better.*

• *Next, try to do the cartwheel to rhythm. Count four for each cartwheel, one count for each hand and foot. Be sure to do them to both sides.*

PAIR EXERCISES

Pair exercises, such as the pushes, pulls, and balances, are fun and are good training for team sports. You simply *have* to pay attention to your teammate.

114. THE VW

• *You can use the wrist hold or hold on to a wand or pole.*

• *Start close together, facing each other.*

The one with the smaller feet covers the toes of his partner with his own.

Tumbling

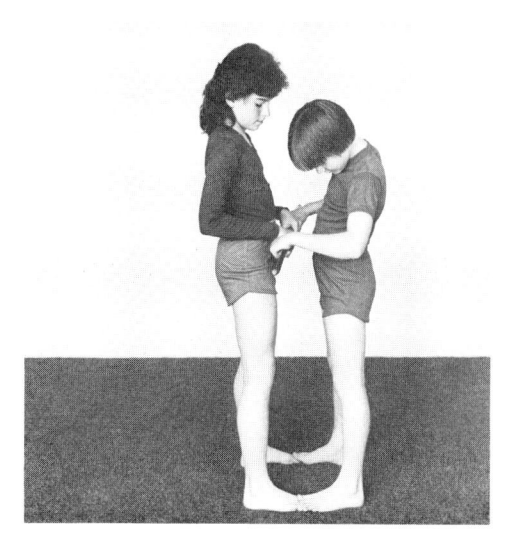

- *Both lean back* slowly *and at the same time. Try to find the exact balance point. If partners are the same height and weight, it is much easier.*
- *When the balance point has been found, drop* slowly *into a deep knee-bend.*
- *Hold for a count of five and then slowly rise to the lean-back position.*
- *Finish together as at the start. Do four.*

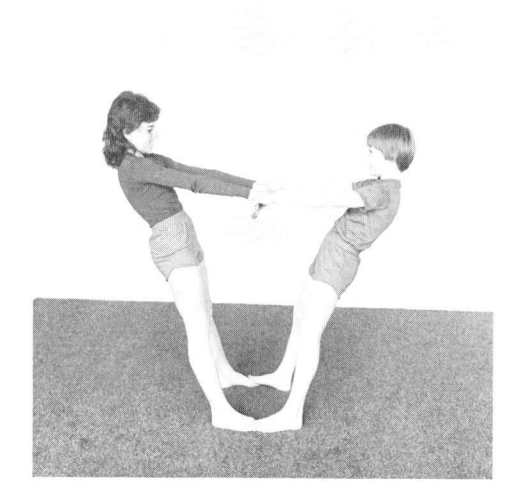

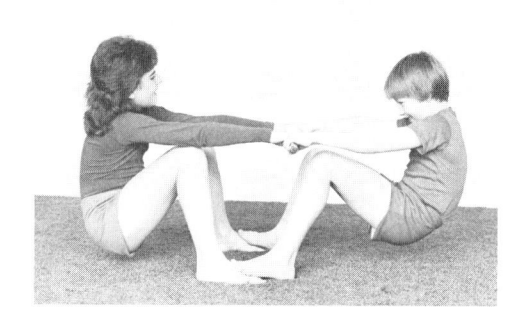

115. BACK-TO-BACK "M"

- *Stand back to back with elbows interlocked.*
- *Walk out away from each other until you are far enough apart to allow sinking all the way to the floor.*
- *Both must bend the same way. If one breaks at the hips and the other doesn't, the descent will be lopsided and incomplete.*
- *When it is possible to sit on the floor, do so and count to four. Then press back up to the standing position. Do four.*

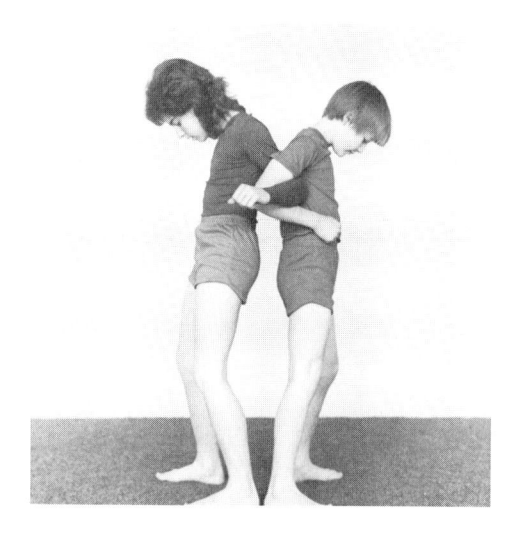

142 Fitness from Six to Twelve

BACK TO BACK "M" *(continued)*

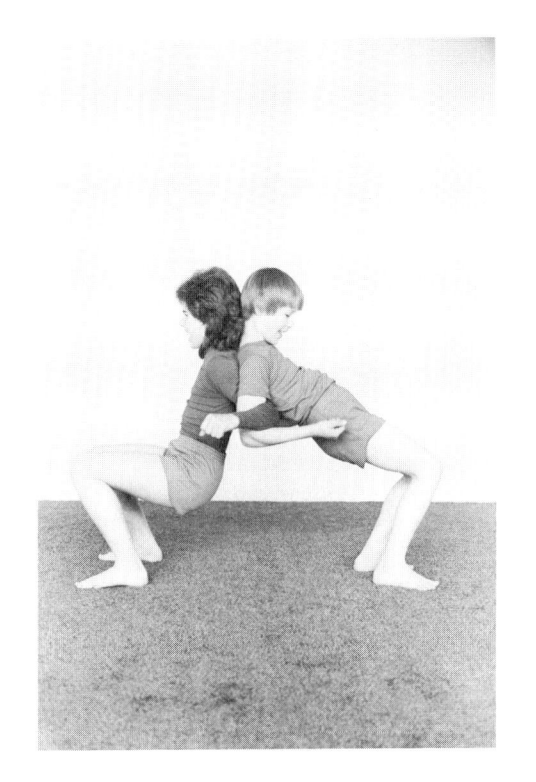

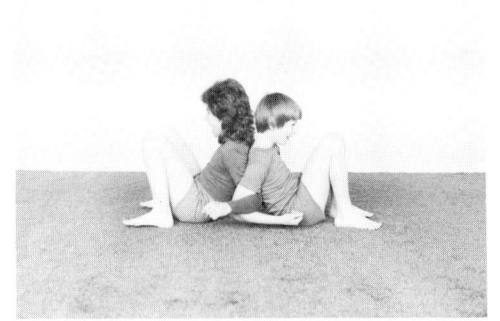

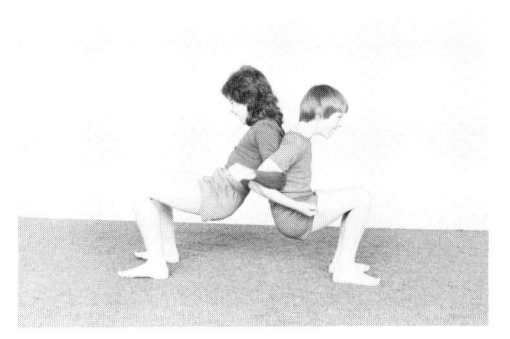

116. LITTLE LIFTS BIG

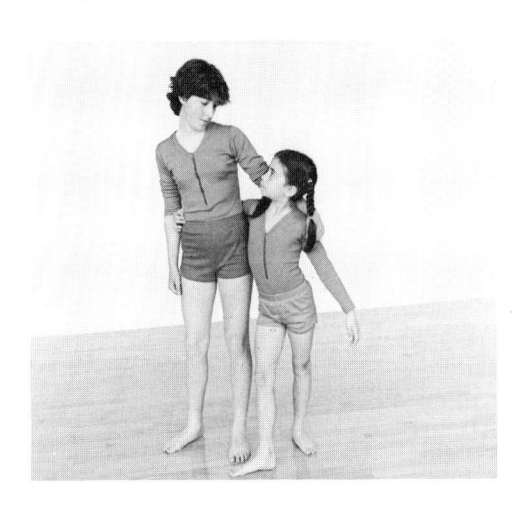

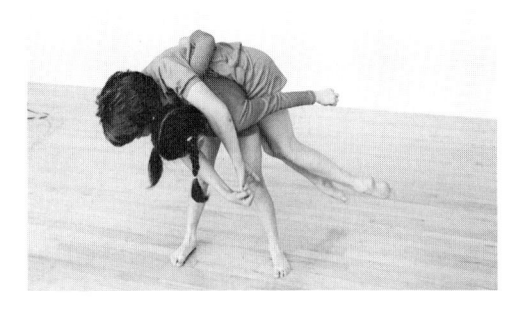

- Little and Big stand next to each other. Little puts her arm around Big's waist, and Big puts hers around Little's shoulders.
- Little then steps way across with her leg

Tumbling

nearest to Big so that both her feet are outside of both Big's feet.

• Then Little swings her hips across to the other side of Big and leans forward. As she does so, her free arm reaches back to steady Big, whose feet have left the floor.

117. BACK-TO-BACK LIFT

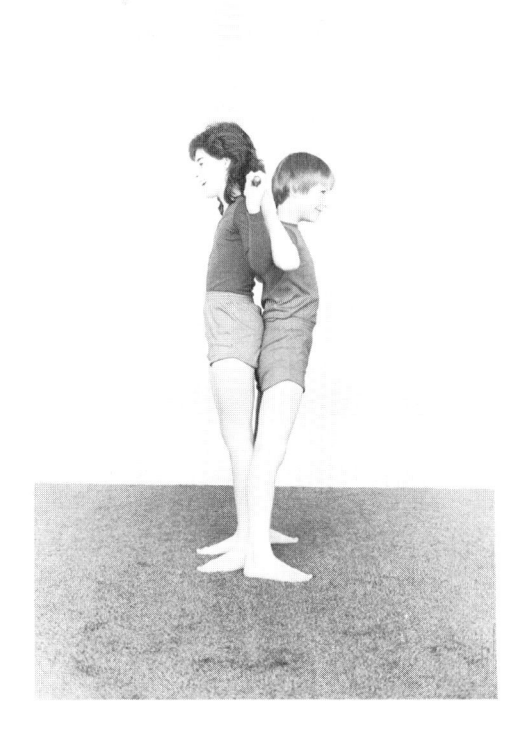

This is best done with the help of a wand or pole.

• Stand back to back holding onto a wand that is between the shoulders.
• There is one trick the lifter must remember. The seat of the lifter must be below the seat of the lifted.

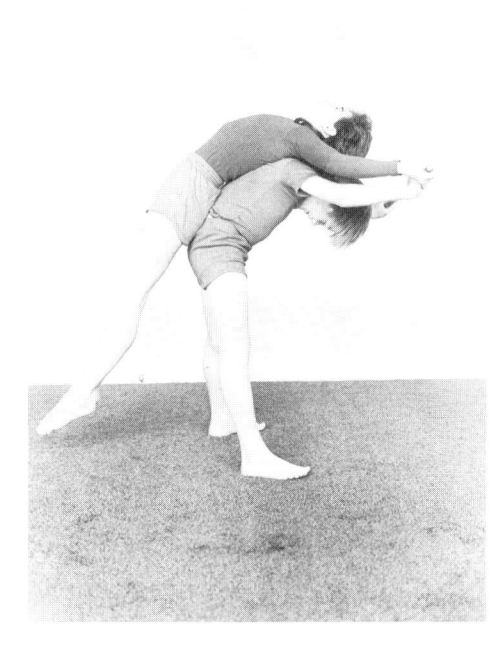

• The lifter bends both knees to slide her seat under that of her partner.
• She then straightens both arms straight overhead and leans forward to lift her partner along her back.
• For the partner's part, the word is relax. Just hang loose. This will be easy if the lifter takes it slowly.

118. THE LAYER CAKE (STUNT)

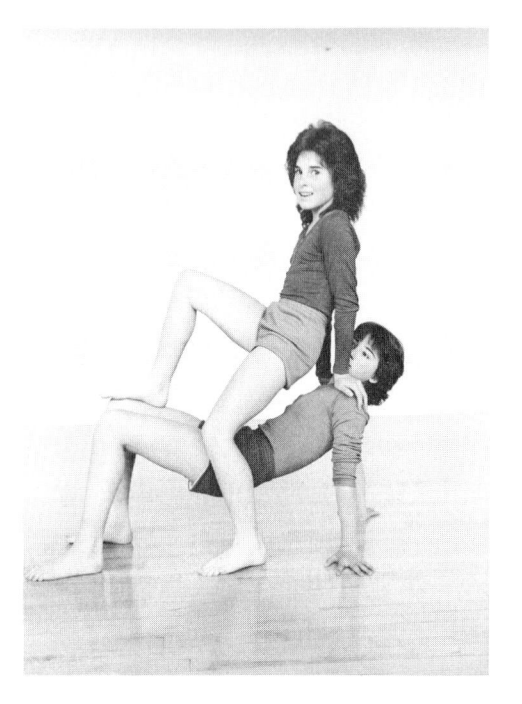

- *The partner who is to serve as support sits down with feet well apart and knees bent.*
- *She leans back on her hands and lifts her torso up to make a table.*
- *The top-layer person faces away from the support and places both hands on support's shoulders.*
- *The top-layer person places her far foot on the support's far knee.*
- *At a given signal the resting foot is brought to support's other knee, and both girls press their bodies up to make two even layers.*
- *To retreat from the finished position, the top layer simply steps down.*

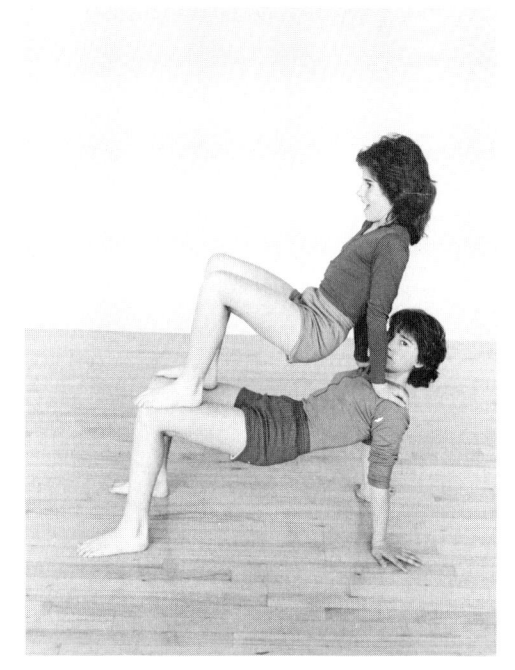

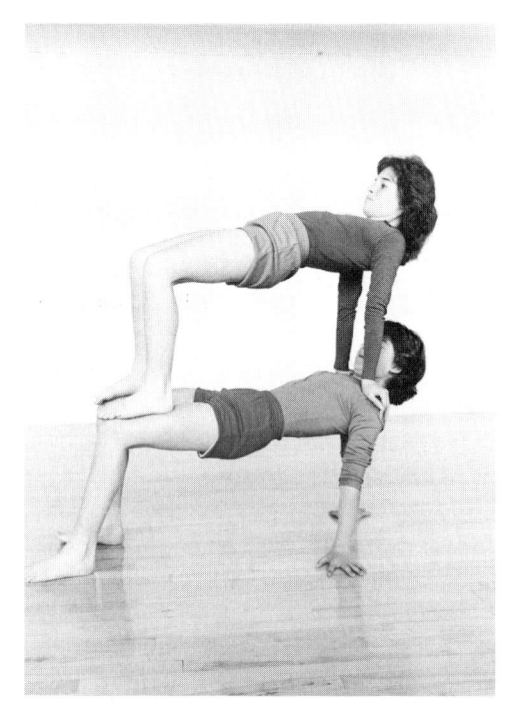

CHAPTER THIRTEEN
EQUIPMENT

Children love equipment and, contrary to what's currently thought, equipment need not be expensive. The major expense is gym mats, which should be light and foldable so that they can be transported by the children and will fit into a fairly limited storage space. They were my first purchase when I started my classes and they made a world of difference, even when I had nothing else. If you are buying mats for a school class, enlist the parents in your fund-raising. A bridge party or tag sale will net you enough for at least one mat for starters. If you are a lone parent, it may take longer, but a cake sale by the participating families can begin the "Mat Fund" and surely there will be some enterprising parents who will dream up other ways. I saved for a year to get my first mat; it was a year spent constantly saying, "When we get our mat, we will . . ." When we finally had it, it was the most treasured mat in America.

The rest of the equipment shown here is very inexpensive. What it requires is the school carpenter or a clever parent, some wood, a length of pipe, and paint. The climate is right today. Parents are beginning to worry about the reports

Fitness from Six to Twelve

on children's lack of fitness and risk of ill health. Millions have been spent on exercise equipment for grown-ups. They will be surprised to learn that children need fitness, too, and there is someone willing to help them get it: us.

THE SAWHORSE

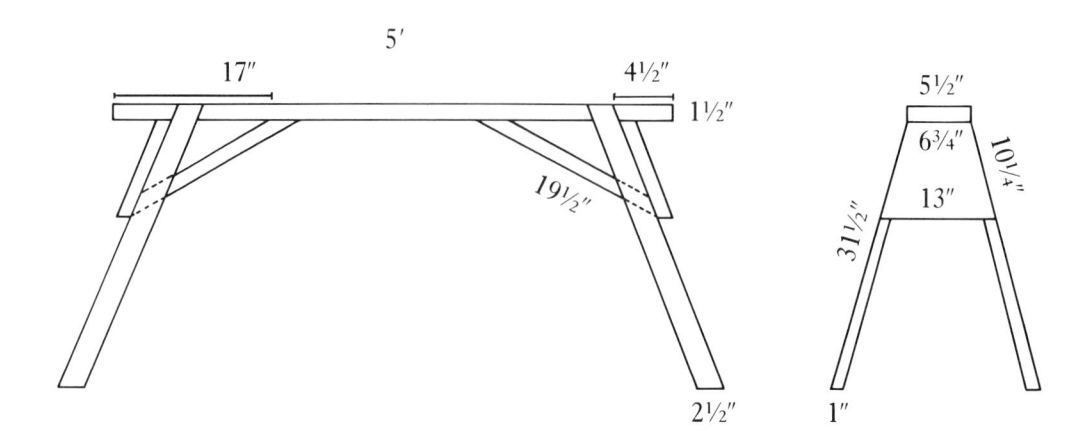

After the mat the sawhorse is next in importance. It has many uses and can be made in varying heights. The first set I had built in 1948 are still in use. They have been used by all ages from toddlers to retired ladies. They have served as a balance beam, hurdles, supports for ladders, narrower beams called railroad tracks, and parallel bars. A hole in each end of the sawhorse can support a 12-foot length of 2-inch conduit pipe that can be used as an even more demanding balancer. Four is the ideal number of sawhorses.

THE RAMP

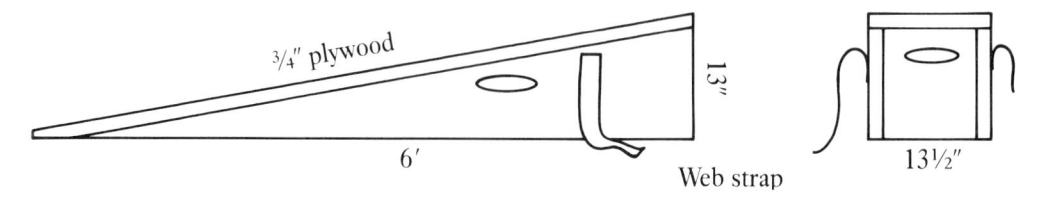

The ramp should be made of ¾-inch plywood, because it takes a real beating from pounding feet. The cross at the high end is made to support the railroad

Tumbling

tracks (see below) in one of three positions. If the horizontal cut supports the tracks, you have either a wide surface (eight inches) or, if reversed, a narrow one supported by the wide one. If the board is placed sideways into the vertical cuts, you have a *really* narrow balance beam.

If you wish to use the ramps as slant boards to increase the workload on the abdominal muscles when doing bent-knee sit-ups, add the webbed straps. Three coats of enamel will give the ramp a good sliding surface. The ideal number of ramps to have is four, but two will do nicely.

THE PARALLEL BARS

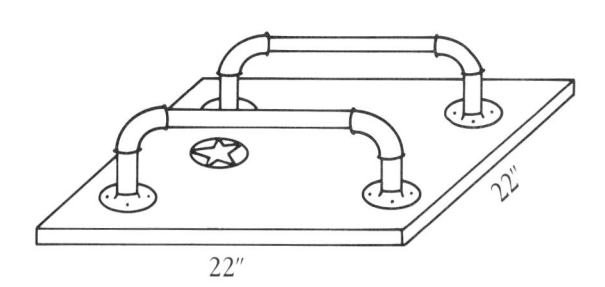

For the bars, use two 14-inch lengths of black iron pipe. The base should be a square of ½-inch plywood, 22 inches by 22 inches. Use railing flanges to attach the pipe to the base. The four support pipes should be four inches long and attached to the horizontal bars with plumbing elbows.

The space between the bars may vary from 1 to 1½ feet. Remember, the whole family, or the class *and* the teacher, are to use the parallels, so consider the widest set of shoulders. Arms can stretch wide to support a body, but they do not do so well when they are pulled in by narrow parallels. Glue a decal of some kind in the center of the board, just inside and close to one of the two sets of upright pipes. This is to catch the child's eye and keep the head up.

RAILROAD TRACKS

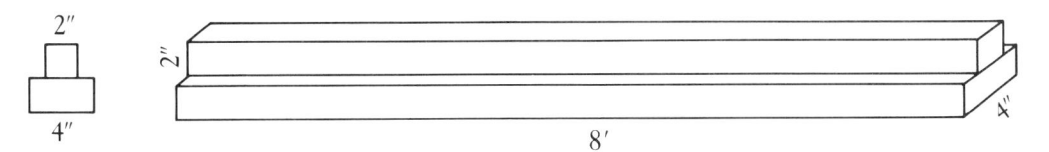

Use sound 8-foot lengths of 2-by-8-inch lumber (which means that your board will be 2 by 7 inches.) To that, screw an 8-foot length of 2-by-2 right down the middle. Round off the edges of the 2-by-2 so that it resembles a railroad track. Use two flat on the floor or a single as one track or one or two stretched from sawhorse to sawhorse.

Secure with holes drilled through the ends of the track and the sawhorse, through which you can thread long bolts using quickly applied wing nuts.

THE STAIRS

If you have a flight of stairs in your house, you don't need to make any. If the apartment house you live in provides clean staircases, again, no need. But if stairs are unavailable to you, have a set made. This goes for schools as well.

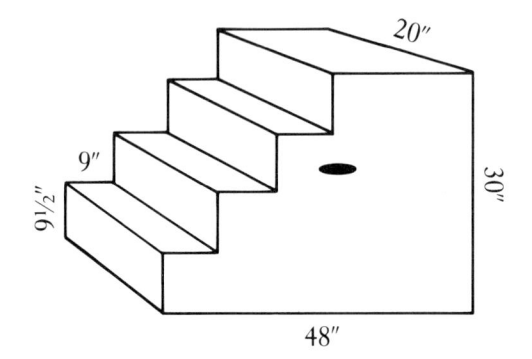

Use ¾-inch plywood and the dimensions given in the drawing. Reinforce all edges and the top with 1-by-1½-inch board. Cut a handhold in either side to facilitate movement. You will need two sets.

A couple of sets of stairs placed back to back can be a great asset to any program. Go up one side and down the other with as many of the floor-progression exercises as are suitable. Train for anything needing leg muscles by climbing and descending to a beat, with ever heavier backpacks. Weight bags are ideal, and if you are an apartment dweller and also a skier, get ready for the season with the backpack and a walkman plugging your ears but driving your legs.

THE DOORWAY GYM

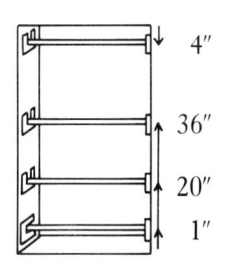

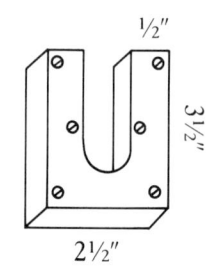

No school is so large that *every* home room would not profit by access to a doorway gym. No apartment is so small (or so posh) that the same doorway gym wouldn't fit right in. A chinning bar used to hang in every "cloakroom" doorway in the "olden days," and every little kid was expected to do three chin-ups. Funny, how much they knew long ago. I can remember my fourth-grade teacher standing with pad and pencil checking us off every Friday noon. If someone who usually could chin suddenly couldn't, she would say, "Tell your mother you may be coming down with something. You'll need rest and fluids. Tell her, remember." By Monday, most of those children *had* come down with something. Years and years later a wonderful physical educator (he really deserved the title), Dr. Frederick Rand Rogers, designed a test at Springfield College. It took a little longer than three chin-ups, but then it was used on college boys. If a boy's strength quotient dropped below a given level, he, too, was suspected of "coming down with something." Most of the time either the boy did come down with something or, if questioned carefully, had overindulged himself the night before.

A chinning bar is good, but limited. A doorway gym is limited only by the imaginations of those using it.

If the door frame is of wood, no problem. If the building is modern and of metal, you have a problem, but it is not insurmountable. Have a carpenter line the door frame with wood.

Next you will need at least five sets of wooden supports for the several lengths of 1-inch pipe you will use. The pipe lengths are the width of the door frame. The supports look like large wooden letter U's and are made from ¾-inch plywood. They are attached with screws to either side of the door frame.

The supports at the lowest level are turned on their sides and will hold the pipe down so that you can slip your feet under it for sit-ups. Or you can lie on your back and curl up like a ball and pull your knees to your nose. When you get really strong, you can pull yourself up onto your shoulders.

All the other sets are put in vertically at the stipulated levels. They can be jumped over, crawled under, climbed like a ladder, hung from by the knees, and used for Pinwheels (exercise 208) and Skin the Cat (exercise 209). Little (or big) ballerinas can use them as barres. People who want to rest head-down can lean a wide plank such as a book shelf against a low bar and do just that. Ladders can be leaned against them and climbed—even on Park Avenue. Ropes can be tied to the highest bar and many of the rope stunts described later on will be possible.

The doorway gym is ideal for the classroom program on page 403.

PIPES

Pipes are just that—lengths of pipe. Their other name is *conduits*, and there are many ways to use them. A 10-foot length of 2-inch conduit can be used flat on the floor as a "tightrope." If you put holes in the ends of your sawhorses large enough to hold the conduit, you have a real tightrope. Ours are 2 inches wide.

If you have two 8-foot lengths and you fasten them side by side and about 18 inches apart from one sawhorse to the other, you will have really big parallel bars that can be swung on, hand-walked on, hung on, and a dozen other things the children will invent. (See Chapter 26, "Swimming")

OTHER EQUIPMENT

There are thousands of pieces of equipment all around us that can be used in classes, large or small, and they can be had for very little money. Children (and grown-ups, too) like to exercise with "things" in their hands. *Frisbees* are colorful and they make noise when clapped together with the music. If you work with the handicapped, you will find that Frisbees tell them where their hands are, and in no time at all their movements become precise.

Then there are *automobile tires*. They are plentiful and can be made colorful with enamel paint. (Allow lots of time for drying and use small car tires.) Children can run through them in a line or they can be staggered, as they are for football training. They can be jumped through, hopped through, and even walked through backward.

A visit to a *carpet* shop can net you enough throwaway samples to make two 6-by-4-inch squares for each member of the class. Exercises can be done sitting. Put the squares under your heels, with your seat off the floor as you rest on your hands, do Russian Forward Thrusts (exercise 96). In a minute your pupils will think up four more "tricks." If you get down on hands and knees and put the squares under your hands, you can "scrub" with the rhythm of the music in all directions. If you put them under your knees, you can do the Apart-Together jumps (exercise 80) as slides. If you stand up, you can skate or run backward or forward or even sideways with the rugs under your feet.

Then there are *hoops*. They can be bought in any toy store and used to create patterns as you go across the floor. They can be lifted, swung, stepped through, and even used as jump ropes.

Blocks, too, are inexpensive. Cut a 2-by-4 into 7-inch lengths, sand the blocks, and paint them with three coats of colorful enamel. Their uses are endless.

One of the problems confronting any teacher—whether in the home with a small group or in a school where some unfortunate teachers confront sixty children in a class—is what to do with the youngsters who stand in lines waiting for a spotter. Blocks, railroad tracks, tires, and so forth provide something for "waiters" to do. Set up an obstacle course around the room, a sort of circuit-training route with which the children are familiar. Then they will have something to do on their way back to the stunts that need spotting, such as jumps off the ramps.

CHAPTER FOURTEEN
EXERCISES ON THE EQUIPMENT

Railroad tracks give practice for balance-beam work later on. The simplest and least expensive example would be two boards, probably 2-by-4s, eight feet long laid side by side. Even one such board could have many uses. If you have a pigeon-toed child, use the exercises (shown later on the sawhorse) on your single board, which you leave out in the hall where all the children can balance on it as they walk down the hall . . . and that means *everyone*, including you. There is an old truism left over from the past: "Monkey see, monkey do." If you want your child to do something, do it yourself. He or she is silently making reels and reels of "tapes" of things you do and say every day. Might as well use this terrific copying machine to get something you want. That would go for children with poor balance, too. In addition, refer to the myotherapy chapter for balance and pigeon toes. *Then* urge the exercises.

If you are going one step further and have had the equipment made, you will be able to provide a nice wide, flat balance beam by pushing the ends of one track into the crosses in the ends of your ramps. This does lift your balancers up into the air a little, but the board is so wide they won't mind.

119. WALKING THE PLANK

The first consideration is slow music. Find something that has a calm, even feeling. This will affect the children's actions and give them better control in the same way that fast, exciting music will throw them into whirls and vaults they would never think of attempting without that stimulation. That's what martial music and tom-toms are for!

• *Start by crossing the plank going forward. At first it is permissible to look down, but as quickly as possible get the little heads up. Feet are sensitive, too, and should be able to tell the brain where they are.*
• *Have them jump off the "plank" into the deep blue sea at the end.*

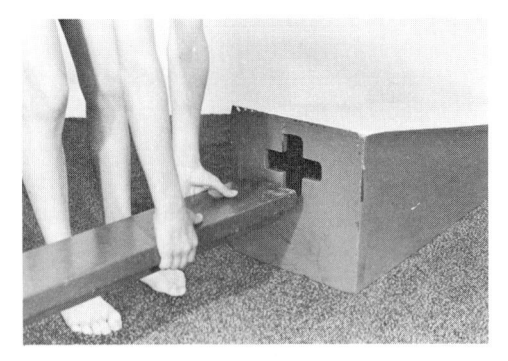

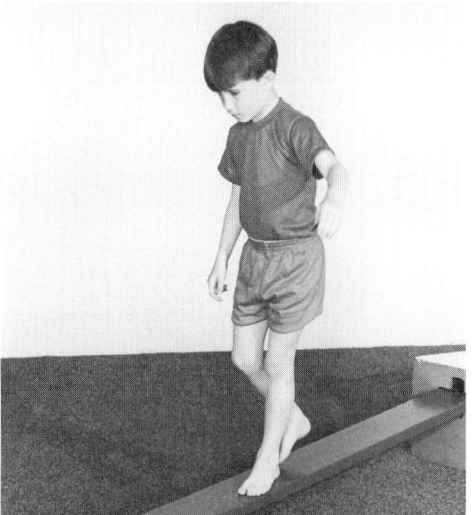

120. BACKING ACROSS PLANK

• *Simply stop at the far end and return, moving backward. This time it is impossible to see where the feet are, so they might as well fend for themselves.*

There are many ways to use this low balance beam. Refer to the exercises to be done on the sawhorse (pages 164–180) and you will find some. In addition, the children will dream up their own.

To make the work more difficult, remove the track from the ramps and turn it over so that the narrow board is on top. Lay a second track parallel with the first with about two feet of distance between. Pairs work well on the railroad tracks. Use a wand as a balance aid.

Exercises on the Equipment

121. ASSISTED KEEL WALK

• *The spotter stands between the two smaller children as they grasp the wand between them.*

• *Step up onto the narrow keel board in the center of the track. It will take considerable concentration to stay there. In addition it will require rhythm, control, and cooperation. All of those things apply to other parts of schooling, and one of the best lessons can begin in your class.*

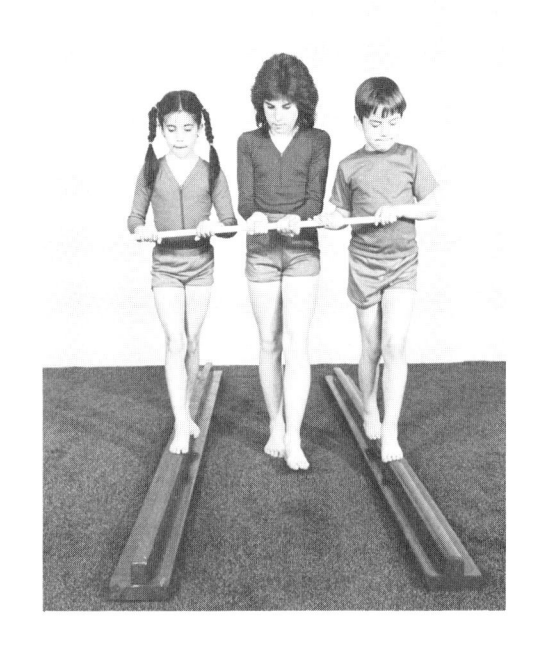

122. TRACK WALK, DIVIDED

• *No spotter is needed for this walk. The children (or you, since you should try these things out first) walk on both sides of the keel.*

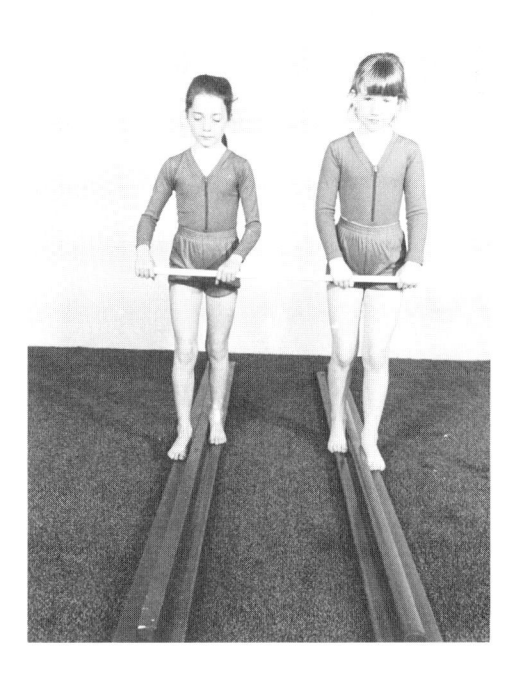

123. BACK TRACK WALK

• *Walk the tracks backward. This can be done either with or without a wand. Have the children take every opportunity to* educate *the muscles of their feet and their sensitivity to the surface under them.*

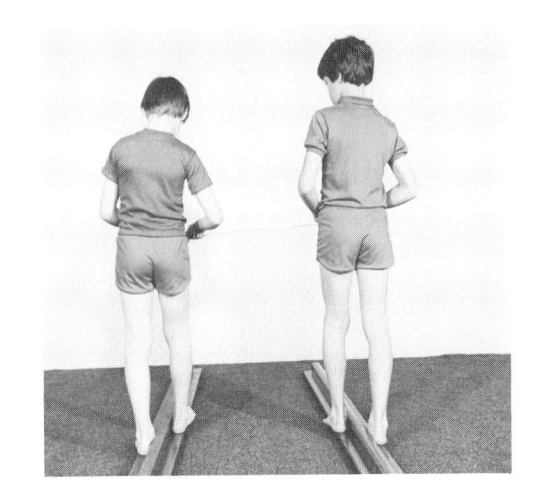

124. KEEL WALK UNASSISTED

• *At this age boys and girls can do equally well (with the girls possessing the edge, if there is one). There will be stars and clumsies of both sexes. Try to match* abilities *rather than ages or heights. Big-boy stars will help little-boy clumsies or even big-boy clumsies until you can bring them up to a better level, but boys rarely want to be saddled with a girl clumsy. Girls rarely care, if the problem is explained. Some boys fall into this category, too.*

• *Watch! Above all watch! You may not know what you are looking at at first, but you will learn.*

• *The two children start out across the keel, and what do you see? The trained gymnast on the left turns her feet out as she has learned to do in "free exercise." The untrained boy heads his feet straight across, as tightrope walkers do. Both are right; but which did you ask for? If you didn't, you now know there are at least two ways to keel-walk. Next time, specify.*

• *The wand is sloping. Where were they supposed to carry it? Did you tell them? That makes two more ways to cross. Add to those, bent-over, hands-overhead, arms outstretched, right or left hand only, and you will begin to see dozens of possibilities.*

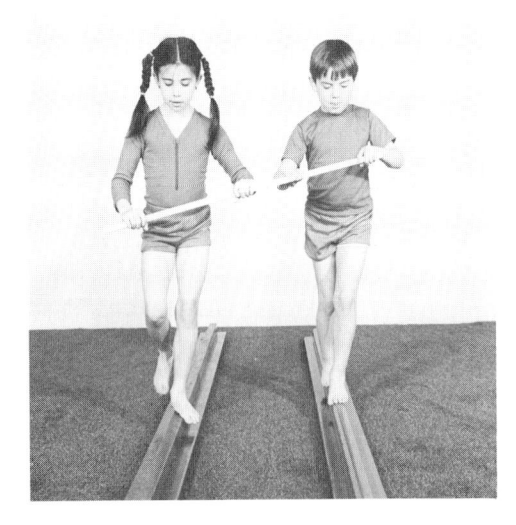

• *Start now to say, "Let's see what you can make up and you* must *give it a name." That's like being allowed to name the new puppy.*

Exercises on the Equipment 155

125. BACK KEEL WALK

• This will need a thoughtful spotter who can provide steady hands and a voice that says gently, "Keep your head up, Johnny, you're doing great." The copycats will copy your way with the children, your jokes, your laughter, and your patience. This is the way to develop assistants.

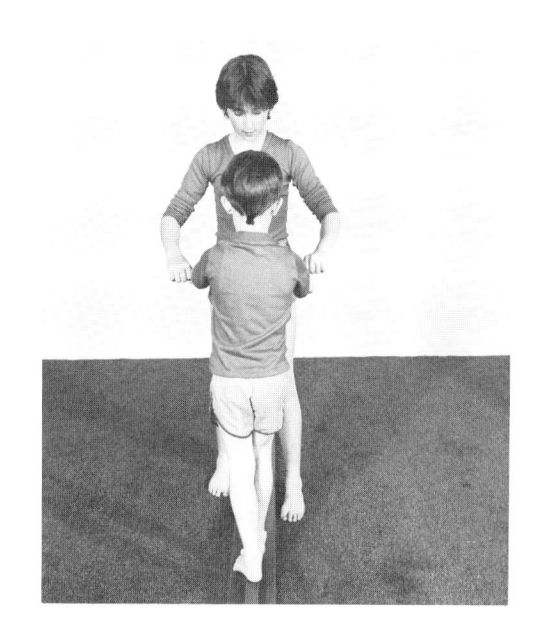

126. KEEL CROSSOVER

Working in pairs has several advantages, and one of the most important is that the children spend less time waiting in line. It's also excellent training for spotters. When you work with someone else in any form of balance training, you are forced to *feel* what the other body is doing and *also what it is about to do.*

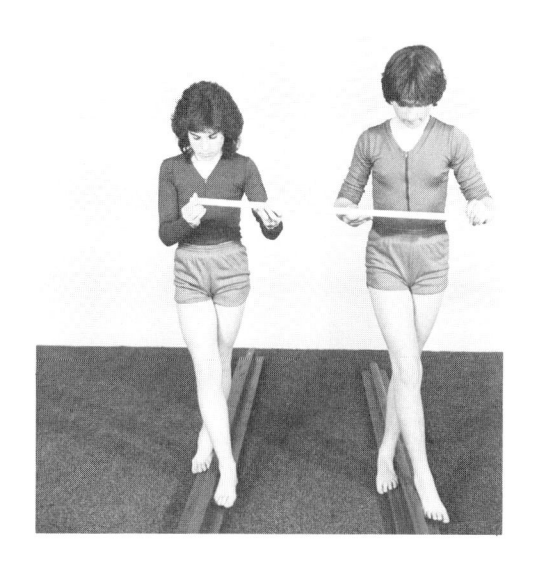

• Place the left *foot on the* right *side of the keel.*

• *Step forward with the* right *foot and cross over to place it on the* left *side of the keel.*

• *Don't take the time to* explain *it; do it.* No one will have trouble following you if they have the musculature and balance. If they don't, look up balance *in the exercise* index and give those people some extra work in that area.

127. BRIDGE WALK

• *Place two tracks parallel to each other, and close, so that even the smallest member of the class can do the stunt.*
• *Place the hands on the keel of one track and the feet on the other and cross by moving first one hand and foot toward the end, then bringing the following hand and foot to touch its companion.*
• *If the floor is slippery, use four children to stabilize the tracks.*

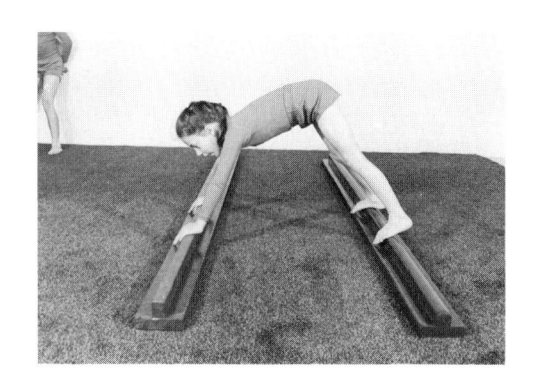

128. BRIDGE WALK, CROSSED HANDS

In this variation of the Bridge Walk the hands cross over each other as the "bridge" moves from one end to the other across the tracks. In both of these exercises, and the ones that follow, be sure to go in both directions, leading with a different side each time.

129. BRIDGE WALK, CROSSED FEET

• *Cross the tracks, crossing one foot under the other.*
• *Next cross using hands and feet at the same time.*
• *Then open it up to, "Let's see what you can do."*

130. TRACK WHEELBARROW

Wheelbarrows are something babies should learn. In my book *How to Keep Your Child Fit from Birth to Six* parents are shown how to pick up the diaper area (pelvis) the first time the baby gets up onto his elbows and then onto his hands. That provides handstand practice. By picking up the thighs and "walking" the baby forward, as little girls "walk" their dolls, a wheelbarrow is achieved. The key to success is the hold at the thighs. That hold, rather than at the ankles, assures *success without strain.*

Exercises on the Equipment 157

- *Place the tracks a shoulder width apart.*
- *The "wheelbarrow" crosses with one hand on each track. The "wheeler" holds at the thighs until both back and abdominal strength are developed to the point where a lower hold will not cause a sag in the back.*
- *Using two parallel tracks four or five feet apart will allow two wheelbarrows to cross hand over hand on one track each. This allows four children to work at the same time.*

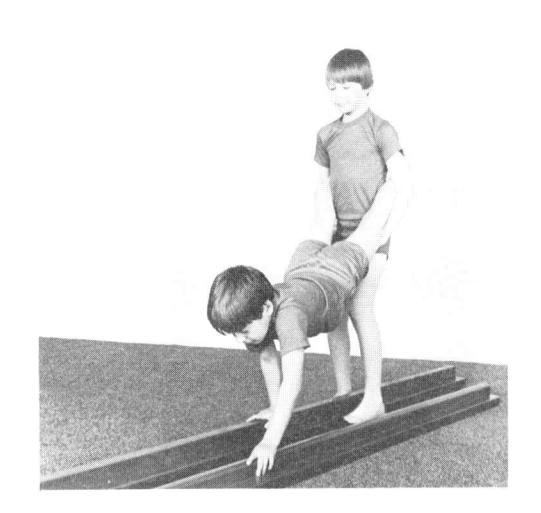

131. ONE-LEGGED WHEELBARROW, TRACK

- *This exercise calls for a strong lower back. The wheelbarrow places hands on the tracks and the wheeler grasps one leg in both hands.*
- *The wheelbarrow must support the free leg herself. Do not let the free leg sag.*

The keel can be raised by inserting both ends into the ramp ends as we did to produce the "plank." It can be raised still higher by stretching the track between the backs of two sawhorses.

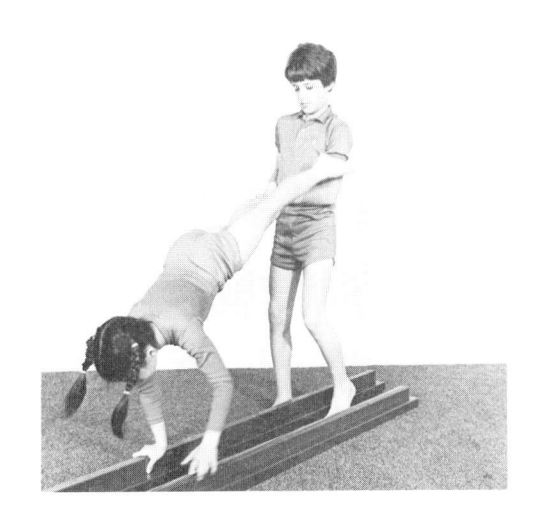

EXERCISES ON THE LADDER

Reading skills depend on a simple basic: *the ability to see . . . and report back to the brain what has been seen.* The ladder is the best teacher of this skill. In reading class, the inability to distinguish between *rat* and *cat* may not seem very important to the little scholar, *but* if you are walking through the spaces between the rungs of a ladder and you don't give an accurate report back to the boss in your head, you fall down and bruise your shin. That *hurts*. It hurts *now*. The pain that goes with not being able to read is a long way off, but a bruised shin cannot be ignored. A child soon learns to pay attention, and paying attention is a habit that can be self-taught. The child who can *pay attention* to instructions has an easier time. The child who can *pay attention* even to boring teachers gets the high marks and does half the work of the dreamer. Nothing wrong with dreaming if you can knock it off long enough to take in the necessary stuff that makes school easier.

Now to developing the habit of *look . . . see . . . and report back*. What you will need is a wooden orchard ladder. They come in pairs, and one has hooks so that it can be lengthened. Keep those hooks on and you will find a use for them with your doorway gym (page 148.)

Children form the habits of a lifetime, the attitudes of a lifetime, the fears and anxieties of a lifetime, before they get to school . . . and during their first few years in school. The *best* nursery school teacher, the *best* kindergarten teacher, and the *best* teachers of the first three or four grades in school are like the very *best* doctor and dentist—barely good enough. What those people do or don't do determines so much of the rest of our children's lives that it's scary. Of course the most important people of all are the ones at home, but more and more parents are working and must employ surrogates. Who are your surrogates?

---

132. SPACE STEPPING

• *Lay the ladder flat on the floor and step into each square between the rungs. You will find that even you have to pay attention. Have the children step in the spaces as you have done. Watch! Does one have trouble? That one needs lots of ladder walking—all the variations here plus the ones the children design.*

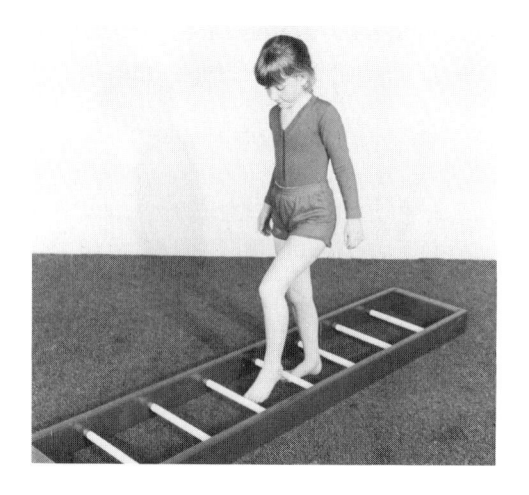

Exercises on the Equipment 159

133. RUNG WALKING

• *Try this yourself before you have the children try it. Walk the length stepping on the rungs on the balls of your feet. If you (or they) use the arches, it will hurt, and it will also not strengthen the feet, which is one of the things you are aiming for.*

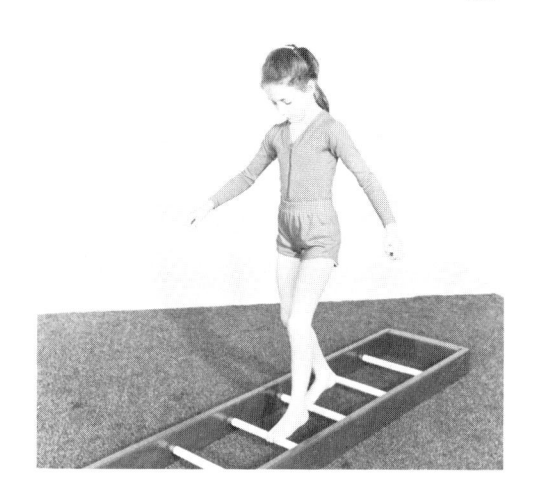

134. LADDER-SIDES WALKING

• *Proceed from end to end on the ladder with one foot on each side.*
• *Little children don't flip ladders over when they walk on the sides. Big kids sometimes do, so put an anchoring child at one end.*
• *As soon as possible, have them do this stunt without looking down to see where their feet are. Blind children can do this very well; sighted children should learn how.*

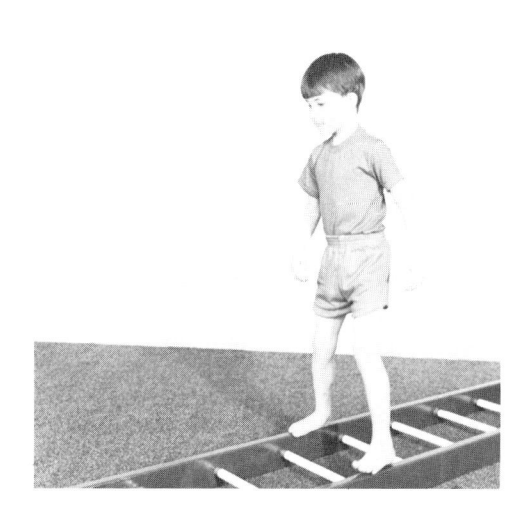

135. WHEELBARROW ON LADDER

• *Wheelbarrows work in many places; the ladder is an ideal surface.*
• *Again, the thigh hold. Pay attention to the beat.*
• *The "wheelbarrow" can use the rungs, the sides, or the spaces for his hands. Whichever way the ladder is used, it compels the children to* look . . . see . . . *and report back—or get bumped.*

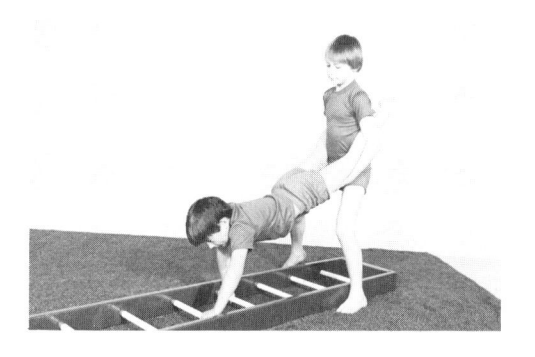

136. HORSE AND CART

There is more to this exercise than meets the eye. First, the horse cannot see his cart and must therefore *feel* how fast he can go. You, of course, are responsible to see that the music fits the need.

All these exercises should begin fairly slowly and work up to a march beat.

• *The "cart" positions herself at the end of the ladder, resting hands and feet on the floor with her back to the "horse."*
• *The cart raises one leg, which the horse holds at the ankle but supports all along the lower leg with his lower arm.*
• *The cart then raises the other leg into the horse's ready other hand and arm.*
• *The horse goes forward, stepping in the spaces.*
• *The cart must go backward holding the rungs.*

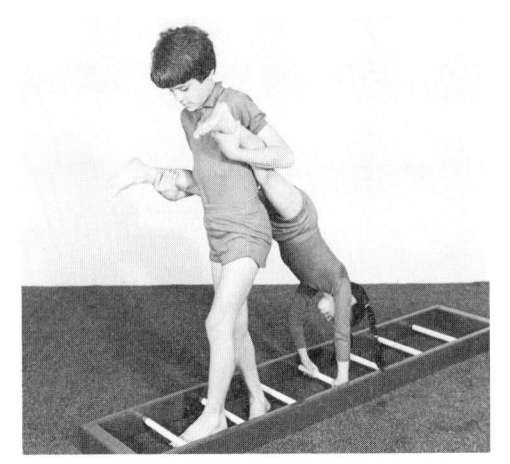

RAISED-LADDER EXERCISES

TO RAISE THE LADDER

Set the ladder ends on two boxes or the ends of two ramps and, later, when legs are longer, on two chairs. Anchor both ends with children.

137. LADDER HIGH STEPS

• *With the ladder raised, little people must not only watch their steps but lift the knees high to strengthen the quadriceps, which will improve their legs for floor progressions.*

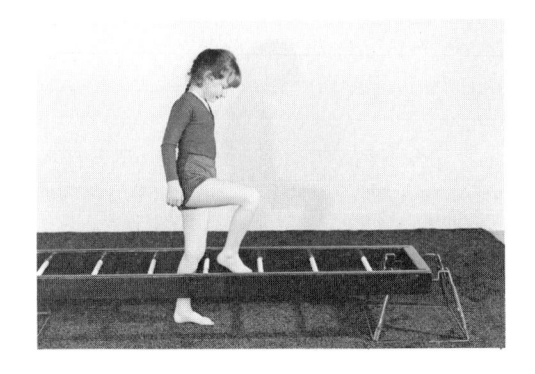

Exercises on the Equipment

138. HIGH-RUNG WALKING

• *Rung walking on the higher level will need a spotter. The spotter holds the walker's hand and keeps with the beat of the music, just as the walker tries to do.*

• *Remember, walk on the balls of the feet, not the arches.*

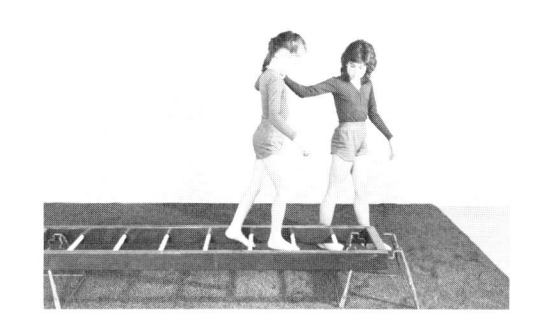

139. CAT ON A LADDER

• *The "cat" goes across the ladder with feet on the rungs and hands on the sides. Later, keep the hands on the rungs as well.*

• *Keep the feet close to the hands and the knees bent.*

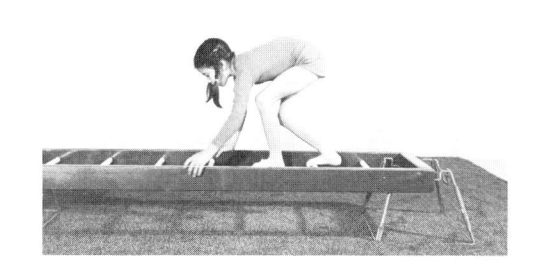

140. MONKEY ON A LADDER

• *The "monkey" holds on to the sides with her hands at first, just like the "cat." She steps forward with a bent knee and then, as she puts weight on that foot, she straightens the leg.*

• *That leg stays straight as the other leg, with knee bent, comes through to take over. This action will involve the hamstrings and the hip.*

• *Later, hold on to the rungs with the hands.*

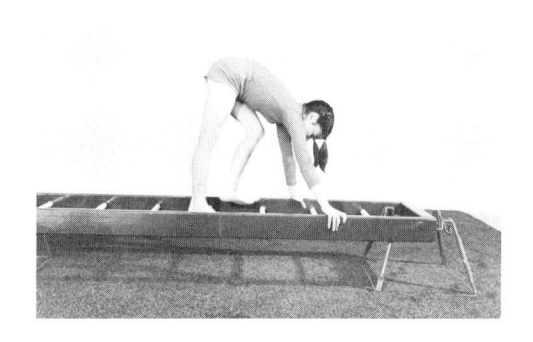

SLANTED-LADDER EXERCISE

Slanted ladders open up a whole new dimension. When you start with a tipped ladder, you can rest the raised end on a box or the end of a ramp or the doorway gym. Anchor it with a sitting child and do *not* walk on the sides—only in the spaces and on the rungs. Keep in mind that in our lives today there are no longer chores to do—no wood to lift and carry, no pails of water to haul, no recalcitrant cows to push through gates, no horses to lead. Sounds good? Your mind may say so, but your body says differently.

Anytime the body heads downhill, whether it be on foot or on all fours, the muscles work harder. It is much easier to climb a mountain than to descend from one. It is easier to go up a leaning ladder than to come down.

141. DOWNHILL ON THE LADDER

Start with a gentle slope. Later (in the section on the doorway gym, page 148,) you can use the hooks on the ladder extension on your movable chinning bar to give you sharper angles.

• *The descender starts at the top of the ladder on all fours, on the rungs.*
• *The spotter keeps a restraining hand on the descender's shoulder to prevent forward falls. This trains the spotter, who may not be needed at this angle but certainly will be needed when the angle increases later on.*
• *Although this is a chest, arm, and shoulder strengthener, this exercise also develops proprioception, an awareness of the relationship of the body to space and pressures.*

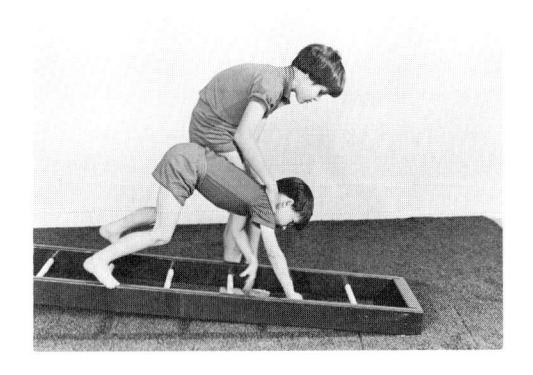

Most pieces of equipment in this book are modified replicas of "obstacles"—attractive nuisances available to most adventuresome children before the 1930s, when our world was altered forever.

Exercises on the Equipment

THE SAWHORSE

The sawhorse represents the backyard fences, the stone walls, and the curbstones just as the railroad tracks represent the real railroad tracks we passed on our way to school. Only "fraidy cats" and "sissies" and "just girls" walked on the sidewalks, avoiding the challenges of "primeval forests," "cliffs," "lions' lairs," "open tombs in old graveyards," not to mention unfinished houses, water-filled ditches, and foundations. Most children knew all about the new houses within their jurisdictions, from under the ground up, long before the owners moved in. Much of the junk lumber piled out back became tree houses or shored-up caves. Was our play dangerous? Probably, but then life is dangerous. Our play sometimes broke our arms and legs, but at least no one was interested in us for the ransoms we might bring. That really began with Lindberg's stolen and murdered child. Our parents didn't steal us from each other; there wasn't any reason for that. Somehow they managed to stay together even when it might have been better had they not. We cut and burned ourselves, but I never knew a single kid to be hit by a car, afoot or on a bike. We smoked (and choked on) Kools but no one stole their mother's Valium or Quaaludes. The most potent drug back then was aspirin. It was said, when I was a teenager, that if you put two aspirin in a Coke and drank it (always in front of the gang!), you would pass out. Did we try it? Of course we tried it. Did we pass out? No, not unless we were allergic to aspirin. (One of my schoolmates was; she got a rash and there was no excitement about that, just itch.) What was different then and now? Opportunity. "Hey! Try this one, it's great." Now, however, you *can* pass out. *You can also die.* Children didn't change; what adults made available did!

So don't worry about the height of the fence or the ladder leaning against the unfinished house. Count on it, a certain percentage of children *will* balance on the one and climb the other. What we can do is to prepare children to handle the obstacles and attractive nuisances so that they don't get hurt.

As to drugs, be aware. Spot the trouble before it settles in. *Know* your children *and see to it that they know you and that they have someone to imitate.* We *are* a drug-addicted society. There isn't another one like us in the world, because we are also affluent. No one can count on spontaneous safety for our children. It doesn't exist on any level. We are at war, and the kids are the "boots." Those were the young, green soldiers, thousands of whom died during their first few days and weeks in Vietnam because they didn't know the ropes, didn't know what to look for, had no way to protect themselves. *We* will have to be the "salts," the ones who have lasted long enough to develop instincts of self-preservation. In wartime they were the only hope of the "boots"; if a "boot" could latch on to a "salt" and copy him in those first terror-filled days, he had a chance. If our children have such people to hold on to, *they* will have a chance. Not all, but a lot of it is up to you.

142. FENCE WALK

The sawhorse is about 32 inches high. That's *very* high for some little people and for lots of big people. Those are (and were) the ones who haven't (and hadn't) had the chance to develop those skills we just discussed. Both little and big people still *can*, however.

• Place whatever number of sawhorses you have, end to end. Help the fence walker to get up any way he or she can. Soon you will teach the right way, but for now, anything goes.
• The walker walks *slowly* to slow music to the end of the "fence." Help the walker to jump off one side or the other, alternating sides. (You started that on the plank with exercise 119.) The purpose is self-preservation, both the children's and yours. *If you know that the children can* jump off *safely to either side, you won't have to worry about them* falling off.
• It would be wise to spot the children at first. Those who feel safe will soon dispense with your helping hand.
• Spotting the frightened child is important. Let him grasp the forefinger of your left hand if it is your right arm that encircles the little waist. You will be able to give less and less support with the encircling arm and the child will let go of your finger when he or she feels secure alone.

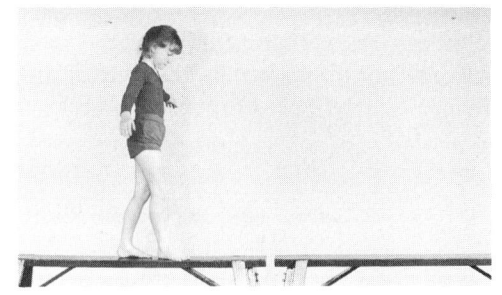

143. PIGEONS ON THE FENCE

• Proceed across the fence with toes turned in, as you did in the floor progressions. You will find that the feet turn in much further on the fence.

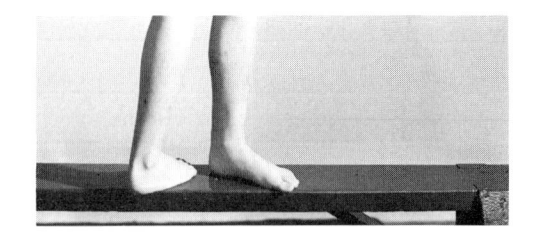

144. TURNED-OUT WALK ON FENCE

• Again, use slow music; the slow beat makes the extremes of turn possible. Try to cover the entire width of the board with the foot.

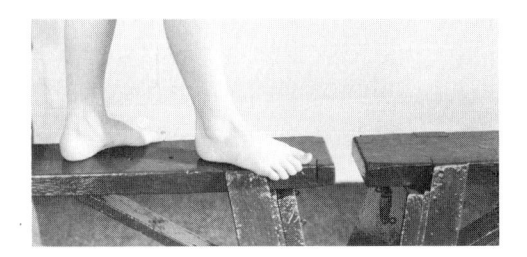

Exercises on the Equipment

145. FENCE WALK ON TOES

At one time I was given the job of teaching a group of athletes (all tomboys) to prepare for a prom and for wearing their first "heels". I put them, wearing heeled shoes, on the sawhorses and also on the stairs. What can be done well under physical pressure will turn out well when emotional pressure is the obstacle.

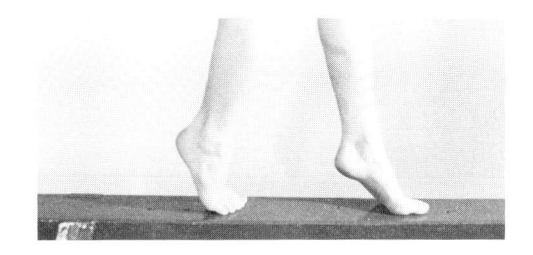

• *Walk the fence on the toes, slowly. The trick lies in tightening all the muscles of the legs, groin, and seat to present as few loose joints to gravity as possible.*

146. FENCE SIDE WALK

You had your first go-round with this one as the Bridge on the railroad tracks (exercise 127).

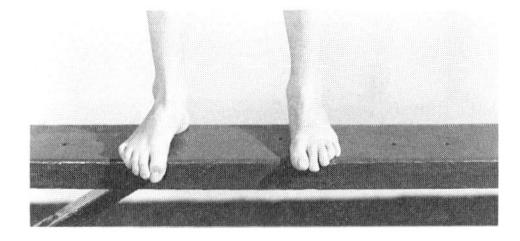

• *Face to the side and step out with the lead foot, being careful to grip the sides with the toes.*
• *Close the space between the feet with the second foot and proceed across.*
• *Spot by standing in back of the walker. If the youngster has more trouble than usual, use exercise 164, the Jump Back, to improve self-assurance. Most falls happen because of fear. "I don't think I can do that" also means, "I know I'm going to fall." Sure enough, your listening subconscious hears "fall," and off you go in order to fulfill your own order. I've done that a time or two. These days I simply say, "I know I can do that well and with style." Sure enough, I can and do.*

147. CAT ON A FENCE

• *Go across the "fence" on all fours like a cat.*
• *Notice the "hands" on the cat; they don't grip the sides of the fence. They have become flat little "paws."*

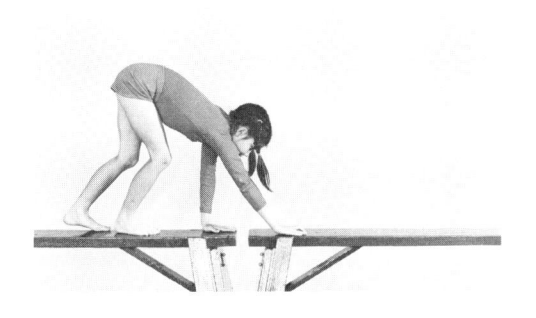

148. MONKEY ON A FENCE

• You have tried this one already also, on a lower level. The child doing it then was a gymnast and has the needed flexibility. The little boy in this picture has not had that advantage. Although young, he is already inflexible and needs training if he is to do well on the playground later.

• As your monkey crosses the fence, try to get the legs absolutely straight and right under the waist. See the section on flexibility (pages 97–106) for help with this.

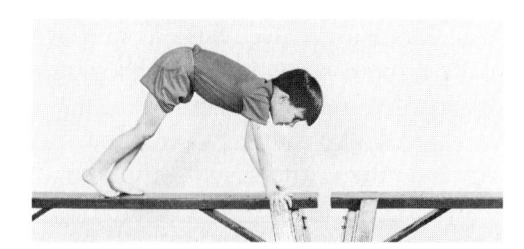

149. HOP TOAD ON A FENCE

• Start in the stoop position with both hands gripping the sides of the "fence."

• Lean forward as far as comfortable to grasp the fence further along.

• Hop both feet forward, close to the hands.

• Later, when the children are stronger, they can stand beside the fence and, gripping the sides, hop both *feet up* onto it. Then they hop forward for two hops and, still gripping the fence, hop off on the other side.

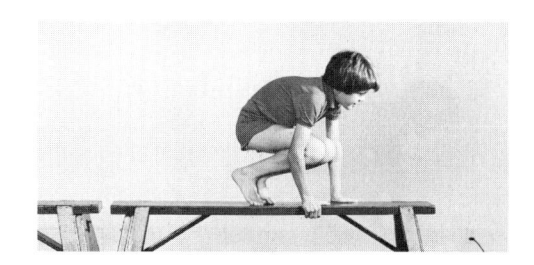

• They then hop up again and proceed forward for two hops. This is an excellent exercise when done the length of the fence.

150. FENCE MOUNT

The Fence Mount should be learned as soon as abdominals and legs are strong enough.

• At first, get on any way you can and sit about two feet from the end with one leg hanging down on each side.

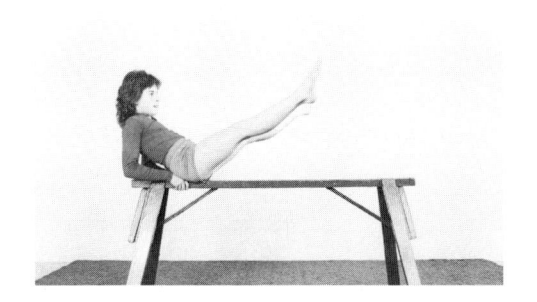

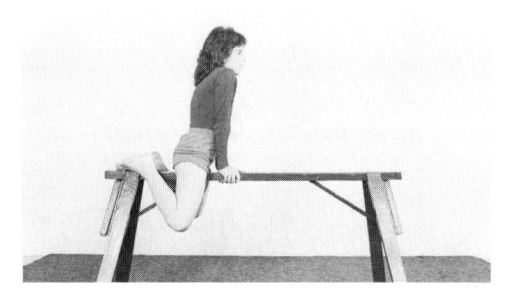

Exercises on the Equipment 167

• Lean back to grasp the "fence" on either side as you swing straight legs up in front.

• Swing straight legs down and back as you lean forward to grasp the fence with both hands.

• At the end of the backswing, bend both knees and hook your feet up on the surface of the fence.

• Be sure that your toes are curled under before you press your seat up. Hold at a half stand to be sure of your balance.

• Straighten both legs while still holding on to the fence. Then stand tall and straight, arms down and head up.

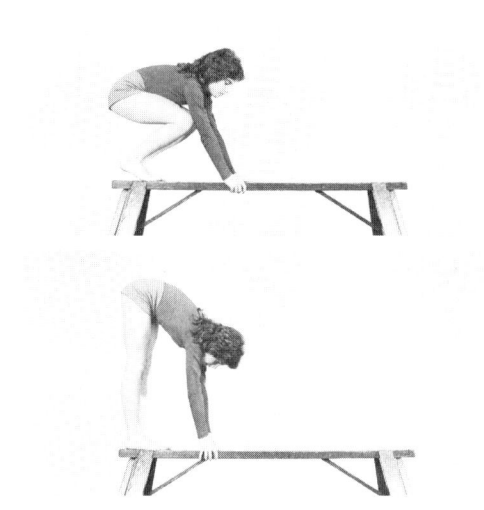

151. WHEELBARROW TROIKA

• The "wheelbarrow" stands at the end of the "fence" and places both hands on it, grasping the sides.

• The two "wheelers" each pick up a leg and proceed down the fence on either side. The wheelbarrow can be held horizontal or the legs can be lifted higher, but they should be kept even.

• To dismount, one of the wheelers reaches under the waist and the other grasps the pelvis. Both legs are then pushed to the side so that the wheelbarrow can step down.

• See that the dismount is done to each side.

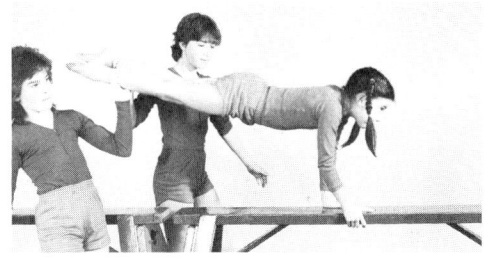

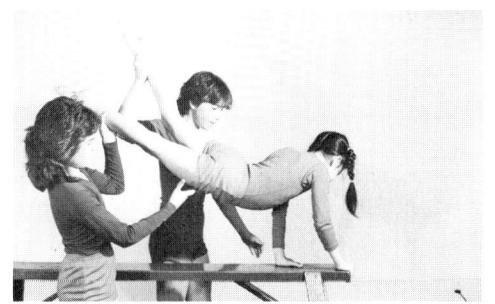

152. ONE-LEGGED WHEELBARROW ON FENCE

• You have already seen this with exercise 135. When the Troika feels safe and looks good, the "wheelbarrow" starts the same way at the end of the "fence," but only one leg is lifted.

• The other leg is thrust to the side by the wheelbarrow and maintained at the same level as the carried leg.

153. UP-AND-DOWN OBSTACLES

• *We begin by placing a wand across the fence about six inches high. The walkers step over the obstacle. As they improve, put several wands in the way, all at different levels.*
• *The next obstacle should force the walkers to duck under.*
• *Lift the wands to neck level and a little higher and lower so that they must duck at different levels.*
• *Lastly, use a hoop. This causes both the*

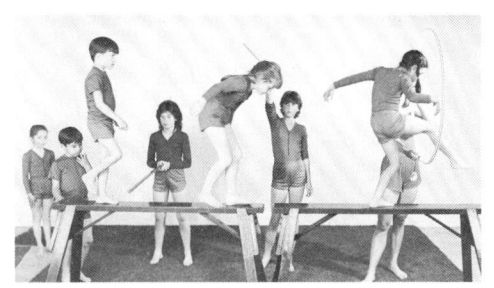

lifted step and the duck under at the same time.

154. DUCK WALK ON A FENCE

Before we start this exercise, you should be assured that there is no truth in the myth that either deep knee-bends or duck walks will cause meniscus injuries. If you want strong legs, you must do knee-bends. This was another of the really incredible falsehoods visited on physical education teachers—and through them on thousands of American children. (See the "Sports in America" section of my book *Myotherapy* [see Sources]).

• *Start on the fence in a low stoop with both legs under you. The level of your head must stay the same throughout.*
• *Extend the left leg to full stretch and place it on the fence in front of you. Lift the leg into position, don't slide it.*
• *Carry your weight forward onto the left leg until all your weight is on the left foot, which is tucked under you. The right leg will be at full stretch behind you.*
• *This is the tricky part: Maintain your*

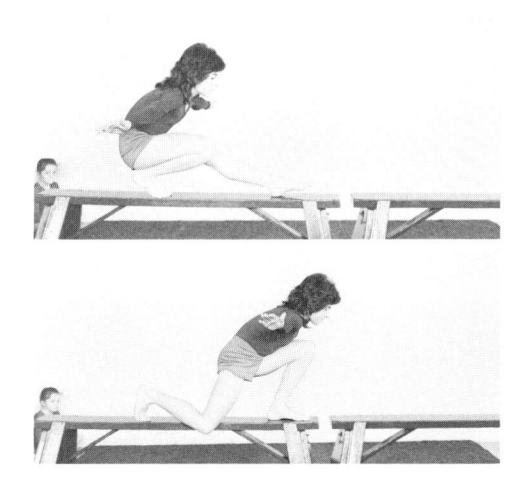

balance on the left foot as you move the right foot off the horse and drop the right leg (still at full stretch) in a controlled arc until you can set it down on the fence in front of you—still stretched.
• *Now it starts over again from the beginning but on the other leg.*
• *Repeat all the way across, trying to keep the movements slow, fluid, and steady. There should be no jerky transitions.*

Exercises on the Equipment

Right about now you should stop thinking of the horse as a fence and call it a balance beam. The regulation balance beam is four inches wide, and although it is one of the main pieces of equipment for girls, very few girls ever see one outside of TV. Their chances of mounting one are virtually nil. If they do get the chance, it is usually long past the time when they can do the most with the least effort. Little gymnasts are about six when they start, and if they already have excellent bodies—strong, flexible, and coordinated—they have a good chance for success. If they don't, but are following the fad of the moment, they stand an almost 100 percent chance of a serious injury. Why are our little ones so deprived? The major reason is leadership. Some will tell you that cost is the reason, but it isn't. Many little girls can prepare on the same inexpensive pieces of equipment you are using.

Then there is the question of little boys. In my school, where we train people to be Myotherapists and exercise therapists, about one-third of the students are men. Most of them have never had even a nodding acquaintance with rhythm, dance, tumbling, or gymnastics. All little boys know is baseball, and baseball does not build bodies. Later, the best and tallest and biggest boys get a chance at football and basketball. Private schools and the rare public school will provide soccer, but all of those games *use* well-trained bodies, they do not provide them. What you can do for little boys in your class is to provide the bodies for whatever they want to do later.

155. STRAIGHT-LEG SIT-OVER

• *Form your group into a line at one end of the beam made up of two or more sawhorses. Let's say they will approach from the left. The children will have to be tall enough to get their seats onto the beam from a standing position.*

• *Sit on the horse as you lift the* straight right leg *over the beam and bring the left over after it.*

• *Keep the legs widespread as you lean back on the right arm to support the lift.*

• *As the first child finishes and gets ready to do the same action with the left leg going the other way, the next child in line gets ready to go over with the right leg.*

• *Use slow music at first until the system has been learned. Later, when they know what to do, you can speed it up to a point where they really don't* sit, *but* slide.

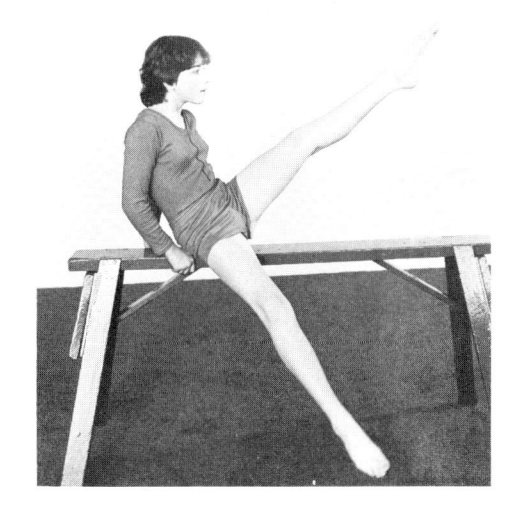

156. SEAT LIFT

• *Approach as you have just done in exercise 155.*
• *Kick the right leg over and lean back as in exercise 155.*
• *Lean forward and grasp both sides of the beam with both hands.*
• *Lift the seat well into the air, hold for a count of four, lower, and, leaning back, bring the left leg over so that you stand next to the beam.*
• *The next child is ready and moves in as you do the same thing on the second horse.*

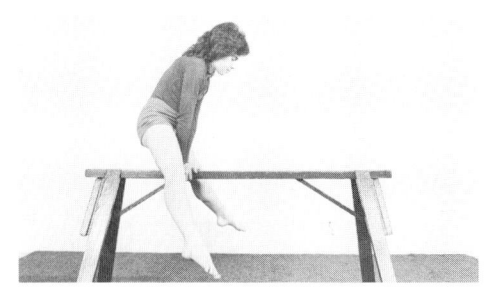

This is the beginning of doing sets of patterns on the equipment.
• *Do a lift on each horse, and everyone try to keep up with the one ahead.*

157. THE MACHINE

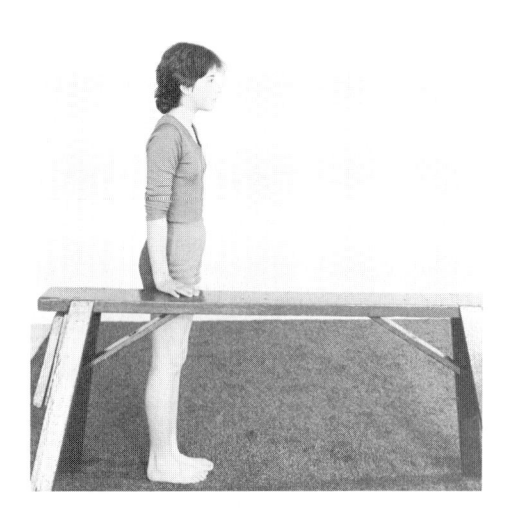

• *Stand on the left side at the near end of the last horse in line and place your right hand on its surface.*
• *Sit on the horse as you did in exercise 155 and lift both legs as you control your balance with both hands grasping the horse in back of you. The left hand now takes over.*
• *Lower the right foot to the floor.*
• *Swing the left foot over, under, and*

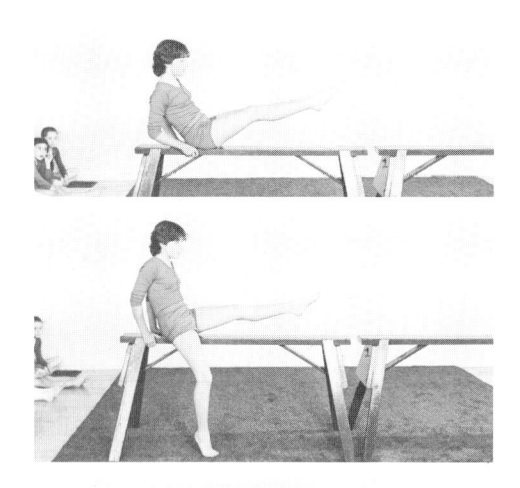

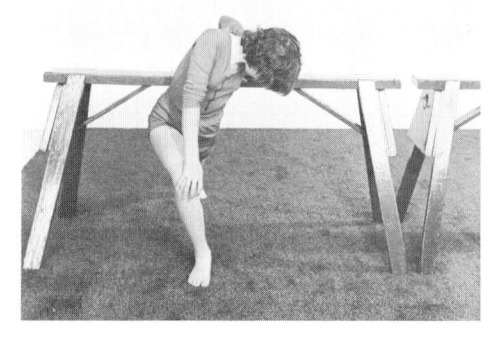

Exercises on the Equipment

across under the horse as far as you can reach to the other side as you turn your back on the horse.

• *Duck* under *the horse.*

• *Stand tall next to the horse you have just circled.*

• *Take two steps forward, ready to repeat the Machine on the next horse as the next child takes his or her place next to the just-vacated horse.*

• *One child follows the one ahead to slow music with a strong beat.*

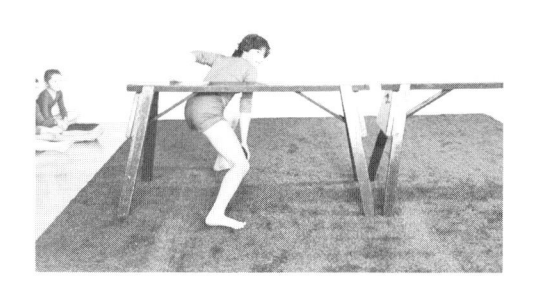

158. TWO-HANDED VAULT, TIGHT

When we say *vault,* a lot of people think of pole-vaulting. Just jumping over the back fence that keeps rabbits out can be a vault, too. This book is only partly for children; *you* are equally important for many reasons. You are the key to their health—and your own . . . and everyone else you love and even those who come to your class, *just for fun.* If you have never vaulted, now is the time to learn. Don't start with the horse; it may be too high. Stay with the little kids on the plank (see page 152). You will soon have the requisite strength, flexibility, know-how, and self-assurance. And would you believe, when you can vault, you will have a better self-image. That also goes for somersaults, shoulder rolls, head-stands, and handstands.

• *Put both hands on a horse and jump both feet onto the horse* . . . and stop right there.

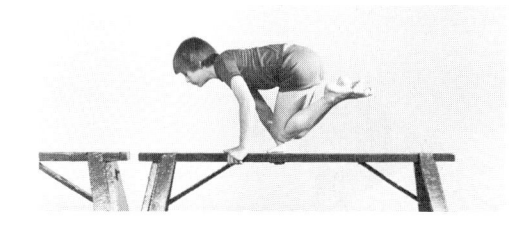

• *Now jump off onto* both *feet on the other side.*

• *Take two steps forward to the next horse and repeat that, leading with the other side. Do two more and you will be ready to vault* over *the horse.*

• *Place both hands on the horse and give a real spring, keeping the knees bent and in close.*

• *Do three more, alternating sides.*

159. TWO-HANDED VAULT, STRETCHED

• *Start the same way, but as you go over, stretch out.*
• *It will be easier if you go over with legs spread wide. If there is a chance that the horse will slide, put a spotter at one end.*

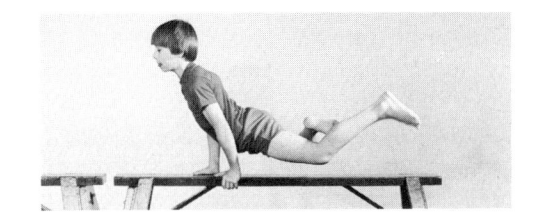

160. ONE-HANDED VAULT

• *This exercise requires the aid of a running approach.*
• *Start about 10 feet back from the horse and take a run at it while readying your right hand. Take off from one foot, but bring them together in the air. Land on both.*

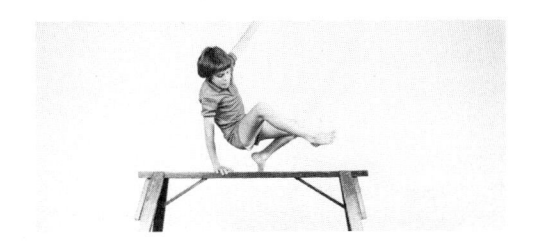

161. ARM AND LEG HOLD

• *Place your right hand at the extreme right of the horse and your left foot at the extreme left.*
• *To slow music, raise your right foot from the floor and, keeping your body straight, slowly bring the right leg through, underneath the supporting left leg, and out the other side. Pause for a few seconds with the leg pointing straight down, toes pointed.*
• *Keep the left arm extended throughout.*
• *Step down onto the right foot and walk to the next horse, where you do the same thing with the other arm and leg.*

Be sure you have both a mat and a spotter for the next exercise. Falling on one's nose assures the tumbler of *two* black eyes—and the teacher of what feels like a heart attack.

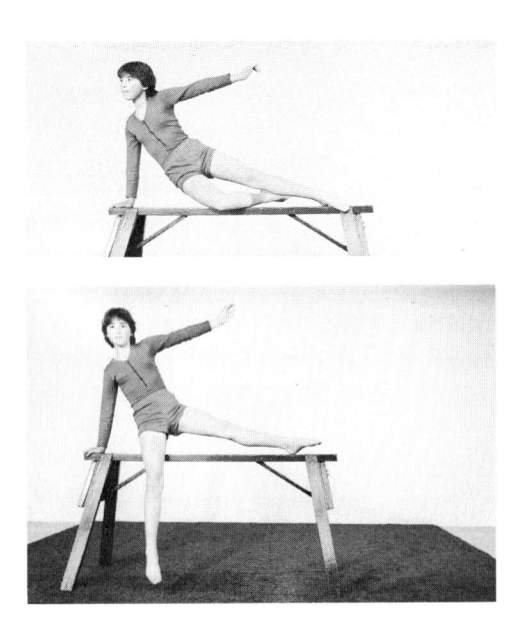

Exercises on the Equipment

162. JUMP TO KNEES

Take a position behind the horse with hands about a shoulder width apart. If they are much more than that, there will be too little room for the knees to slip through.

• *Before you try this one, have a good spotter standing by. In addition, try it on the plank (see page 152) first and do the same for the children. One more thing: Be sure that the child you allow to do it is ready physically. Some children, ready or not, will try anything. Later on in life they will bet a week's wages on the colt Silver Heels because they have a hunch, someone gave them a hot tip, or perhaps they liked the name. The one who hangs back until he or she knows all the ins and outs of each exercise and every stunt is probably going to turn into an accountant. Accountants and some (many) children are perfectionists.*

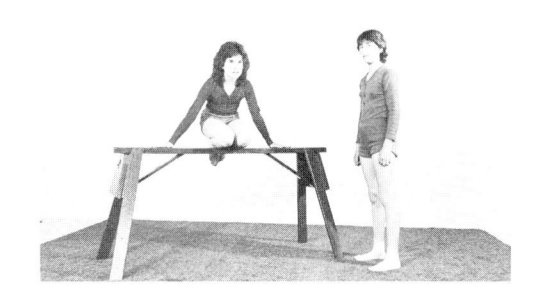

• *Press down hard on both hands and jump the body up to rest on both knees. The one who does it best will jump the seat up so high that there are several inches between knees and horse and then let the knees down slowly.*

• *Jump back down, walk around the horse, and proceed to do the same stunt on the next. This builds arm, hand, and back strength—and self-confidence.*

163. JUMP TO SPRADDLE

• *When the Jump to Knees (exercise 162) is predictable, jump to the knees first.*

• *Holding on with both hands, place one foot and then the other on the ends of the horse. Straighten the legs so as to get the feel of their ultimate positions. If the leg flexibility (see the section on flexibility, pages 97–106) is such that the spraddle is easy to achieve and hold, the stunt will be easy.*

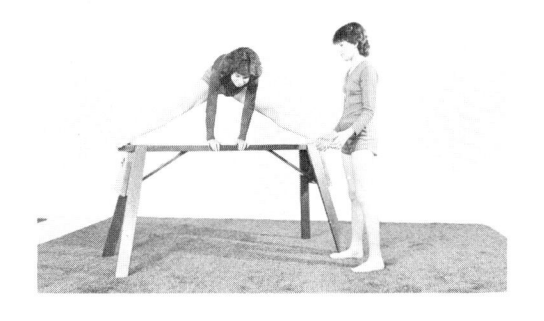

What went up must come down, and you want it to come down under control. If you have been having the children jump off the horse or balance beam and plank from the start, they will have no trouble jumping off forward, but what about backward? Have you thought about those who *may* have trouble seeing things as most people see them? A great many dyslexics have to wait until they start to fail in school before someone wonders whether or not those clear, beautiful eyes are doing the job they were intended to do. *Watch!* Prepare them for anything.

164. JUMP OFF BACKWARD

• *Start by standing behind the horse. Place both hands on the horse's "back."*
• *Do four knee-bends and proceed to the next horse and repeat.*
• *When the body understands where it is to go and what it is to do, climb onto the horse standing tall.*
• *Jump off backward and catch the fall with both hands on the horse's back and drop into a knee-bend. Stand and hold. Start early to teach the children to* hold *a "finish" to each stunt, as the Olympic gymnasts do. This prevents a sloppy stunt* and a sloppy attitude.

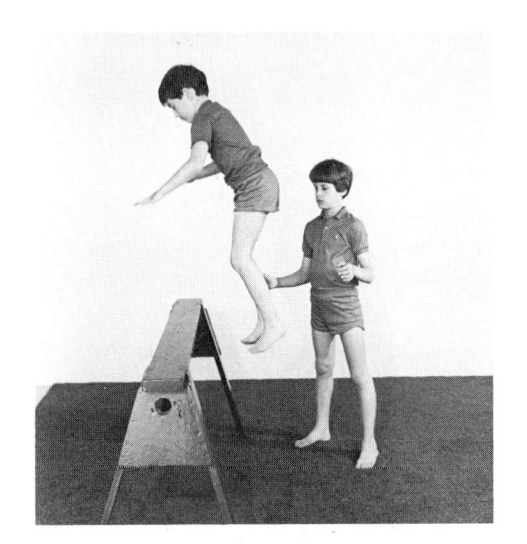

165. JUMP COMBO

This stunt combines several exercises, the knee-bend, the spraddle, the "start-pause," and the "finish."

• *The children start by standing in a line, ready to go.*
• *The lead child addresses the horse by stepping up to it and stands at attention for the "starting-pause."*
• *He or she places both hands on the horse and jumps to the spraddle position, stands, and brings first one foot to the center of the horse and then the other.*
• *Jump off frontward into a deep knee-bend or squat.*
• *As that child steps forward with arms and head lifted and back arched (they've seen that a hundred times on TV), he or she prepares mentally to take two steps forward to address the next horse in line.*
• *The next child in the line is warned by the "finish" to be ready to step forward to address the first horse as the leader steps forward to the second horse.*

This sort of stunt, like exercise 157,

Exercises on the Equipment

The Machine, once learned should be put to music. Again, that will be your responsibility. The beat must be both clear and slow, just as the music for vaults should be fast and a little manic.

Whenever you can, put two and three children on the equipment at a time and teach them how to do exercises as a team. This will free you to spot the scary stunts and yet keep *all* the children busy most of the time. For example, put them into pairs. Set up an obstacle course around the room so that as they finish their handstands or jumps (which you are spotting), they can return to the start via the following exercises for duos and triples.

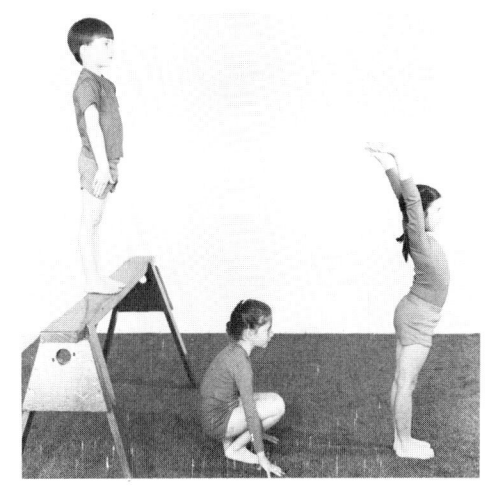

166. THE MANTLE

- *Place both hands on the horse and jump up to take all the body's weight on straight arms. Feet should clear the floor.*
- *Start with four and work up to sixteen.*

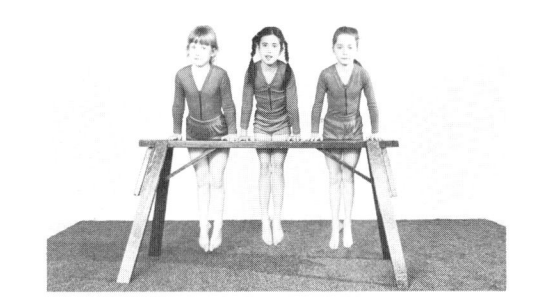

167. PULL-UP, BICEPS

This kind of "chin-up" was suggested for girls, since they were so "delicate." It has many uses, but cannot replace a real Chin-up (page 202).

- *Lie on the floor under the horse. Reach up to grasp the horse's "back" with palms facing toward the face.*
- *Hang with arms at full stretch and body straight and stiff.*
- *Pull up until you can see over the horse.*
- *Start with four and work up to sixteen.*

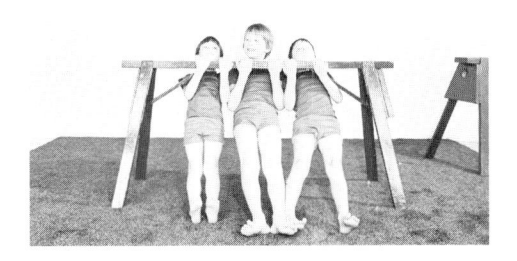

168. PULL-UP, TRICEPS

By the simple expedient of reversing the hands, an entirely different set of muscles, the triceps, in the back of the upper arm, will be strengthened. If you ever intend to go rock climbing, this exercise is a must.

• *Lying on the floor as before, reach up to grasp the horse with the palms facing away. Start with four and work up to sixteen.*
• *You can also alternate the biceps pull up, exercise 167, with triceps pull up as a separate exercise.*

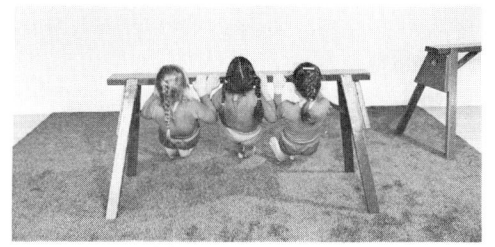

The next two exercises require some sort of cover over the back of the horse. An old blanket will do.

169. CHEST LIFT OVER HORSE, PRONE

• *Lie prone over the back of the horse, far enough forward so that you can hang down to rest your hands on the floor. Your partner weights both of your legs in the horizontal position.*
• At first *hang the upper body down so that the upper torso is vertical.*
• *Lift the upper body to the horizontal and hold for a slow count of four. Lower and repeat. Start with four and work up to eight.*
• *As soon as the back strength has been developed (exercises 3, 4, and 5 will help), carry the hands behind the neck.*

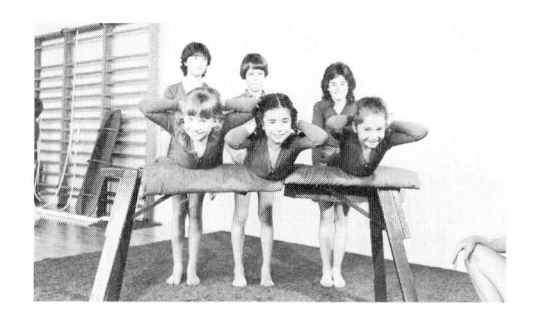

170. LEG LIFT OVER HORSE, PRONE

• *Slide forward so that both legs can hang straight down with bent knees. The partner holds the shoulders.*
• *From the bent-knee hang, extend both legs straight out until they are parallel with the floor.*
• *Retract and extend the legs four times at the start and work up to eight. Later, weights can be placed on the ankles.*

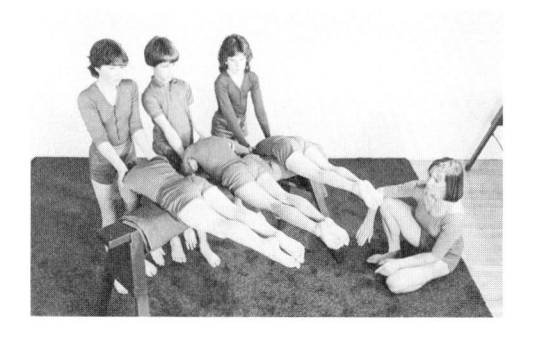

Exercises on the Equipment

At first, the next exercise will require two spotters per child. When abdominal exercises have made the abdominal muscles strong, the spotter checking the descent of the upper body can be dispensed with.

171. LEAN BACK ON HORSE

• Sit on the horse facing the spotter, who will weight the legs . . . and I mean really weight the legs.
• The second spotter stands behind the child about to lean back with arms stretched out in front as in the first abdominal corrective (pages 26–27).
• It is the spotter's job to see that the exerciser does not lean further back than the horizontal line.

• The exerciser, with arms resting on thighs, holds that level position for a count of four and then sits up again.
• Start with four and work up to eight; then do the same exercise with arms folded across the chest.
• Finally, do the roll back with hands behind head.

172. BACK BEND ON HORSE

• Roll out to the horizontal. With the second spotter holding the shoulders, but without support unless needed, *lower into a back bend*. If the abdominals are strong, there will be no difficulty going either down or up. If a lack of flexibility prevents a nice arch, practice with Back Bends (exercise 111).

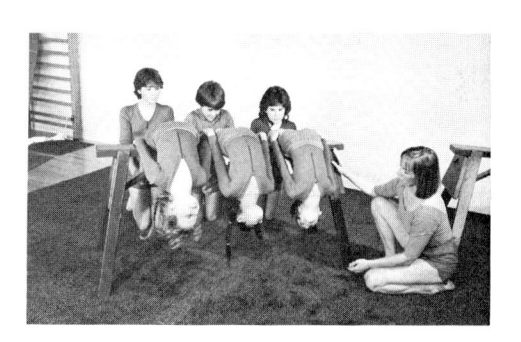

173. BACK WALKOVER FROM HORSE

This follows naturally after Back Bend on Horse (exercise 172).

• The spotter may have to unweight the legs a little, especially if the children are rather short. This will make it possible for them to put their hands on the floor as they hang in the back bend.
• When the hands are firmly set, the shoulder spotter puts one hand on the front

of the child's pelvis and the other under the waist. The child should look at the floor to aid proprioception.

• The leg spotter pushes one of the back-bender's legs right over her head, to land on the floor right under her nose.

• The other leg follows right along.

• At first both legs will land on the floor at the same time, but in time one will come down first; as the back-bender stands up, the second leg will touch down about a foot further back.

• That should cause the child to end in a standing "finish."

There are two things to remember about all these exercises: There are almost always easier exercises that *prepare* the body for the harder ones. And there are always harder ones—and then sports—waiting to use what you are developing. Usually, in school sports, the best players get to play and the ones who can't perform well get to watch. Not in *your* class. Everybody gets a chance to develop, and the competition is the best kind for beginners: *self*-competition. Nobody loses and everybody who works to improve, wins—and so do you.

The next exercise is really easy once the children have learned headstands and handstands. It is a balance and control improver.

174. TEAM-OF-HORSES, SHOULDER STAND

The spotter must be attentive. You will need some padding laid over each horse's back. The horses are parallel and just wide enough apart to permit the passage of a little head.

• *Kneel with one arm on each horse and push your head down between the horses.*

• *Place the shoulders on the two horses and lay each arm flat along the sides of the horses, palms up. The arms must be straight and the palms up in order to flatten the shoulders. This allows most of the weight to rest on the deltoid muscles in the upper arms and protects the bones of the shoulders, much as the padding on the horse does.*

• *Rest the full weight on the shoulders as you grasp the sides of the horse with both hands.*

• *Rise up onto both feet, keeping them as close to your face as possible.*

• *Tilt the torso back and lift the weight*

Exercises on the Equipment 179

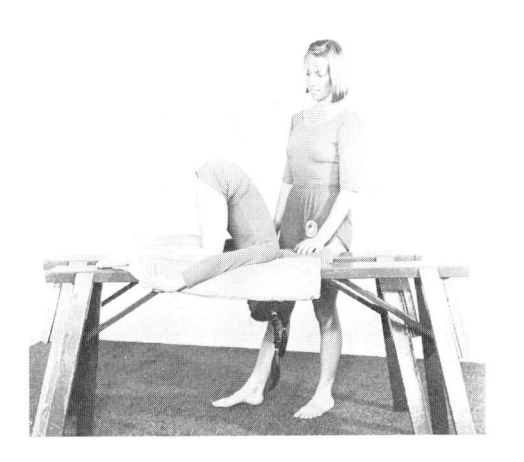

from your feet. This will allow you to stay curled as you slowly straighten into a full shoulder stand. The spotter watches to see that you don't tip sideways.

- *Hold the shoulder stand for a slow count of four. Check for straight, tight body and pointed toes. Remember the position of the head in the handstand—tipped back, facing the floor.*
- *From the full shoulder stand position, tilt the body back slightly as you start to lower straight legs downward. Hold for a count of four at the halfway point.*
- *Lower until the toes touch the horses and then go down further to rest one knee on each horse.*
- *Withdraw the head; with one hand on each horse, jump both feet to one side and stand for the "finish."*

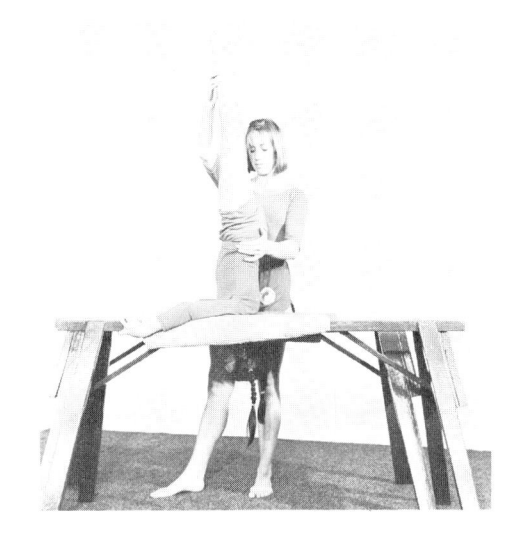

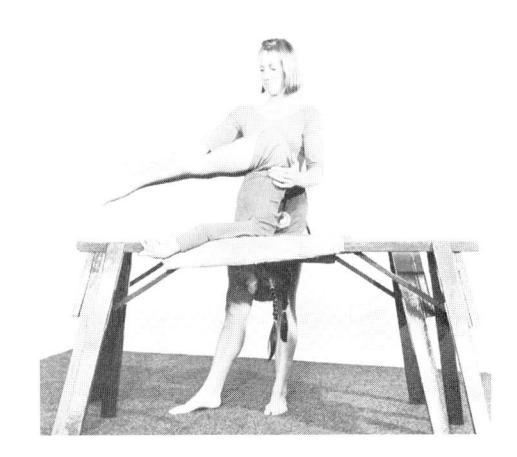

This book does not try to make gymnasts out of all of you. It does *prepare* your bodies so that you can do difficult stunts safely. Always keep in mind that if you want to learn a sport correctly, get a teacher who specializes in that sport . . . and *never* stop taking lessons.

175. MOUNT SERIES A

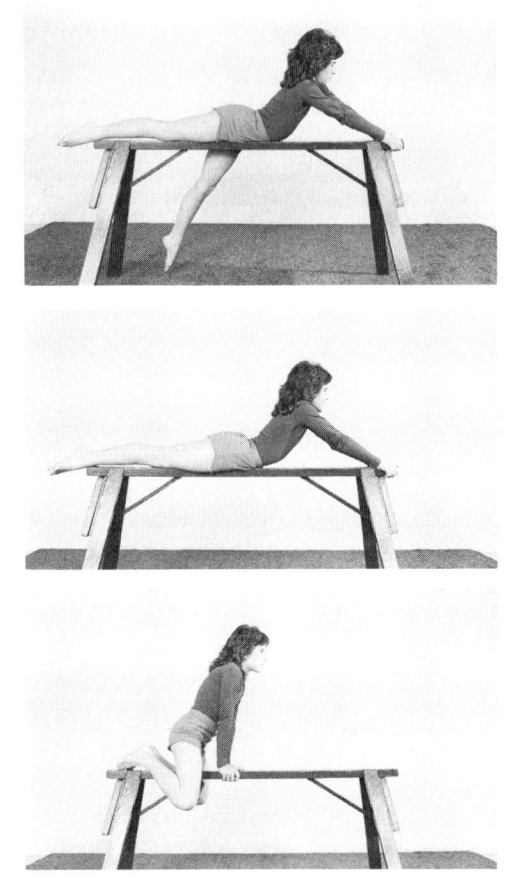

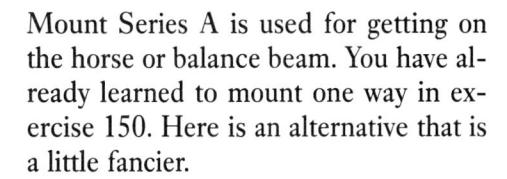

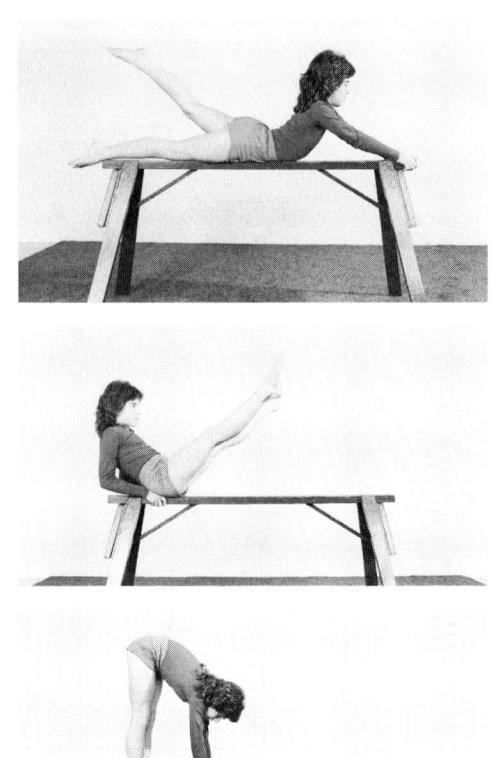

Mount Series A is used for getting on the horse or balance beam. You have already learned to mount one way in exercise 150. Here is an alternative that is a little fancier.

• Stand on the left side of the horse, grasping both sides of the front end.
• Lay the right leg on the horse, keeping the leg straight and the toes pointed.
• Swing the left leg back and *up*, arching the back.
• Lay the left leg flat on the horse while maintaining the arch.
• Press the torso back as the straight legs drop to either side of the horse. Catch your weight on both hands, which have moved to a spot on the horse just behind your seat. Kick both legs up and hold the V for a second.
• Swing the legs back and bend both knees as you hook your feet onto the horse behind you.
• Curl the toes under as you press up into a straight-leg stand *without* letting go of the horse.
• Stand straight. You are now ready for all manner of balance stunts on the horse or balance beam.

Exercises on the Equipment

176. PREP FOR SCALES

Using a broomstick, mop handle, or pole (which can be purchased from a lumberyard), three little people can practice balancing on one leg at a time.

* *It will take two spotters, but very little strength.*
* *Stand on the left foot and draw the right knee up only as high as the one who can do the least. This is always the rule in duos or triples. Solo work is just that—solo; each can do his or her utmost. But when it's a team, then all should try for uniformity.*
* *Stand straight and stretch the right leg back and up as far as is possible for the weakest team member. Do four with each leg and work up to eight.*

The children will think up dozens of duos and triples—just be ready to catch them.

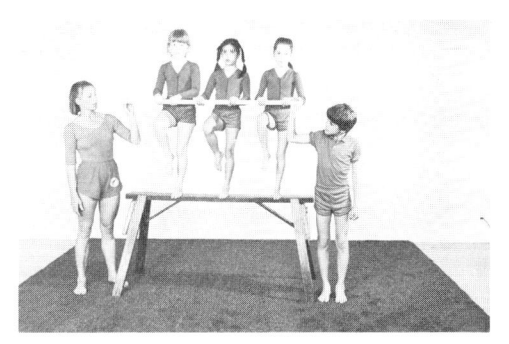

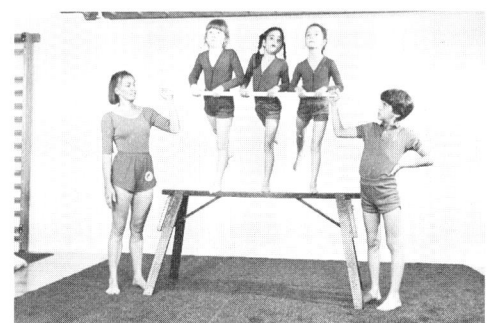

RAMPS

Ramps are substitutes for the hillocks we ran up and jumped off in the golden age of childhood when today's grandparents were America's children—the days before school buses, TV, drugs, and people who couldn't be trusted with little children or big children either. In those days we had a game called "Follow the Leader." The chosen leader took off like a cross between Peter Pan and the Pied Piper. Over, under, along, in, out, and around, the leader whirled and gyrated with the whole gang in his wake.

One of the first things you need to know about ramp jumping is that you should *take off* from one foot, but always *land* on two. Then, if one foot doesn't find a smooth spot for the landing or is twisted in some way, the other foot can carry the weight and prevent a sprain. But if you *should* take a spill and sprain something, see the section on immediate mobilization (page 432).

177. WALK-UP

In order to establish the habit of "one-foot takeoff, two-foot landing," teach it as though performing for slow-motion movies.

• Start the waiting line about ten feet behind the ramp.
• From the beginning let it be understood that no one takes off without a "Go!" from you. Hopefully you will have a "gatekeeper" who will see to it that the rule is obeyed. You, the major spotter, should stand about five feet from the high end of the ramp and be fully aware, from the first minute, that there is a good chance that one of the kids will think he's Superman and fly straight at your chest, headfirst.
• Walk up the ramp as though you really are in that slow-motion movie. Kids think that's great fun. At the end of the ramp place one bare foot right at the edge, with your toes curled over that edge, just as you would place both feet on the board for a racing dive.
• Jump off from that foot and land on both, with soft knees.
• Practice "Indian landings." Indians can't be heard when they walk through the forest or jump off rocks. See how quiet you can make those jumps. That will teach control even as you develop the strength that is needed.

178. RAMP SOMERSAULT

Before you start the excitement of ramp jumping, use your ramps for something slow—a somersault.

• The spotter kneels at the high end as a "caterpillar" slides on his stomach all the way up the ramp. He uses his arms to accomplish this, and when he reaches the end, he pulls himself over the ramp edge.
• The caterpillar then places his head on the mat in front of the ramp. The spotter directs the head to a spot as close to the ramp

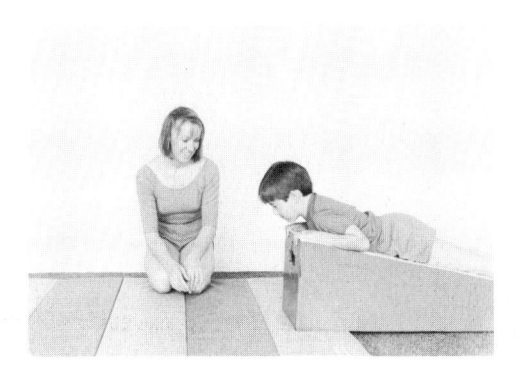

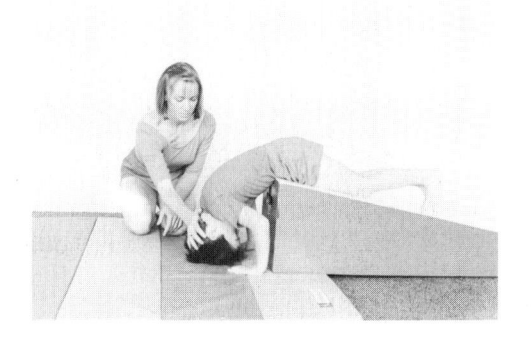

Exercises on the Equipment

as possible as the caterpillar wiggles himself further over the edge.

• As the caterpillar slides over the edge, keep pressure on the backs of the thighs so that he will remain rounded and not come down flat on his back. You will have need of this rounded somersault connected with the ramp a little later.

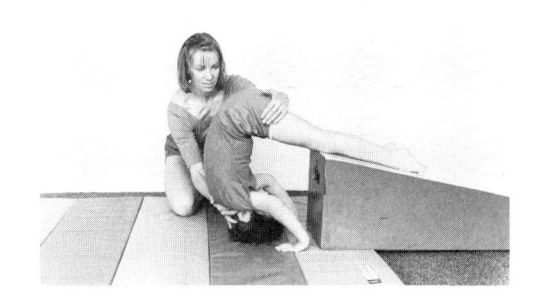

179. ROLL DOWN A HILL

There will be no hang-backs when you put two or three ramps side by side and drape a mat over them to make a hill.

• Start by lying across the top of the ramp or hill and simply roll down to the bottom, trying not to roll off either side.
• This can get pretty hilarious as rollers roll into each other, but the chances of getting a bump are very slim.

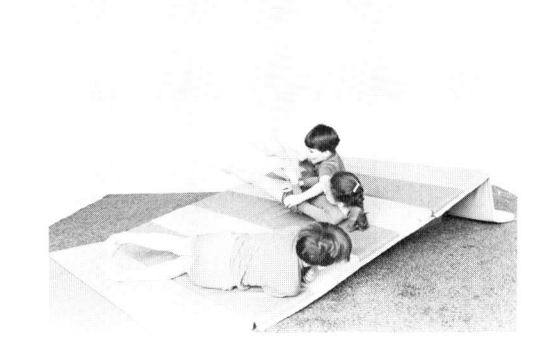

180. RUNNING JUMP

• Start this without music and practice until you are sure that all the children can run up the ramp, take off on one foot, and land on two . . . softly.
• The next habit to develop is that of getting out of the way immediately when the stunt is finished. That way you avoid not only collisions but having fifty or sixty flying pounds land on top of someone.

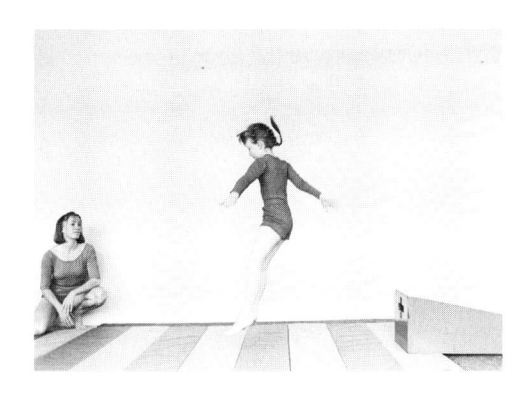

181. JUMP OVER A DOWEL

You will always have to be two steps ahead of the children, and the next step to just jumping is jumping to exciting music. The wilder the music, the higher the jump will be. That's good. But at the same time, the wilder the music, the wilder the kids. For that you must be ready. What do you do when it gets *too* wild? Put on some slow music and crawl or duck-walk around the room for a few minutes.

After adding music, you add obstacles.

• *You need a spotter to take your place while you set the height of the dowel. For the little ones who barely jump down without a sprawl, the dowel could be held an inch out in front of the ramp. For the best legs in the room it might be as high as your head. You have to be the judge . . . how to challenge yet not endanger?*

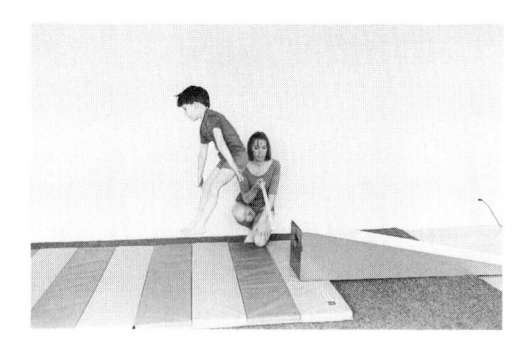

182. TOE-TOUCH JUMP

You can use the dowel with this one, or just run and jump.

• *Run up the ramp, taking off from one foot. Try at the top of the jump to pull bent knees up as high as possible and touch the toes.*
• *Land on both feet.*

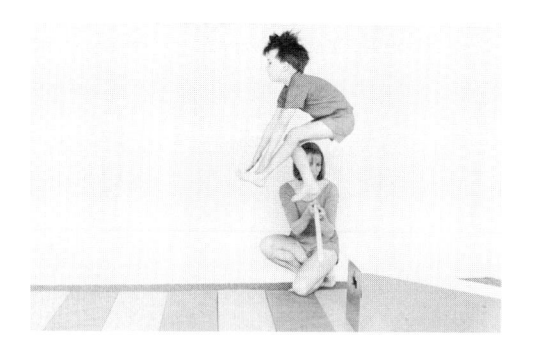

183. PEOPLE-JUMPING

Children love to dare, and jumping over the teacher is very daring indeed. The first time I ever tried this was in 1947, and my teachers and I have been doing it ever since. Once, a small person who felt he might not clear me used *me* as the takeoff ramp; no one else ever failed to clear the human obstacle. Not only that, the children jump much higher than either you or they think they can.

Exercises on the Equipment

• *Kneel down in front of the ramp (having given your spotting job to the most responsible child in the room). At first, get down as far as you can. Just your presence there is enough to pull little legs up. In time you can kneel higher, then stand bent over, and for the best there will come a time when you can stand erect. At that time, stand a good distance from the ramp and face the "kangaroo." Then, if he or she isn't quite up to it, you have time to duck.*

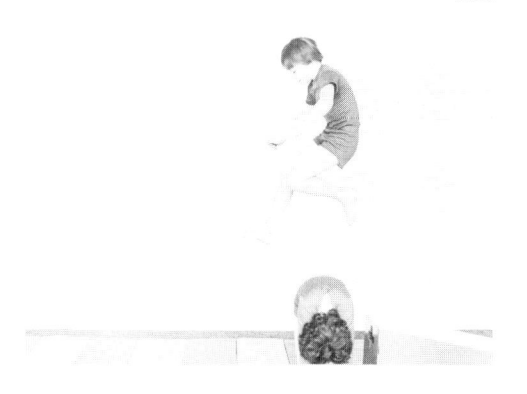

184. RETRACT LANDING GEAR

• *As the "speeding bullet" takes off, it becomes a "plane" and retracts the landing gear in order to miss either a high steeple, a jagged tor, or wires. You can give the children ideas at the start, but they will soon present their own. If you listen closely, you will know where the next generation's novels will come from.*

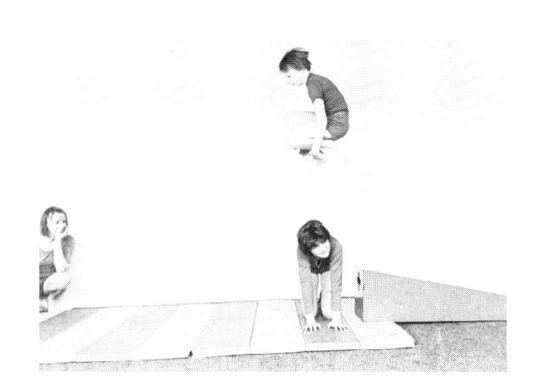

185. BIRD LANDING ON LAKE

The Japanese give fanciful names to their exercises. If you have ever read any haiku, you know that Japanese children are taught to see and, more important, *look for* beauty in everyday occurrences. Should we do less for the wonderful minds of *our* children?

• *Make your straight-legged flight with arms outstretched look like a bird (or even a plane) coasting in to land.*

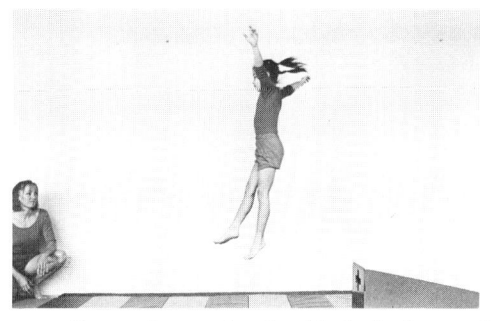

• *Remember to land with both feet and soft knees.*

186. JUMP OVER STEEPLE

Believe me, if you tell the children to jump spread-legged over the top of a tall steeple, they will go high and spread wide. Children still have magic eyes . . . they still *see* the steeple. Just in passing, children *feel* the slap that is thought, even though not given physically. Try to remember that when your patience is tried beyond endurance. Remember, too, that there is such a thing as "looking daggers." When one of the children in your class is sullen or recalcitrant, look with *your* magic eyes and see if there aren't the scars of old dagger wounds on a little heart.

• *Run up the ramp and spread legs as wide as possible as you jump.*

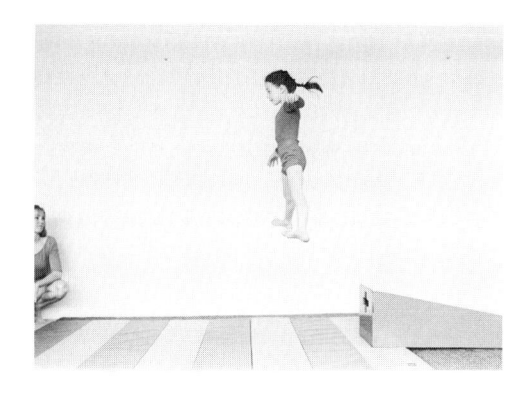

• *Remember to bring your legs together and bend both knees slightly when you land.*

• *Later, when they have had plenty of practice, combine the Toe-Touch Jump (exercise 182) with Jump Over Steeple to make a Widespread Toe Touch.*

187. THE LEAP

Leaping into space is no problem for children; they watch that kind of thing on TV all the time and half of them don't know the difference between what they see and "reality." The problem will be to get both feet on the ground for the landing and to do the stunt in good form.

• *Run up the ramp and, with arms outspread, leap off with one leg leading.*
• *Land on* both *feet and keep running to the end of the mat.*
• *During the leap, try to point the toes.*

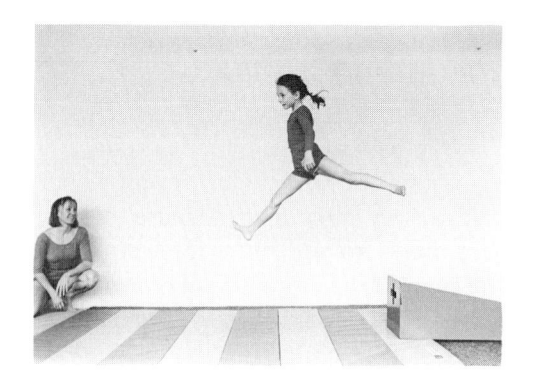

Exercises on the Equipment

188. RAMP TURNS

• *Walk up to the end of the ramp and place your* left *foot on the leading edge with toes curled over the edge for stability. (You will not need the toe grip later on.)*

• *Advance the* left *arm and reach back with the* right. Think: *"In my right arm is a basketball. Without bending my arm I will hurl that basketball across the room into the corner on my* left."

• *Don't think of turns. Don't think of succeeding. All you think about is that ball flying hard into the* left *corner of the room.*

• *Lean your weight back on the* right *leg and get set.*

• *Throw! At the same time jump off the ramp. The momentum of the throw will carry you to the* left. *It may be only a little way to the left, but to the left you will go, landing softly on* both *feet.*

• *With practice you will make a quarter turn, then a half, a three-quarter, and finally a full turn. Don't hurry. Never hurry. You are not teaching stunts, you are patterning muscles.*

• *Always alternate sides; otherwise you will be favoring one set of muscles over another, and even doing the same thing to certain spots in your brain.*

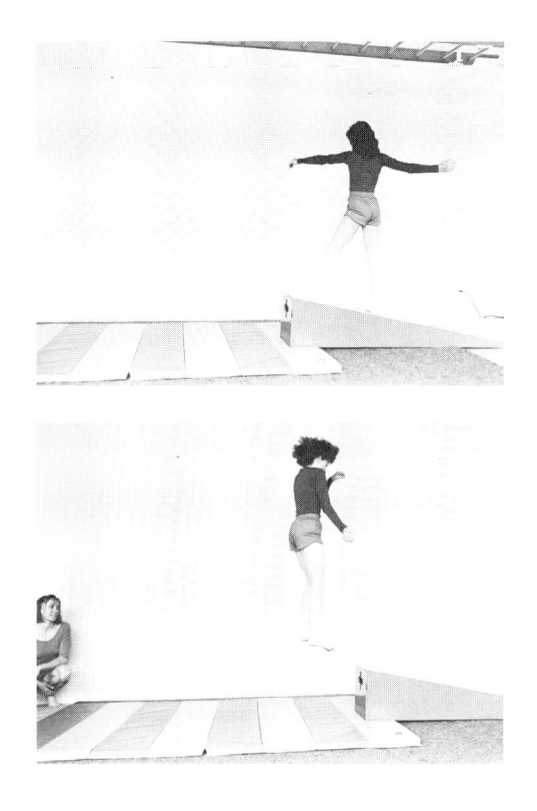

189. THE HILL CHALLENGE

Now we are back to the hill, but this time with more developed bodies and a better sense of proprioception. Try to see how many ways there are to use the hill. The easiest was the Roll Down a Hill (exercise 179), but now you aren't looking for "easy"; you are looking for "interesting" and "inventive."

• *Address the top of the "hill" and place your hands and one foot on the edge. Tuck your head down close to the "hilltop" if not on it.*

• *Push off with that right foot into a somersault and then add a second when you reach the bottom.*

• *Alternate feet.*

Do forward shoulder rolls, backward shoulder rolls, anything that comes to your mind and theirs. Theirs will be the most fruitful, because whereas you will be seeing a mat over a few sawhorses, they will be seeing a hill of green grass or golden wheat. Perhaps they will see a slide into a Time Machine or out of one. You will be seeing children; they will be seeing sprites, gnomes, slithers, and dragons. What does a dragon do on a hill? Ask them.

Don't forget the music. You can change children into almost any form at all with the right music. *Don't* stick with the pop stuff, though its heavy beat has definite uses. Go to the library and listen to all sorts of music. Listen to Grieg, Strauss, Rachmaninoff, and the modern Russian composers like Kabalevsky and Prokofiev. Listen and, as you listen, *see.* Music calls up *things, people* and *places.* You may not know what to do with Indian, Japanese, or African music, but *they* will. *Watch!* You may get the thrill of a lifetime as you discover that many of them come into this world with an advanced musical education, just as many are true artists until someone tells them what they *ought* to draw or makes them copy.

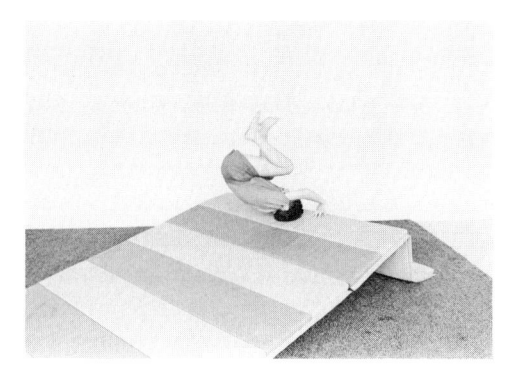

Children are not just a national resource. Until we "educate" them to be like everybody else, they are a national treasure.

CHAPTER FIFTEEN
MAKING AND USING WEIGHT BAGS

Not too long ago, when America's fitness pendulum was at the opposite extreme from what it is today, weights were considered the exclusive property of the "muscle beach boys," and their use was frowned on by both the true athlete and the nonathlete. Weight lifters were considered "odd" or "narcissistic egotists." Of course weights weren't at fault, but the goal was certainly considered suspect. Weights can be used for building huge, bulging muscles. All it takes is determination and persistence. Those muscles, however, are self-limiting. Strong they may be, but they lack *flexibility,* and as we keep saying, it takes *both* strength and flexibility to turn in a good physical performance.

Today things are very different: We have gone overboard the other way (which is the American way). Now weight emporia are on every other street corner, and if you don't speak the weight-training lingo and have the right clothes and attitude, you are not considered "with it." Women as well as men visit these places where sweat and strain is a way of life. Nothing wrong with that if you know what you want and how to get it. Mostly these people know neither of these things and are dependent on "athletic directors" who don't know either. The price is paid in disappointment and pain. This is *not* going to happen to you.

There are all kinds of weights, and the best are free weights. That means barbells and dumbbells. For a long time the chrome machines have had the edge, but so many people preferred free weights and got so much better results, that now, the machine emporia are putting in free weights as well. You can do better than that. True, you could go out and buy a set of barbells, and that's fine except that their very presence in gleaming stacks is a temptation to lift too much too fast. Then, too, they take up a lot of space, and if dropped on a small (or not so small) toe, they do an excellent job of squashing it. In addition, they have very limited uses.

Weight bags are a very different thing. They can be used one way or another with most of the exercises in this book. As most joints are put through ROM, which means full range of motion, the *whole* of the muscle being exercised gets into the act rather than only limited sections of it. A set of weight bags can serve the whole family in almost every way, including recovery from injury. (See the chapter on Myotherapy.)

The entire family can use a set of weight bags, from the one-year-old to the ninety-year-old great-grandpa, the parents, both athletic and unathletic (but figure conscious) siblings, and the ex-dancer aunt, who is married to the ex-football player uncle and who both suffer from "arthritis." Of course the ex-football player and his current football-playing nephew will want two extra five-pound weights because of their extra musculature!

The family will need two five-pound weight bags, two two-pound weight bags, and a couple of one-pounders for those starting out. I have always bought yellow denim or sail cloth for the one-pounders, red for the twos, and royal blue for the five. Little people, using yellow can't wait to graduate to red, and those using red think that royal blue is just their color. In time it is.

Whatever colors you choose, you will need a total of three-quarters of a yard of 36-inch-wide fabric. And you will need sixteen pounds of lead shot (hardware store). You will also need half a yard of cotton rope (yard goods store, where you get the denim) or nylon rope (hardware store).

Your material should be cut into rectangles. You will need two that are 10 inches wide by 12 inches long. These will make up the two five-pound weights. Then you will need two rectangles that are 9 inches by 11. They will make up the two two-pounders. Finally, you will need two rectangles that are 7 by 11 for your one-pounders. The remaining rectangle of 20 by 15 inches will make the bag for storage.

To make the storage bag, simply fold the rest of the material (with waste cut away) in half, stitch two sides, and hem the top. When the weights are inside, wrap the cord twice around the neck of the bag and tie closed. To use the weights as barbells, you will need both weights and a wand or ¾-inch dowel 36 inches long.

Making and Using Weight Bags 191

HOW TO MAKE WEIGHT BAGS

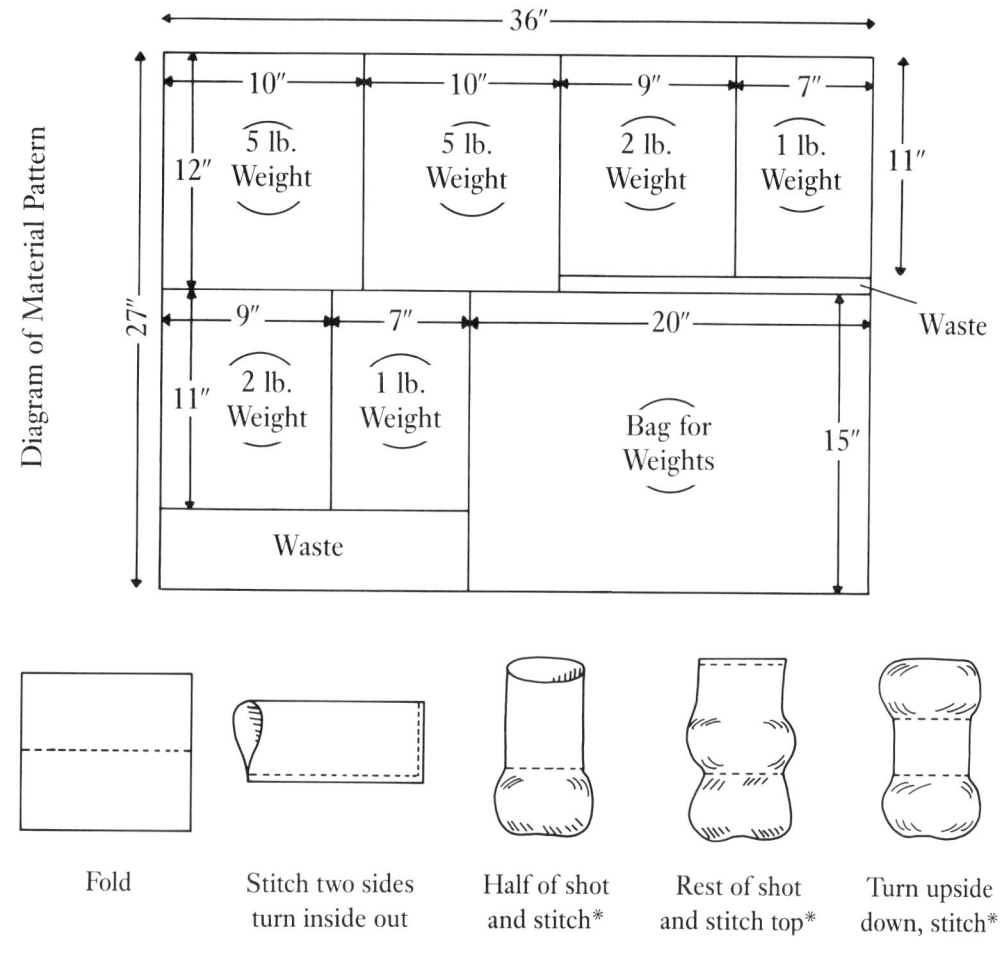

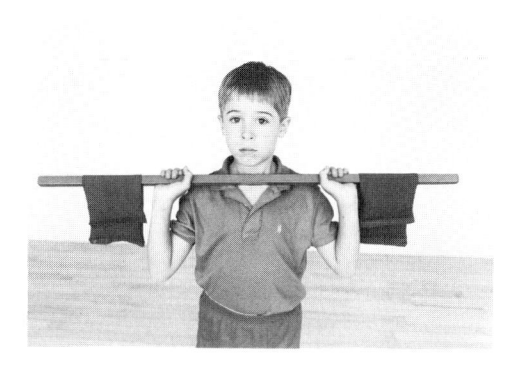

Diagram of Material Pattern

36"
27"

10"	10"	9"	7"
5 lb. Weight	5 lb. Weight	2 lb. Weight	1 lb. Weight

12" 11"

9"	7"	20"
2 lb. Weight	1 lb. Weight	Bag for Weights

11" 15"

Waste

Waste

Fold — Stitch two sides turn inside out — Half of shot and stitch* — Rest of shot and stitch top* — Turn upside down, stitch*

*Use pins to hold shot while stitching

Emphasize to the child at your house and all the youngsters in the class that bulk is not what they should be after, but rather *definition* and *performance*. Also, it isn't what you can lift this week that counts; it's the difference between what *each* child lifts now and a month from now. That will depend entirely on how much time and effort is put in each week.

Explain that bulk is what Mr. Universe has in the way of muscles: very large. (And incidentally, very costly when it comes to muscle pain.) Definition is what the runner, swimmer, biker, dancer, and skier have. You can *see* the muscles, but they are mostly long and slender, well formed, and not at all bunchy. You get that kind of muscle and the strength that goes with it by doing many repetitions with comparatively light weights—*and by stretching warm muscles.*

190. MILITARY PRESS

• *Lean down and keeping knees relaxed, grasp the dowel with hands facing your legs.*
• *Keeping your pelvis tucked under, stand erect, bringing your dowel to chest level with elbows* down. Yes, I know there is a lot of talk about lifting from the thighs, and so on, and if you were lifting the piano, you might need such leverage. But to lift two five-pound weight bags, I doubt it. The reason we Americans have to spend so much time worrying about our leverage is that we lack muscle. What you are doing is building strength so you don't have to think about leverage.
• *Raise the dowel overhead and follow it with your eyes. Tighten every muscle you can find all over your body. At the same time, push those weights up as high as you can.*
• *Lower the dowel and let the arms hang at full stretch, the dowel in front of your thighs.*

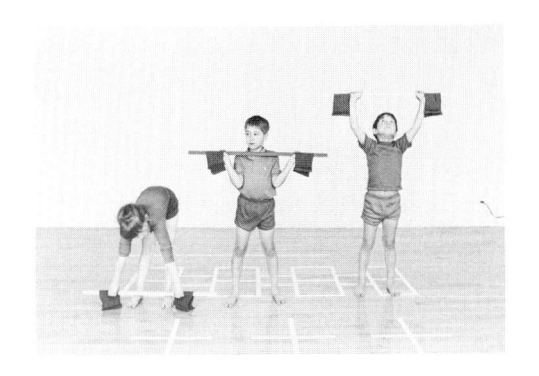

191. REVERSE CURL

• *Without setting the weights down, bring them to chest level. The palms will be facing out, which gives the exercise its name.*
• *Do two repetitions* slowly. *Then set the weights on the floor and reverse your hands.*
• *Stand erect with arms hanging straight down.*

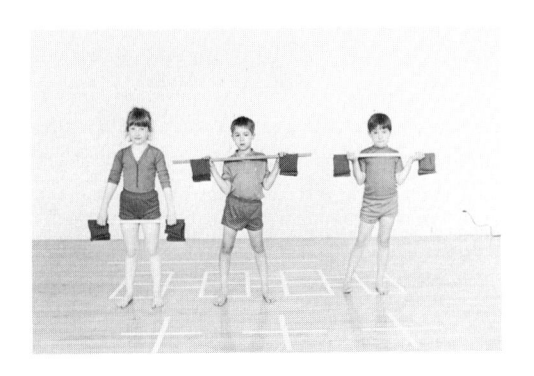

Making and Using Weight Bags

192. CURL

• *Curl your arms in, bringing the dowel to your chest.*
• *Lower the arms to full stretch and repeat the curl.*

These three exercises, one Military Press, one Reverse Curl and one Curl, comprise a "set." *You* should do three sets. The scoring will be based on *your* lifts. If you have five pounds on each end of your dowel, your score will be quite impressive.

193. BENT-OVER ROW

• *Spread the legs wide and keep the knees straight.*
• *Lean over to pick up the weighted dowel.*
• *Keep the back level as you raise and lower the dowel with arm strength only. Do ten.*

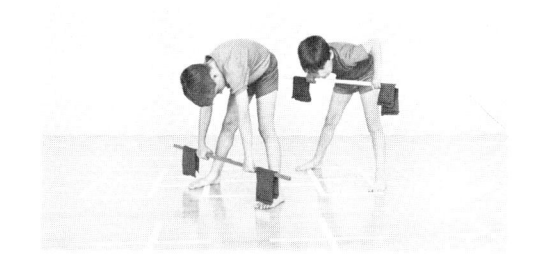

194. WEIGHTED KNEE BEND

Weight lifters doing deep squats with enormously heavy loads on their shoulders have unquestionably injured their knees. Such people were part of a study that convinced physical educators that *deep knee-bends injured knees.* Ask the children to do a deep knee-bend with weights on a dowel placed behind their necks. Then ask them to put the weight down and do a free knee-bend. Then ask them what the difference was. Almost every one of them will be able to tell you that one of the bends was done with weights and one without. Unfortunately the man doing the study wasn't able to make that distinction, so he condemned *all* knee-bends for everybody, including children. Also unfortunately—but this time there was a price—we sent that generation to Vietnam without the benefit of strong leg muscles.

The other group who participated in that study were football players—American football players. The players had not built the necessary leg strength as children, so they began to hurt their knees as soon as they went out for football in seventh or eighth grade. By the time they had hurt them continually (football does that to knees) through high school, their knees could stand very little stress. Sure enough, the coach, who knew very little about preventing injury, had them *duck-walk* around the field *after* practice, and many of them fell over with knee injuries that showed.

Now ask your children which sex plays football. Most of them will say boys. So why weren't girls allowed to do knee-bends? Next ask them how many football players on a team. Most of them will tell you eleven. So two school teams would mean twenty-two boys playing and injuring their knees. Ask the children how many kids there are in school who *don't* go out for football. They will range between three hundred and a couple of thousand. So why couldn't *they* do knee-bends? When you hear (or read) *any* new "discovery" about exercise, ask yourself, "Does that make sense?" Most of the time it won't. Look at the training of dancers and gymnasts. Those are two sports that build both strength and flexibility. Those people look and move the way almost all healthy people *could* move. Both the muscles and the potential are there in every one of us. Your *body* will tell you what you can and cannot do. Don't trust people who compare apples and oranges and sell you the results—lemons.

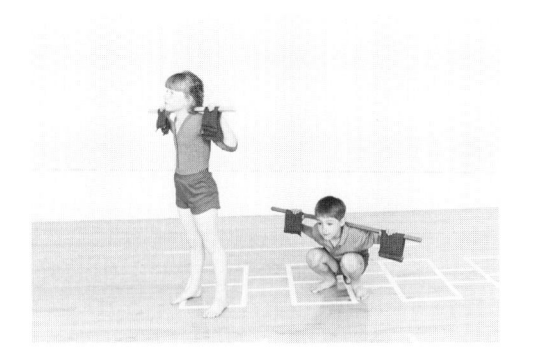

• *Stand with the feet apart and place the weighted dowel behind your neck.*
• *Drop slowly into a deep knee-bend with knees open.*
• *Rise to the standing position and rest a second. Do three.*

195. SUPINE PRESS

• *Lie supine holding the dowel at shoulder level just above your chest.*
• *Raise the dowel to full stretch and lower. Do three.*

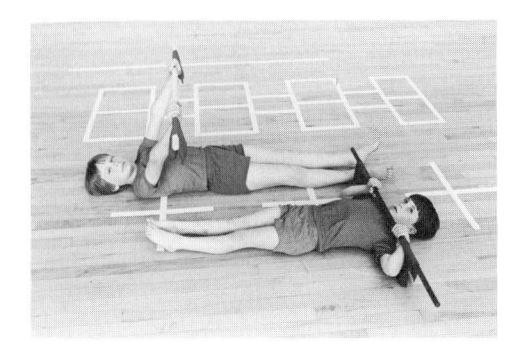

Pipes, Ropes, and Rings

196. PULL-OVER

• Take the weights off the dowel and hold one in each hand.
• Still supine, raise the weights straight up. Keeping the arms straight, *lower to the floor above your head.*
• Keeping the arms straight all the way, carry the weights in an arc above your face and down to your thighs. Do three.

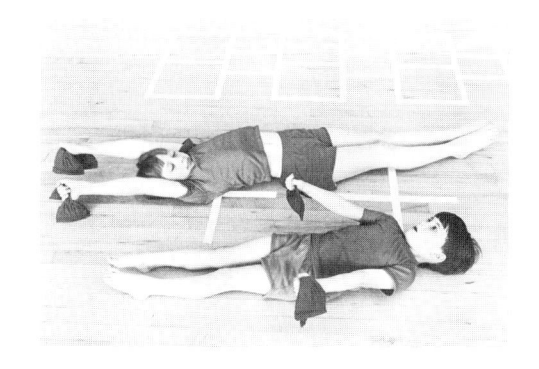

197. LATERAL STRETCH

• Start with the arms at chest level and cross them over the chest.
• Open arms at full stretch to the side. Do not *allow the weights to touch the floor.* Cross and open three times.

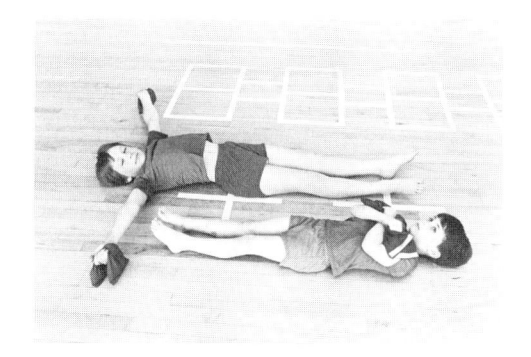

198. KNEE-TO-NOSE STRETCH, SITTING

• Sit with outstretched legs.
• Hang one weight on each ankle.
• Bring the right knee to the nose and then stretch the leg full out.
• Place the leg on the floor and do the same action with the left leg. Alternate for ten.

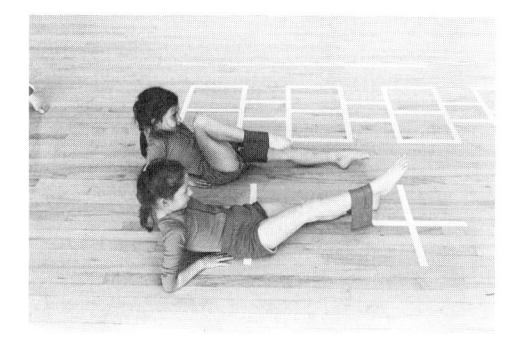

199. PRONE ARM-AND-LEG LIFT

- *Lie prone with weights in your hands.*
- *Raise first one arm and then the other as high as possible. Do not roll the upper body from side to side.*
- *Alternate for ten.*
- *Now change the weights from the hands to ankles.*
- *Raise first one straight leg and then the other. Alternate for ten.*

All weight work should be done to slow music so that every part of the muscle gets an equal workout. If you notice a jerky movement, look for a weak spot in the muscle. Cut back on the reps or weight until the movement can be done smoothly and build up from there. *No one should have to struggle.*

Make a work sheet for each child and encourage them to increase the work load from time to time, but never more than two pounds at a time. Surely there will be those who can do as well as you; they should be allowed to, and to surpass you if they can, but this is not a contest except against the self and what that self could do a month ago and the month before that. *Fast* development is like cramming for an exam: You may pass the exam, but what you studied will not stay with you for future use.

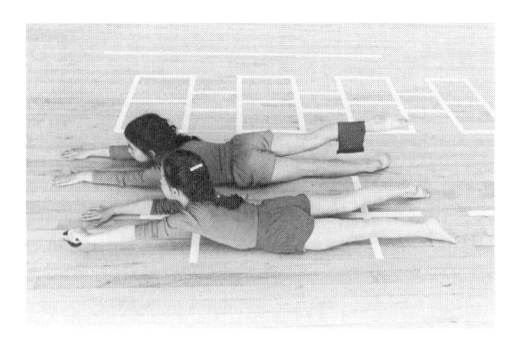

Take great pains to help with work sheets, making new ones and recording each performance. Ask for changes in strength and be sure to notice and record posture improvement. Make the children self-aware.

Sample Work Sheet (Yours)

Date	Exercise	Number of Reps	Weight (in pounds)	Total Lift (in pounds)
	Opening Set of 3	3	10	30
	Bent-Over Row	3	10	30
	Knee-Bends	3	10	30
	Supine Press	3	10	30
	Pull-Over	3	10	30
	Lateral Stretch	3	10	30
	Knee-to-Nose Stretch	5 each	5 each	50
	Prone Arm and Leg Lift	3 each	5 each	50

Day's total lift: 280 pounds   Time spent:

CHAPTER SIXTEEN
PIPES, ROPES, AND RINGS

Pipes have many uses, are not expensive, and, depending on your ideas, are easy to store. We use 2-inch conduit for balance beams, skin the cat, knee hangs, and so on. Pipes can also be used as ballet barres. An 8-foot pipe can stand in the closet; a 12-footer can lie against a wall and not be too noticeable. Have holes cut into the ends of your sawhorses for a beam 32 inches high, and into the stairs for one 28 inches high.

200. FLOOR BALANCE BEAM

• Lay the beam on the rug if that is your exercise surface. If your floor is cement (the garage), or tile (the "all-purpose" room), or polished wood, you will need to rest each end on a couple of towels, blankets, or carpet samples.

• Have the children balance on the pipe as they cross the room. Forward is a good start, followed by backward. You can vary this by changing the rhythm.

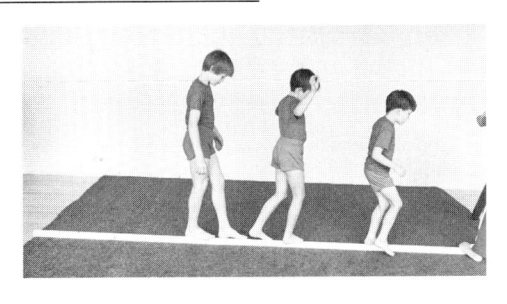

201. LIMP ON PIPE

• *Walk across with one foot on the pipe and one off. Don't forget to limp with the other leg too.*

202. ON-ON-OFF-OFF

• *Take two steps on the pipe and two off. Then give the children a chance to make up some crossings of their own.*

203. RAISED PIPE

Raise the pipe by putting it in the holes at the ends of your sawhorses.

• *Use a spotter at first as the children cross. In no time at all you will discover that they can walk that kind of tightrope without any help.*

204. PIPE, WALK AND TURN

• *Walk across with the spotter on your right. When you reach the end, be sure that your left foot is advanced.*
• *Turn on both feet at the same time, facing the spotter. The spotter will be able to help you change hands and regain your balance. Walk back.*

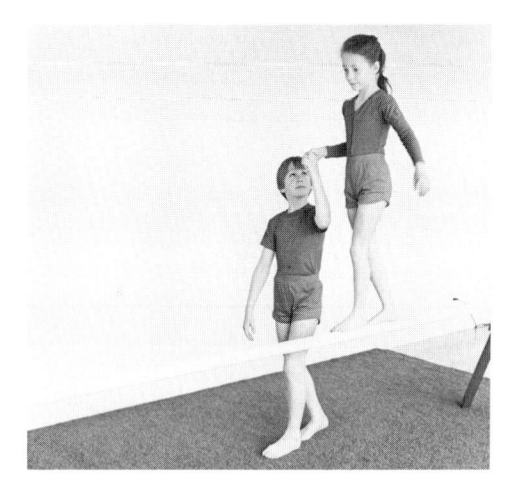

205. HANGING TRAVERSE

This is the way that rope traverses are done in rock climbing from peak to peak. The only difference is the height. If you can get from one end to the other a few inches above the floor, you can get from one place to another above a three-

Pipes, Ropes, and Rings

hundred-foot chasm. It is good for the ego and self-assurance to know you could if you had to.

• *Grasp the pipe in both hands and between your legs and GO!*

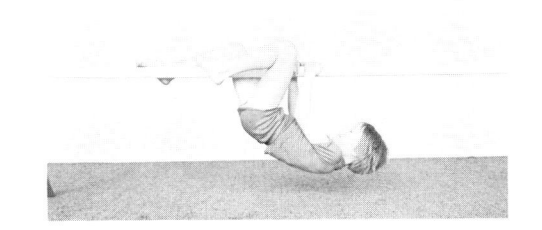

206. KNEE HANG

• *Sit on the pipe with your seat well back and your weight supported by your thighs.*
• *Bend forward until you are jackknifed and have a good hand-hold.*
• *Let your body fall backward as you turn on hands and knees.*
• *Stay curled up and let go with your hands. (Spot at the back of the neck.) If space allows, slowly uncurl and hang free from the knees.*

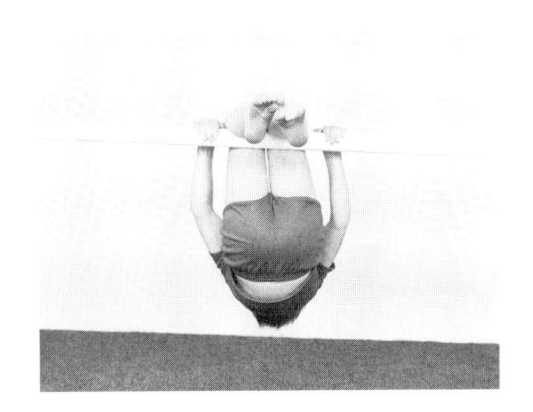

207. HAND-SUPPORTED STAND-DOWN

Little children will be able to hang with just their hands touching the floor. The spotter holds the lower legs in place over the pipe. Older children will find their heads on the floor.

• *With hands or head and hands on the floor, get ready to stand first down, then up.*
• *Let first one leg leave the pipe and then the other. Gather both feet in close to the face and stand up. Hold for a "finish."*

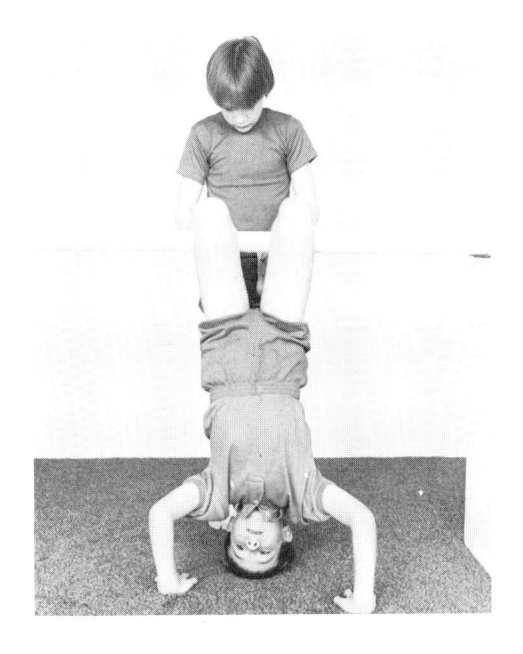

208. PINWHEEL

• *Face the bar with hands holding on about an inch from each side.*

• *Jump up to do a Mantle as you did in exercise 166.*

• *Tip forward and bend at the pelvis with both knees bent.*

• *Keep going until your feet have gone over your head and landed on the other side.*

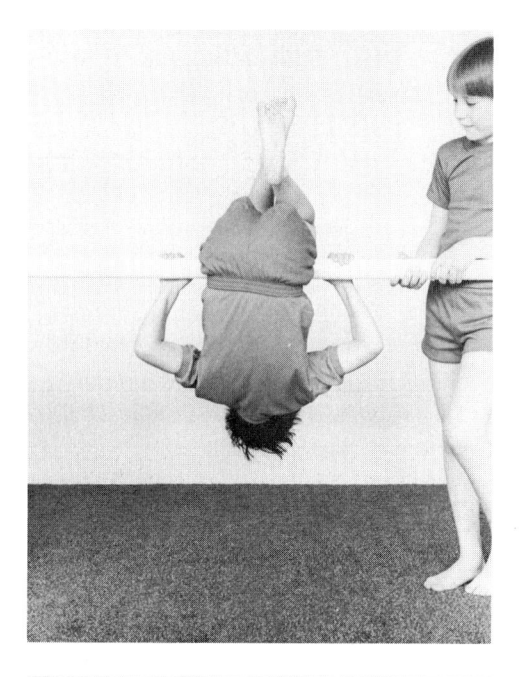

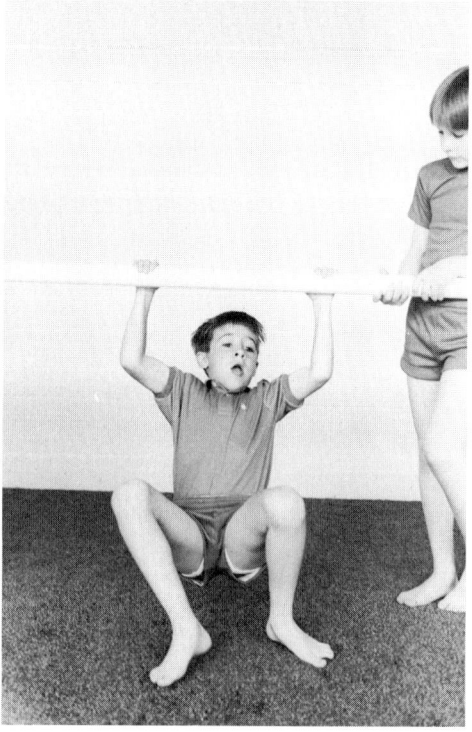

Pipes, Ropes, and Rings

209. SKIN THE CAT

• Sit on the floor under the pipe after you have completed the Pinwheel (exercise 208).
• Stick both feet through the hole created by your two arms and head.
• Push all the way through until your feet drop to the floor behind your head.

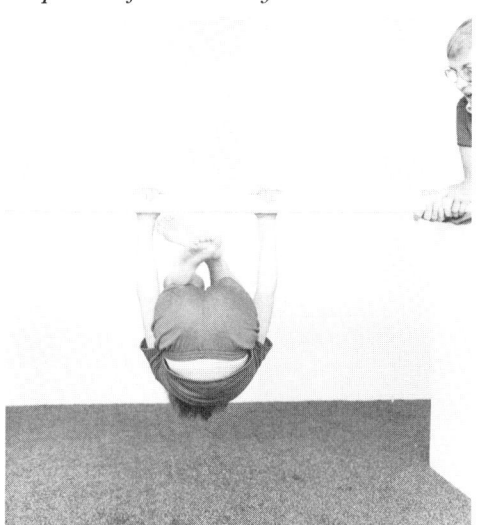

• Then give a little bounce with both feet to get your seat in the air.
• Slide your feet through the hole and you will land on the floor the same way you started.

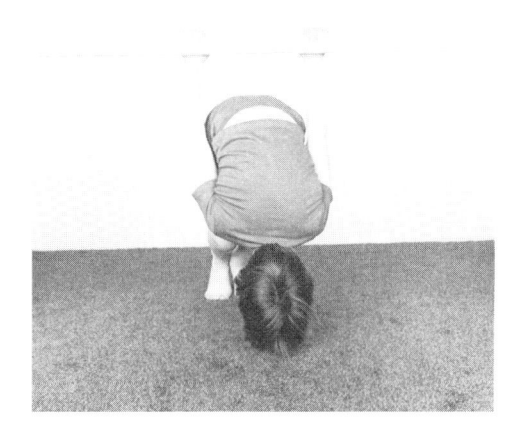

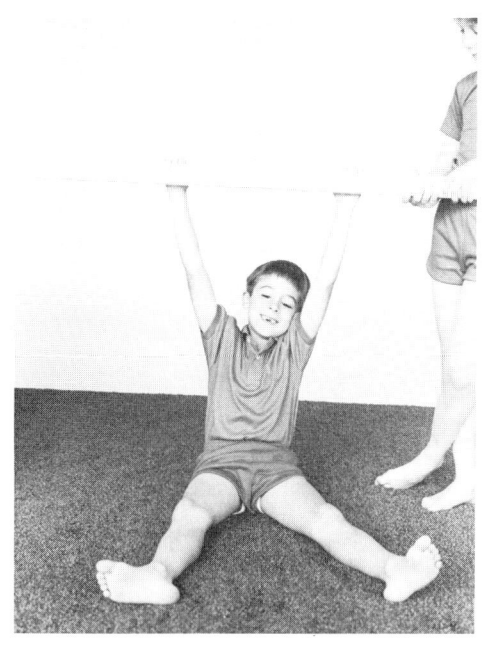

Such exercises are good preparation for doing these stunts from hanging ropes. They teach the needed proprioception ... and the courage to be other than right side up with both feet on the floor. In addition, being upside down is *fun*. One summer at the training program where we develop exercise therapists and Myotherapists, there were two young women who had never done anything in their lives that even whispered of tumbling. One was a professor of music and one had worked in special education for the handicapped. *Both* were musicians. *Both* had rhythm. We started with the backward shoulder roll, which is the safest for people who have never tumbled. That's because the spotter has complete control, so that before the tumbler knows what has happened, it's over and he or she has done it. The music professor burst into tears. "I've always *wanted so much* to do that and I never got the chance until it was too late. And now I did it and it was *easy*." As a child, she'd been a proper little girl and *never* kicked her feet over her head to reveal probably very pretty underpants. Her school had either gone down the primrose path of progressive teaching, which meant games, or was too poor or uneducated about fitness and its relation to academic studies to provide real physical education. For whatever reason, she gave everything to the piano. All her emotions poured out at the keyboard, which is a wonderful release, but *never* enough for the body. Roughly 75 percent of the students at music schools have developed muscle spasms and severe pain *from working at the instrument. If your child is taking music lessons of any kind,* see the chapter on Myotherapy (page 411).

The next exercise is another of those that are controversial in America only. Girls were supposed to be the weaker sex, and most women have been *conditioned* to believe that, accept that, and live by it—and teach it to their daughters. Before you read another book, go down to the library and pick up Ashley Montagu's *The Natural Superiority of Women*. That will scotch that myth forever. Girls can do most physical, mental, and artistic things boys do. Chin-ups were one of the things supposed to be beyond girls, those and push-ups. Nonsense!

210. CHIN-UP

If you are going to use the pipes for this, stand two strong children on each staircase to hold your pipe. You will do far better to install a doorway gym (see page 148). That will make it easier for you.

Pipes, Ropes, and Rings

• *Use a level (doorway gym) that the children can just reach by standing on tiptoe. With palms facing in (that works the biceps), pull to a chin-up with the chin over the pipe. Lower slowly to the floor.*

• *Now reverse the hold so that the palms face* away *(this contracts the triceps). Pull the chin to above the pipe and then lower.*

For girls the accepted chin-up was done on the sawhorse (see exercise 167). The heels were resting on the floor. Disgraceful! Not for you. *You* are fully aware of the studies that show that children live up to expectations, both the positive kind and the downers.

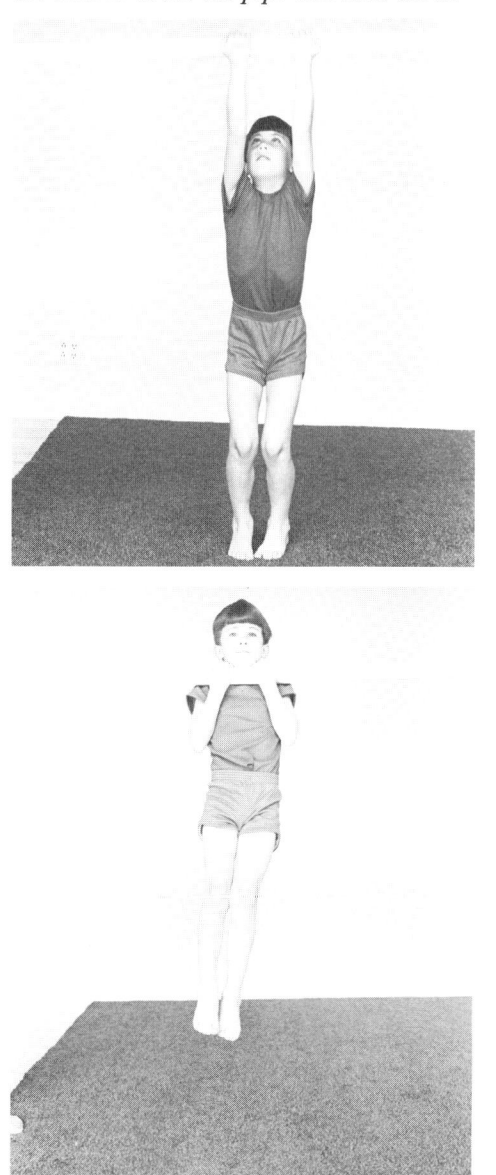

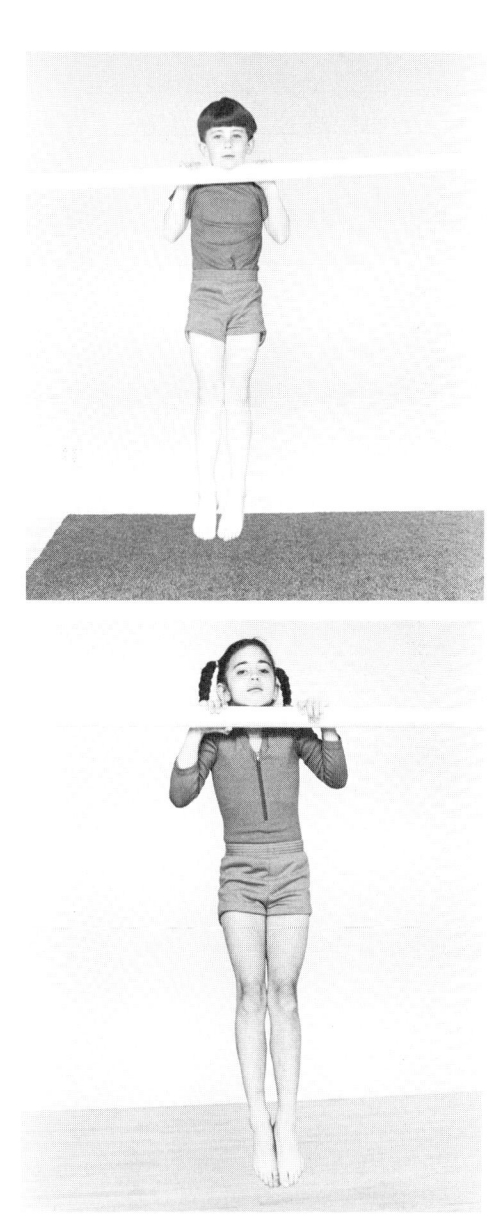

211. ONE-HAND CHIN-UP

• *Hold on to the bar with one hand and grasp the wrist with the other hand. Pull up and let down as before. Alternate hands.*

But suppose you can't do a chin-up, what do you do then? Simple: You do a Let-down.

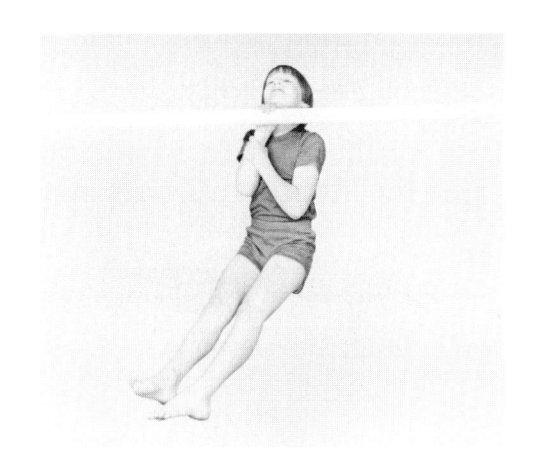

212. LET-DOWN

• *Climb onto a box or a chair until you are high enough to hold on with both hands and rest your chin on the bar. Maintain that hold for a slow count of five and then step back on the box and back down to the floor. That's step number one.*
• *Step number two (after about a week of daily five-second holds) is to hold on for ten seconds.*
• *A week later, lower yourself with a* slow *Let-down. Try for a ten-second lowering, but be satisfied if it's an express trip in two seconds. Just hang on and repeat it daily.* When you can let down in ten seconds, you (or they) will be able to do a chin-up. There really is no such thing as "I can't," but there's no such thing as an Olympic gold medal either if you haven't taken the time and spent the effort in practice.

When you have used your arms enough, how can you use the pipe for more exercises, ones that will work the legs but rest the arms? You turn the pipe into a ballet barre. On page 205 you will discover how to *prepare* for ballet classes.

But if you have a class of boys, you may prefer to skip that and just use the parts that would help with the inflexibility that's common in children who engage in speed and contact sports only.

---

213. PIPE PLIÉ

• *Explain that this exercise is to stretch the calf muscles, which are needed for running and skiing.*

• *Stand facing the barre with legs straight, heels together and feet turned out.*
• *Bend both knees into a turned-out half*

Pipes, Ropes, and Rings

knee-bend, which is called a plié *in ballet circles.*

• *Check to see that the toes are covered by the knees. If toes can be seen peeking out from the outside of the knee, the foot is pronating, which is wrong. That foot must be "patterned" into the right movement so that it can build the needed strength to keep it there.*

• *Start with sixteen pliés and refer to the pliés on the blocks for more (see page 223).*

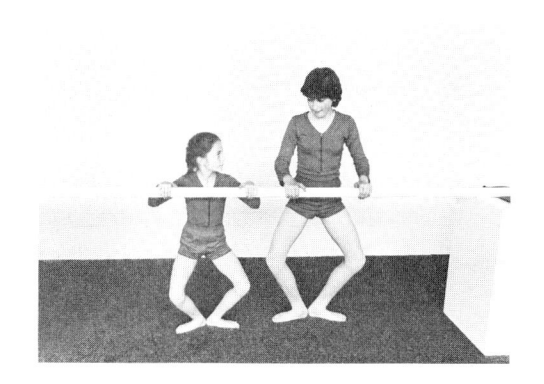

214. PIPE, HAMSTRING STRETCH

Your little boys have seen runners do this before setting out on a run, so they will accept it as normal procedure. It is anything but! *You* are stretching warm muscles that have already done many exercises to loosen them. Those muscles are soft and pliable. The runner usually does his or her stretching *before* the muscles are warm. He often leaves a tense situation to go out and run. That means that the muscles are not only cold, they are taut with stress. *You* will never do that because you know that cold muscles tear a little every time that's done to them; eventually, they become badly injured. Explain this to the children because they are in grave danger from their trainers if they are good athletes and from themselves if they are not. In the first instance, the teacher or coach rarely knows about warm-ups or thinks that jumping or running is a warm-up. In the second, the children will try desperately hard, whether they have cold muscles or not—and they hurt themselves.

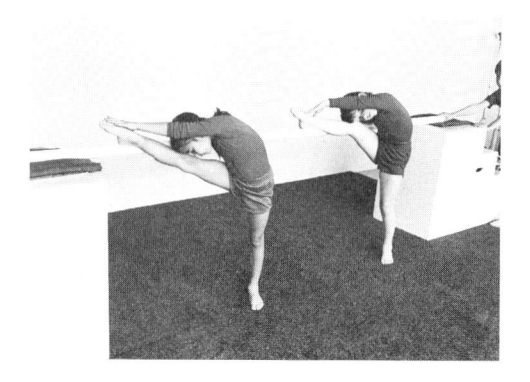

• *Stand facing the barre and place the right ankle on it while keeping the left leg straight. The height of the barre is important. The one the children (or you) are to use should be level with the crotch at first. As the stretch improves, the barre will have to be raised.*

• *Lean over the right straight knee and grasp the ankle.*

• *Pull the head down toward the knee in easy bounces.*

• *Do eight bounces and change legs and direction. Do four sets* after *the legs are warm.*

> If you are reading this book piecemeal and haven't come to the part on ballistic versus static stretch (page 97), read it. It applies right here.

PARALLEL PIPES

These pipes are much narrower (see page 149) and have many uses. The children can do push-ups on the parallels and handstands and slide-throughs, in which they grasp the pipes and walk their feet through. The following exercise is both easy and useful. It develops many muscles and yet the assistant is always in complete control. If the child is very new or very weak, grasp at the thighs instead of the ankles. That's a good habit anyway. Make it easy and safe until *you* know the ability of the person you are working with. Nobody likes to fail, and it takes many successes to wipe one failure out—so avoid them.

215. THE PUMP

- *The child addresses the parallel standing straight and still. With that firmly in his or her mind, you assure him or her that you will not be surprised if you receive a kick to your groin.*
- *The assistant stands a few feet behind the child.*
- *At the signal "Go," the child places both hands on the parallels and raises one leg. The assistant grasps the ankle, knee, or thigh, depending on the ability of the child.*
- *The other leg is then lifted into the assistant's waiting hand.*
- *"Bottoms up," is the signal for the child to raise the bottom high.*
- *"Arch down" tells him to let his body sag down while keeping the* head up and arms straight.
- *Alternate up and down for four at first and work up to eight. As that becomes easy,*

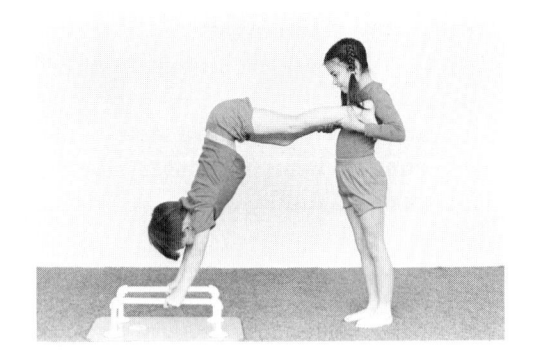

Pipes, Ropes, and Rings

slide the supporting hands further down the legs, which puts more pressure on the torso, arms, chest, and shoulders.

• *At first it may be necessary for the assistant to raise her arms in order to help the "pump" get his seat in the air, but that will pass.*

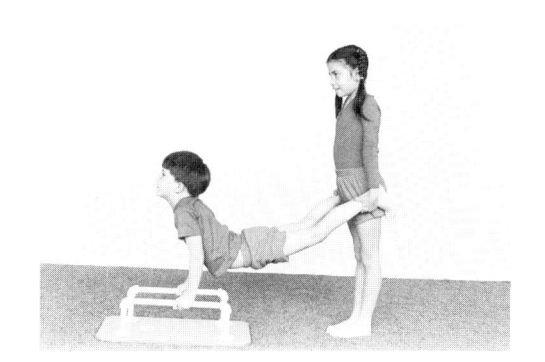

THE HORIZONTAL ROPE

In many places where people hold classes there is little height and no supports in the ceiling for vertical climbing of ropes. That is true of most of our homes and "all-purpose rooms." That is no excuse for giving up on rope climbing or preparing the children for upper schools where there *might* be rope climbing. Few things are more embarrassing than to be given the order to "climb to the top, touch, and slide down" if you can't even get off the ground. That won't happen to your children if you will invest in a ½- or ¾-inch nylon rope (hardware store). Tape both ends and then hold the ends over a flame. This will melt the strands together and prevent unraveling. Tie one end to a board that is wider than the window at the end of the room. Stick the board out the window to rest horizontally against the house. Close the window to keep tension on the board. That's *one* way to anchor the rope.

Fasten the other end around two strong students at the other side of the room from the anchor. You now have a fairly taut *horizontal* rope.

216. OVERHEAD PULL

• *Lie supine with your head toward the anchor.*

• *Reach up and pull yourself with alternating long, reaching arms to the anchor end.*

• *Try to keep time with the fairly slow music, hand over hand.*

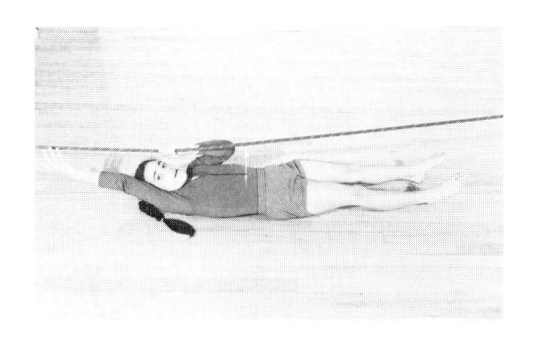

217. FISH ON A LINE

• Start the same way, supine, head toward the anchor. Keep the legs tightly together, turning you into a mermaid.
• As you pull with your right arm, swing your mermaid tail to the right.
• As you pull with your left, swing your tail to the left.
• Swish that tail from side to side. Stay with the music.

218. SITTING ROPE-TUG

• Face the anchor with straight legs straight ahead.
• Put the arm nearest the rope over it.
• Pull yourself hand over hand to the anchor end.
• Bare legs do not slide well, especially if damp with sweat. Go to the rug store and ask for throw-away samples. They make good sliders to sit on.

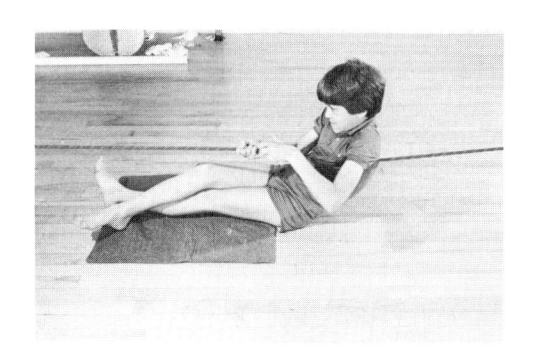

219. THE CABOOSE

• The "engine" lies on the floor as in exercise 216.
• The "caboose" lies prone, holding onto the "engine's" ankles.
• The "engine" pulls the "caboose" to the end, and then they change places.

Suggest that the children dream up some other ways of using the rope; you may be surprised.

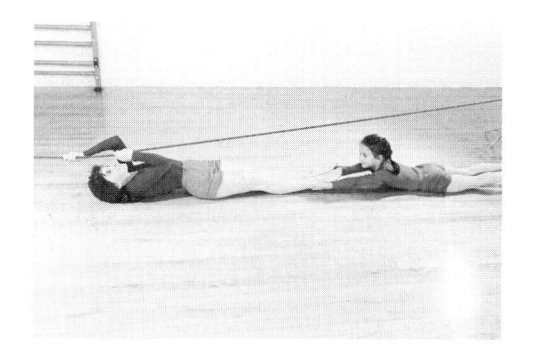

VERTICAL ROPES

You may be lucky enough to have access to Vertical Ropes. Almost all elementary schools in other countries do. Most of our elementary schools don't even have

Pipes, Ropes, and Rings

a gym. When they do, they throw balls around, for the most part. The symbol of American sports is a ball; large or small, it's still a ball. Even *blind* children must play ball—one of the few things they can't do!

220. CLIMB TO SIT/STAND

As with other equipment you have introduced, vertical ropes also have an easy way to start, a way *everybody* can feel good about.

• Lie supine under the rope with its end dangling over the tops of your thighs.
• Sit up to reach for the rope and hold it tight to your chest.
• Let yourself back down to the lying position via the rope.
• Pull back up to the sitting position three times. That may be all some of your charges can do. Remember, nothing *they do builds arm strength. We sent kids just like them to Vietnam. Criminal!*
• As soon as possible, have them begin lying supine as before, but this time pretend that the body is in a plaster cast neck to toe. Only the arms are free.
• Have them pull themselves to the standing position without breaking at the knees or hips.

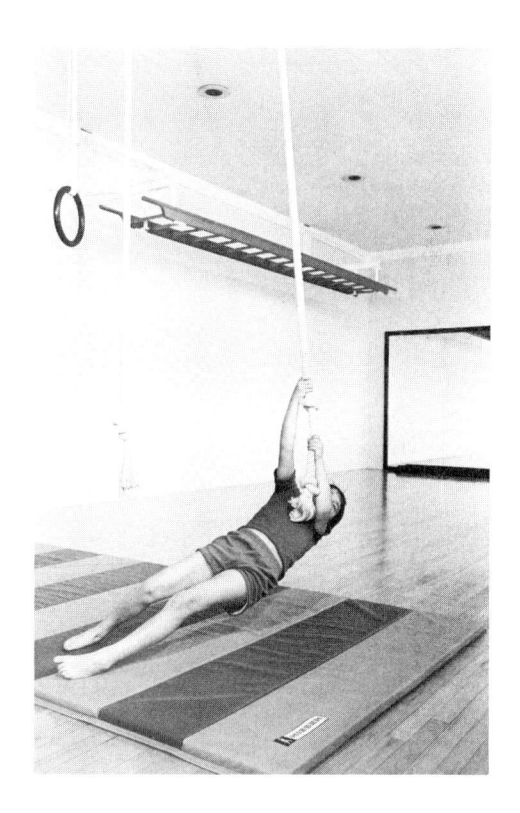

221. ROPE CLIMB

• Grasp the rope above your head as high up as you can reach.
• Stand on the left foot and hook your right a whole circle so that the rope passes all the way around the leg and drags across the instep.
• Keep the rope over the instep by turning the foot up to trap it.

• *Pull up with both hands and pull up both knees.*

• *Trap the rope by stepping on your right instep where the rope lies, with your left foot. Clamp down hard to keep it there.*

• *Using the foothold on the rope, straighten your legs and reach high again with your hands.*

• *Some children are so weak that climbing is out of the question, but if they can merely hang on and swing, that's a start.*

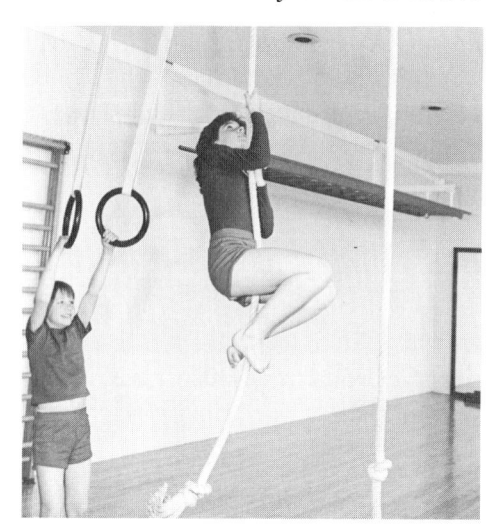

TWO ROPES

222. CONTROLLED UPSIDE-DOWN HANG

• *Address the ropes and grasp both a little above your shoulders.*

• *The spotter controls the climber by holding the near hand on the rope, the other at the shoulder. Bend the knees slightly to be ready for a hand to let go. (It almost never does, but be ready.)*

• *The climber kicks the feet up overhead* outside *the ropes and bends the knees. Hand, knee, and thigh pressure on the rope makes it possible to stay there for a few seconds.*

• *Unhook the legs and let the legs fall to the floor in front of the face. That completes a Back Flip on the ropes.*

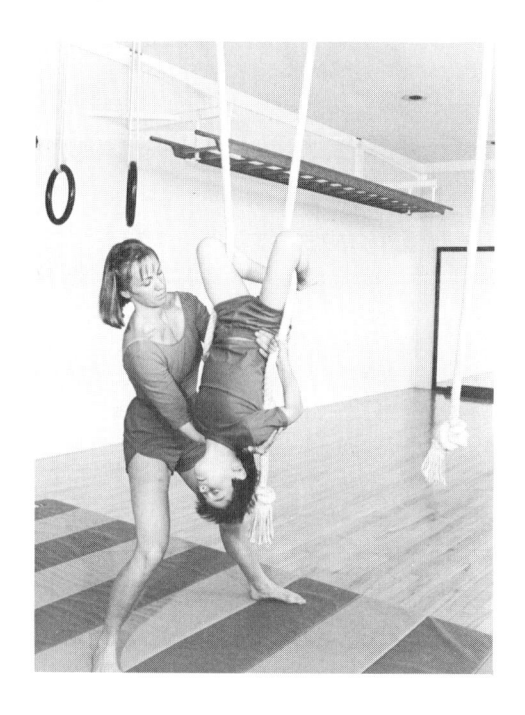

223. CONTROLLED BACK FLIP

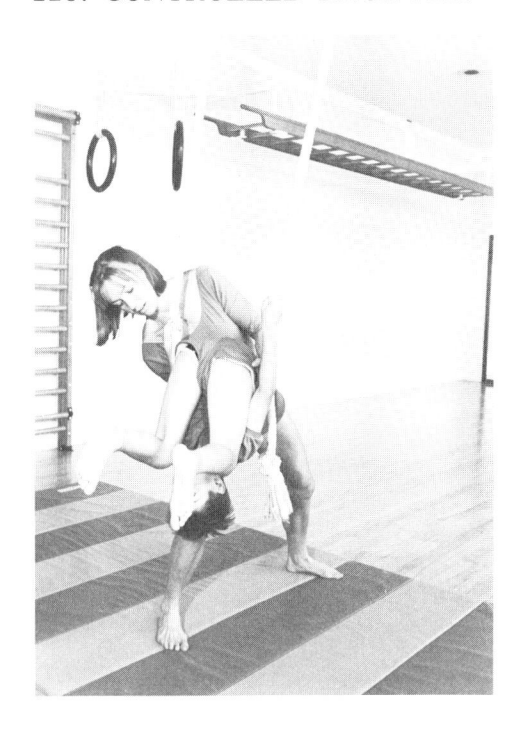

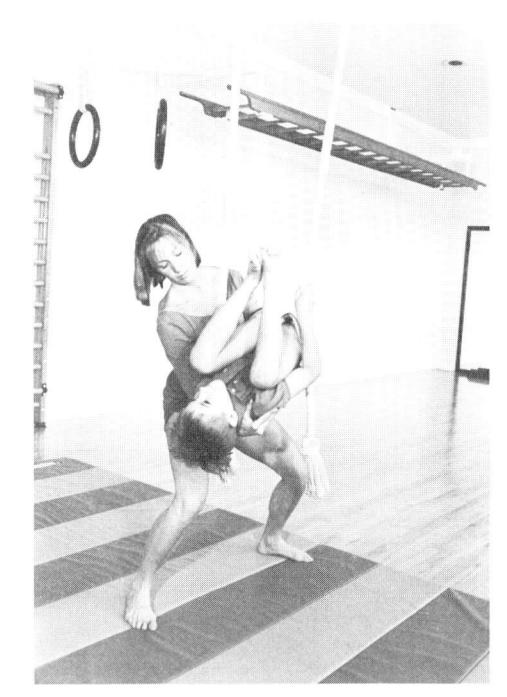

- *Address the ropes as for exercise 222 and spot the same way.*
- *Jump the legs up and over as you stay curled. The trick to getting over lies in the strength of the abdominals and the ability to look where you want to go.*
- *At first form should not matter too much; just get over. The legs have a life of their own. Try to stay curled.*
- *As the feet touch down, they may be too far back, which means that the curl was lost too soon. They should be right under the nose when the rope is still.*
- *Push off and carry the legs through to land on the floor where you started. That is a Front Flip on the ropes.*

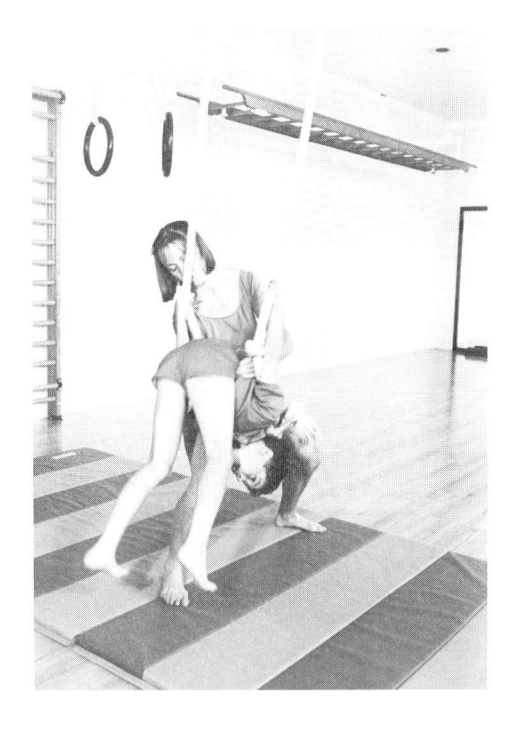

224. INTERRUPTED BACK FLIP, SOLO

• *Start the Interrupted Back Flip as you just did in the last exercise. However, since this time you are on your own, the push-off will have to be harder, the arms straightened at the same time as the kickoff, and the head tipped back at once. Say those things to yourself before you take off.*

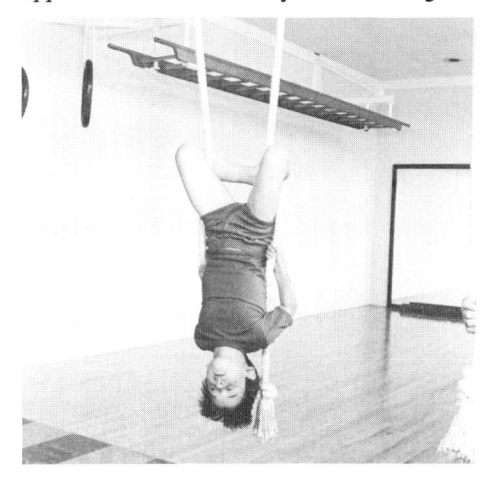

• *Start trying to straighten the legs out as they unhook from the rope. They should land right under your nose. The knees bend and immediately straighten to start you into your curl and over.*

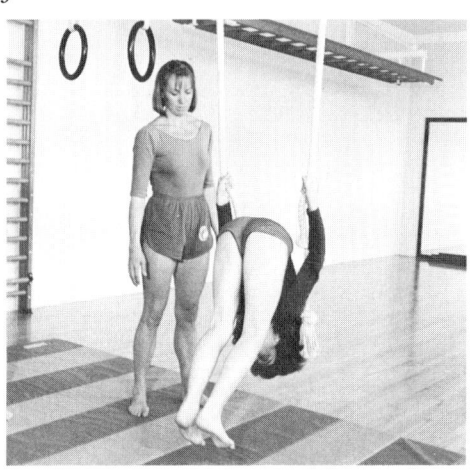

225. UPSIDE-DOWN HANG AND CLIMB

• *Grasp the rope at waist level, tip your head back, and kick up both feet over your head.*

• *Grab the rope in your feet by overlapping them.*

• *Straighten your body and hang for a count of ten.*

• *Loosen your legs around the rope and drop your feet to the floor.*

• *When your arms are strong enough, you will be able to climb* up *the rope while upside down.*

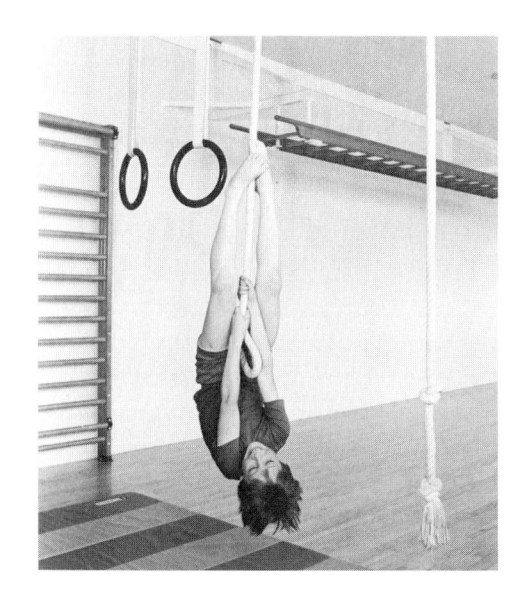

RINGS

Some gyms have rings such as you see here. Most do not, but there are less expensive rings to be had in sports stores and they can go in your doorway gym (see page 148).

226. RING SWING

- *To build strength in the hands for rings, swing on them. You don't have to tell kids to swing on rings; that's the very thing they want to do, so let them. At first it will be all hit or miss. When they get tired of that, show them where to go from there.*

227. TWO-HANDED TWINS ON RINGS

- *Two children each take a ring in their two hands.*
- *They should stand back as far as they can on tiptoes.*
- *Then, on your command, "Retract landing gear and swing forward," they bend their knees and swing.*
- *When they reach the other end of the swing, they should both let go to land on both feet. Stop and "finish." Have both walk away at the same time, one in each direction.*
- *In the meantime, the next two have caught the rings and are ready to swing forward, and so on.*

228. TWO-HANDED SWING OVER POLE

- *Start the swing as above. The difference this time lies in an obstacle. Have a child on each side of the pole; hold it six inches off the floor.*
- *The swingers will have to retract the landing gear way up to get over the pole.*

229. SIAMESE-TWIN SWINGERS

- *Each child takes a ring in the hand away from his or her "twin."*
- *They then hold hands with the near hands and repeat both of the foregoing exercises.*

230. UPSIDE-DOWN HANG, RINGS

• *Kick the legs up as you straighten your arms and tip your head back. (This young fellow forgot the* head back *hold, which is why his body is bent.)*

• *At first it may be necessary to kick up fast and grope for the ring straps with wandering feet. Soon you will be able to curl and straighten slowly, keeping feet together and toes pointed.*

• *Curl up to come back down at first, but as soon as possible keep the legs straight and bring them down that way to the floor.*

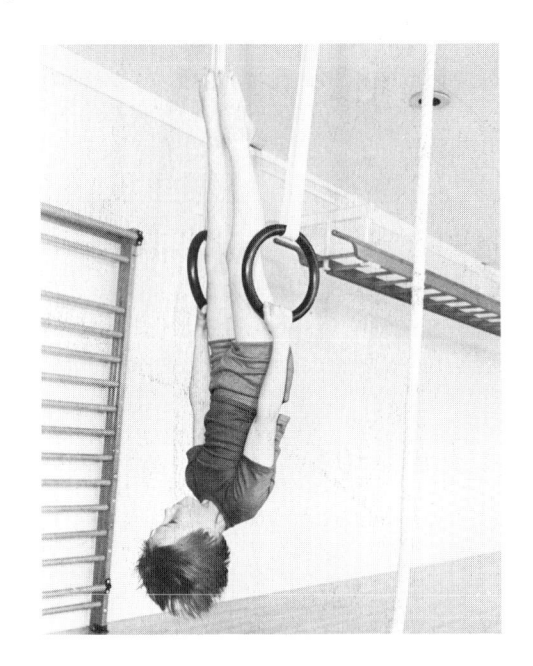

231. BIRD'S NEST

• *Grasping the rings firmly, kick both feet into the rings as you curl.*

• *The spotter should control at the shoulders.*

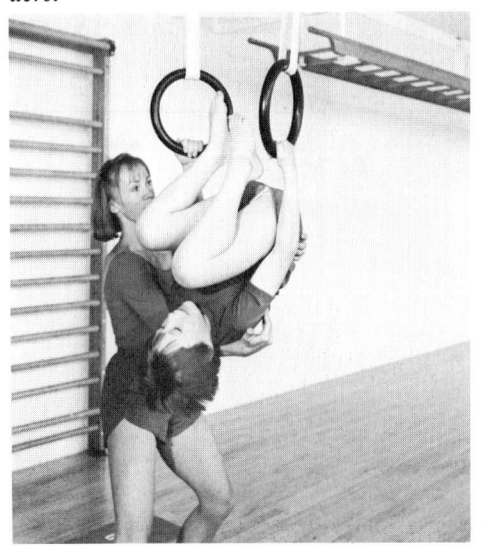

• *Keeping the feet* in *the rings, turn inside out and lift the head.*

• *Turn right side out and come down.*

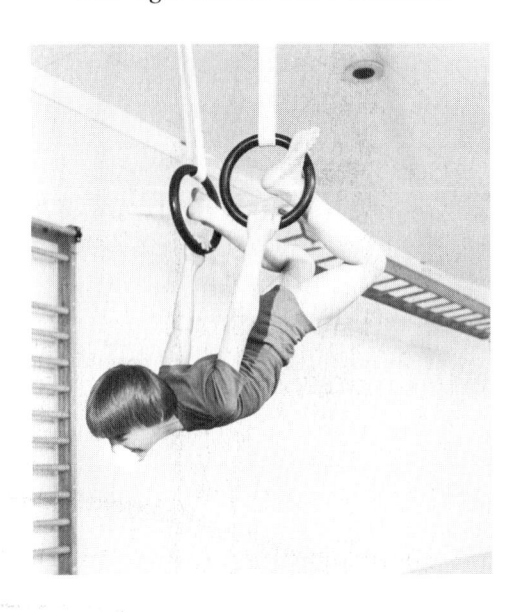

232. FLYING BIRD'S NEST

- *Kick up to put one foot and then leg into each ring. Sit up, using rungs as a seat.*
- *Pump to swing as you would in a regular swing.*
- *When you have the rings swinging nicely, grasp the rings firmly and sit back so that you are held in the rings by hands and knees.*
- *Slide the legs back so that your feet are engaged in the rings.*
- *Turn inside out as the rings swing forward.*

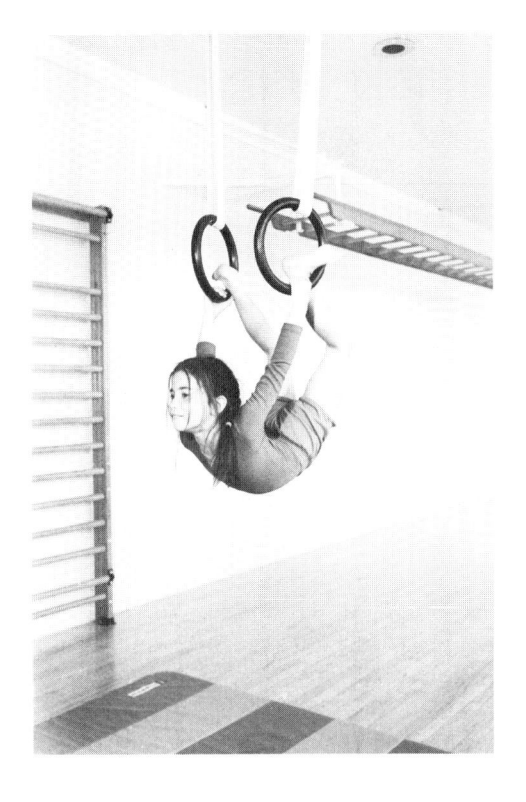

CHAPTER SEVENTEEN
THE GARAGE OR BASEMENT GYM

Most people today have garages or basements, just as once upon a time most folks had nice spacious barns. Barns usually meant haylofts and rafters. If *we* had such structures, *we* would use them a little differently, but then we have a different need. The children who lived next to such barns were well exercised by nature and need. Today when we test around the country we find that the children who still live in rural areas are usually stronger than suburban and city children. There are still chores for the children to do, which does make a difference, even though the school bus and TV have invaded rural areas, too.

You may think that my constant harping on earlier times is unrealistic; after all, we can't go back, nor would we want to—but everything has a price. The price of progress and labor-saving devices is the need to find other ways of keeping our body-machines in good order. *Everyone* knows that even the best Rolls-Royce put up on blocks and never driven will soon have rust spots, a moth-eaten interior, and a dead battery. Rolls-Royces need to be used, tuned, dusted, polished—and driven. So do people. If you have a garage or a basement, you have a place to do just that.

What you will see here can be done

The Garage or Basement Gym

on the gym floor, as I did for these pictures, using tape. Tape means that you can take it off if you want to. Paint means that the patterns you put on the floor stay.

The first time I made a garage gym, I pulled all the junk out and laid it on the lawn. It's the same thing you do when you move. I separated what I *had* to keep and split the rest between Goodwill and the junk heap. What was left could be stored in the corners of my then-empty garage.

I painted the floor with two coats of royal-blue deck enamel and let it "cure" for a month. (Whoopee! That gives you an excuse for not doing it. Where can you put the car for a month? You'd be surprised what you can do if you really have a reason. You'll find a way.)

Next come the patterns. Tape is easiest, unless you have a friend who loves to paint straight lines on floors. You need three patterns. One is the still-familiar hopscotch pattern of two boxes, one box, two boxes, and so forth. The next is a simple straight line over near one wall. The third is a set of crosses about two feet long, horizontal and vertical lines crossing in the middle. That's it for floor patterns. All the equipment we have used so far can fit in your garage if you have one large enough for a car. (The stairs might not make it, but that's all. In that case you can use the in-house stairs.)

There is one secret to making a success of a garage or basement gym: No one can ever use it unless you are there. If it is used as a rainy-day playroom, the children will get used to the patterns, and they will lose their specialness. What does that tell you? What that *should* tell you is that *you* are the most important person in that child's or those children's lives. "Watch me, watch me, Mommy and/or Daddy" is a universal cry. You still have that power while they are six, but it is waning fast at twelve. Make the most of it. At twelve, and often before, peers become far more important than you. That's why we have drug addiction. "Cool George" knows so much more than you do. Don't despair, it was the same for you at twelve. It will take another ten to forty years for them to discover how much you know. The one thing you can be sure will last (maybe long enough) is a good body.

233. WALKING THE LINE

• *Here we go with eye training. Walking the line means* Look . . . see . . . report back to the brain. *Walk the line to slow, then faster and faster music.*

• *Keep the feet straight on the line, not turned out or in.*

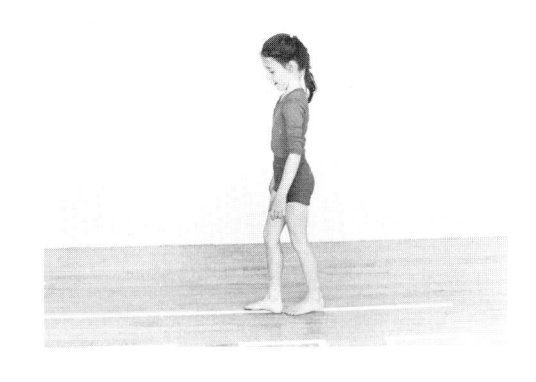

234. PIGEON TOES

• *Turn the feet inward as far as possible. This strengthens the anterior tibialis, the muscle that works to help flat feet and is constantly overworked in anyone who has a long second toe (see page 435).*

• *Note what the little girl in the picture is doing: turning her hands in to match her feet. Break that habit.*

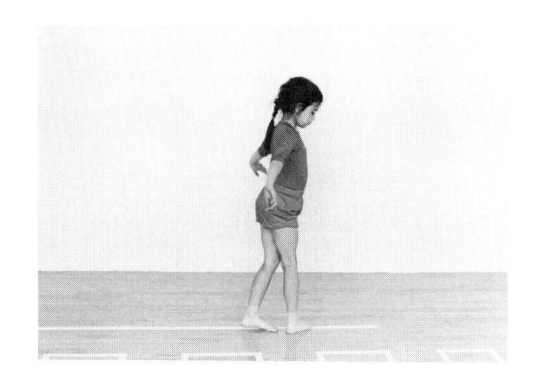

235. TEN-PAST-TEN WALK

• *Turn the feet out as far as possible as you walk the line. You can get them much farther out if you will bend the knees slightly and tuck the pelvis under.*

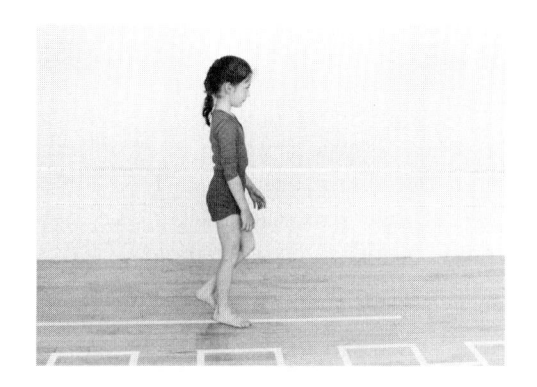

236. CROSSOVER

• *Cross the right foot over to the left side of the line with the foot turned out, the toe just touching the line.*

• *Then cross over with the other foot. This is especially helpful for pigeon-toed people (see exercise index).*

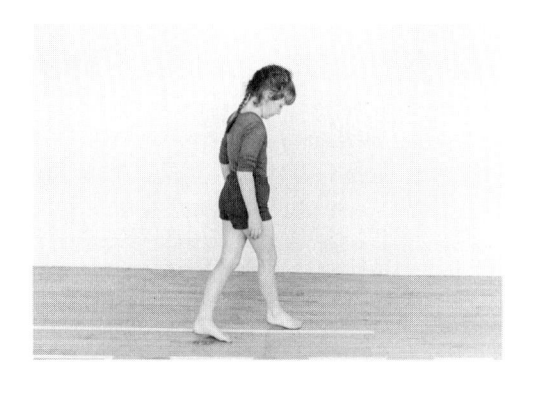

237. HOPSCOTCH

- *Have the children go through the hopscotch pattern the way they do at school; if they do it at school. If not, you may have to teach them, because children no longer teach each other games, and sidewalks are not chalked for them. There aren't many sidewalks left, unless you live in the city; but can you let your little children out unsupervised?*
- *Now put music on and have them go through the pattern again, staying with the music. Slow, medium, and fast will each net different forms.*
- *Try it backward to slow music and don't pick up the beat until they can do it without missing a box or stepping on a line—or looking back.*
- *Now do two jumps in each box.*
- *Next, one-legged jumps into every box. Don't forget the other leg!*
- *Look at the chapter on floor progressions (page 435) and see what would work with this pattern.*

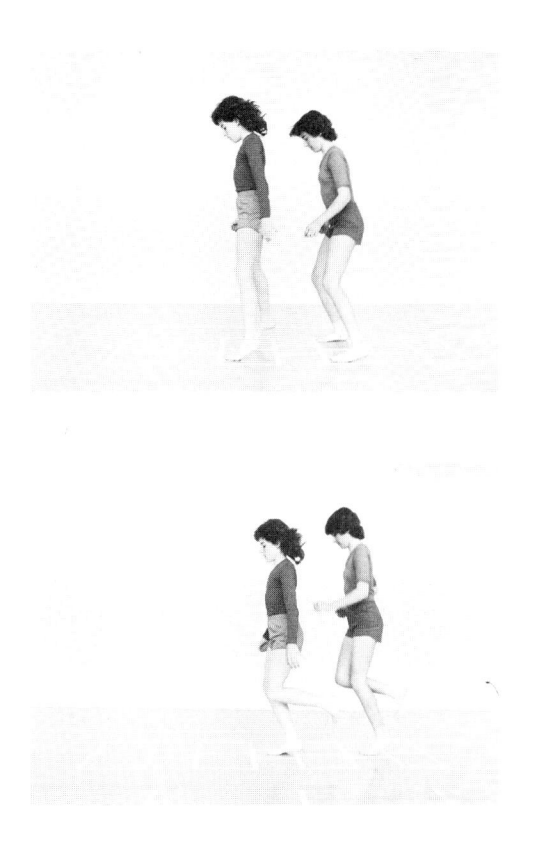

238. DOUBLE JUMPERS

- *Three set out together and endeavor to stay together. One each to a line, but the single center boxes go to the leader, who can set and hold the beat.*

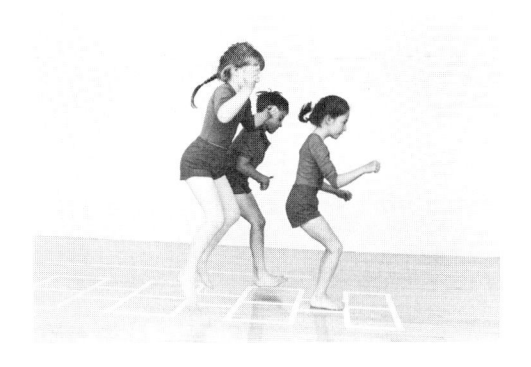

239. CROSSES FORWARD AND BACKWARD

• *Stand in the first two boxes provided by the crossed lines. Jump forward and backward over the horizontal lines.*

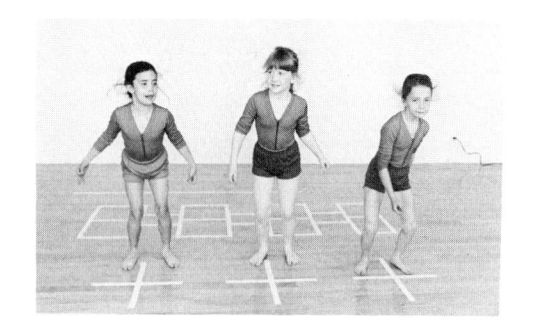

240. CROSSES SIDE TO SIDE

• *Jump from side to side over the vertical lines.*

241. CROSSES CLOCKWISE AND COUNTERCLOCKWISE

• *Jump into each of the squares, first clockwise, then turn and go counter clockwise. If you are using ¼ time, jump eight times clockwise and on the eighth count, jump to the other direction and go around for eight counts that way.*

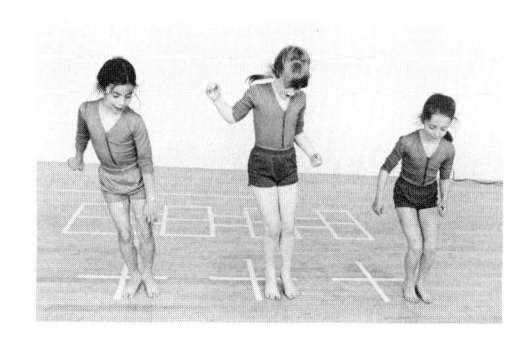

242. CROSSES ON ALL FOURS, FORWARD AND BACK

• *Place your hands a little way ahead of your cross and jump your feet forward and back over the line.*

• *Keeping your hands where you have just placed them, jump both your feet from side to side, first in one set of squares and then in the other.*

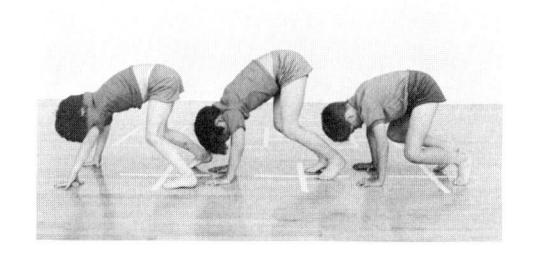

The Garage or Basement Gym

RAILROAD TIES

Railroad ties are made from 3-foot lengths of 4-by-4 lumber that have been sanded and enameled. Mine have two sets of handles on each of two sides, which make them even more versatile.

243. WALKING THE TRACKS

• *Lay two sets of ties parallel and about 16 inches apart. They can then be walked on, one foot on each of the rails of the narrow-gauge railroad you have made.*

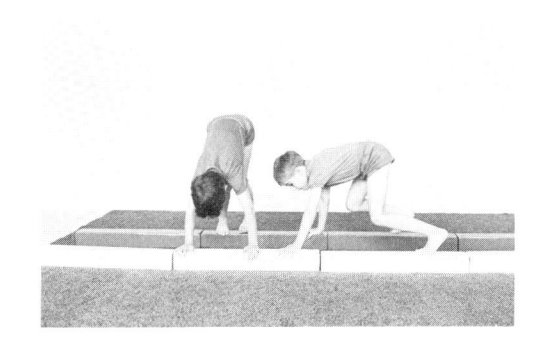

244. WHEELBARROW ON THE TRACKS

• *Use the tracks for wheelbarrows. (See the section on railroad tracks, page 147.)*

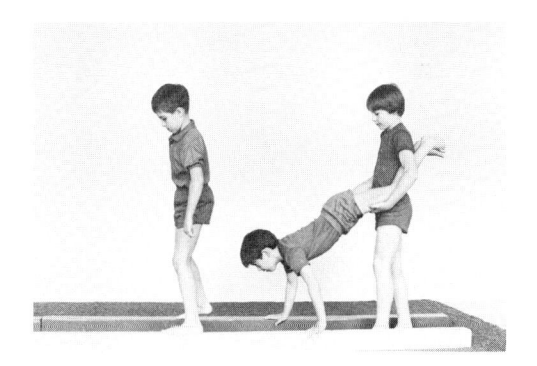

245. FOUR-FOOT TRACK WALK, FORWARD AND SIDE

• *Place the feet on one track and the hands on the other and proceed along the narrow-gauge railroad to the end.*

• *Walk forward on all fours, left foot and hand on one track and right foot and hand on the other.*

246. FOUR-FOOT MIX-UP

• *Walk your feet along, one foot on each track.*
• *Walk the right hand on the left track and the left hand on the right track.*

• *Change to put one hand on each track but the feet crossing over.*
• *Do both backward.*

247. BALANCE BEAMS

• *Use one or both tracks as balance beams.*

(See the section on the sawhorse, page 163.)

248. RAILROAD TIES

• *Place the ties crosswise like real railroad ties (from which the idea came) and walk them in pairs, using wands or dowels to make teamwork easier. Walk backward and then sideways.*
• *Lengthen the distance between the ties a little at a time.*

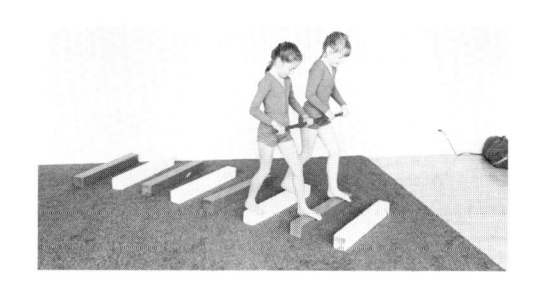

249. DOG ON THE TIES

• *Just cross over the ties as a dog would. Pay no attention to which foot matches which hand.*

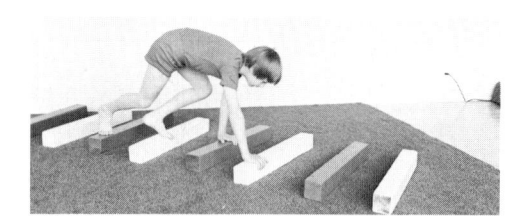

250. RIGHT, RIGHT, LEFT, LEFT

When they know others are watching, many people will become tense when told to walk across the floor. As a result they interfere with nature which holds that as we step forward onto one foot, the *opposite* arm swings forward. That maintains balance. That student will stride forward onto the right foot and at the same time thrust the right arm forward. He or she knows something is

The Garage or Basement Gym

wrong because it doesn't *feel* right. But, as with many beginners learning a new skill, the student doesn't know what is wrong. The cure lies in making an exercise out of the *wrong* movement, doing it so often that the entire class gets used to a new *feeling*, right foot . . . right hand, left foot . . . left hand. *Then* set out with feet and hands in opposition.

• *Step forward on the right foot and punch into the opposite corner of the room with the right hand.*

• *Turn the entire body as the left foot is brought forward and the left hand punches toward the corner.*

• *Proceed in this manner across the floor, making half-turns with each step and hard punches with each hand. Subtle movements come much later.*

• Now *do it the natural oppositional way: Cross the ties with right hand and left foot advancing, then left hand and right foot.*

BLOCKS

Blocks are easy to make. Just cut a 2-by-4-inch piece of lumber into 7-inch lengths, two to a child and two for you. Sand them and give them three coats of enamel. They can be used as balance beams, stepping-stones, percussion instruments; for pre-ski training (see page 337), single foot balance, and ballet work.

251. BLOCK BALANCE

• *Turn the blocks outward slightly so that the foot standing on them is always turned out.*
• *Place the right foot on the block like the first little girl.*
• *Place the left on the floor behind with a strong turn out.*
• *Pick the foot up and bring it forward and place it on the floor in front, as the third girl is doing. Be sure the turn-out is strong.*
• *Do eight such changes with the right foot and then eight with the left.*
• *After these changes become easy, try to turn the knee out as the leg is brought forward or moved back, like the middle little girl. Do eight to a side. Then have the children make up block exercises. Use all the blocks you have and see what they come up with.*

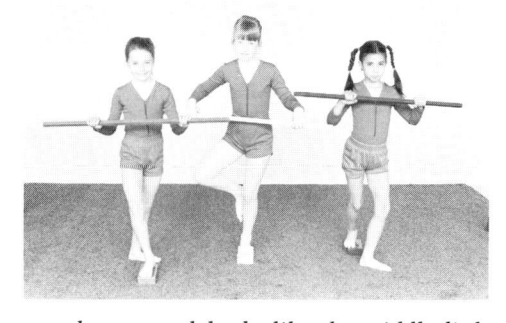

THE REBOUNDER

The rebounder is a fun gadget that everyone enjoys. Children like the *feel*, grown-ups see it as a way to get or stay fit—and everybody likes to jump on the rebounder to music. Rebounders are sold in sporting goods stores and in large department stores.

252. THE JUMP

- *There's nothing to this; just get into the middle and jump. When you've found that it's easy, then do it to your favorite music.*

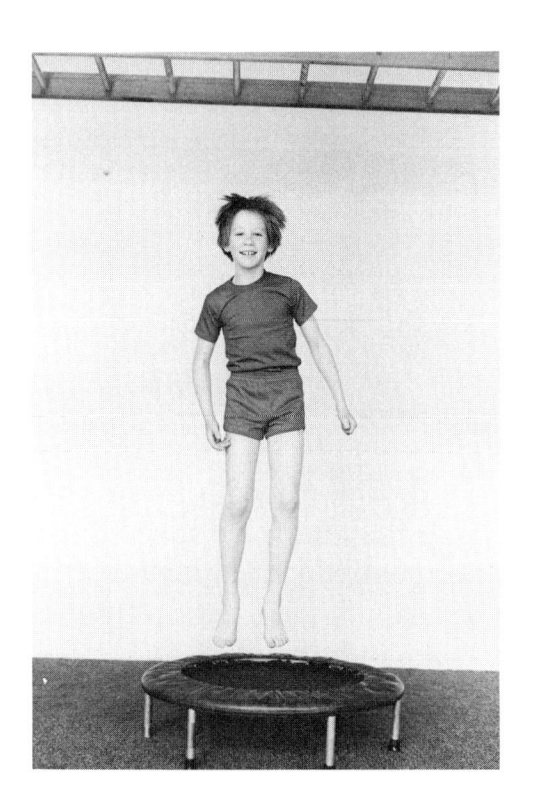

253. JUMP TURNS

- *Make small jump turns at first so that it takes six or eight jumps to get around. As you feel more secure, lessen the number of turns for a complete revolution. In time you or one of the children will be able to jump a few times and then make a complete turn in one jump.*

254. REBOUNDER RUNNING

• *Run in place and keep the beat. To make this more difficult, bring the knees up high in front.*

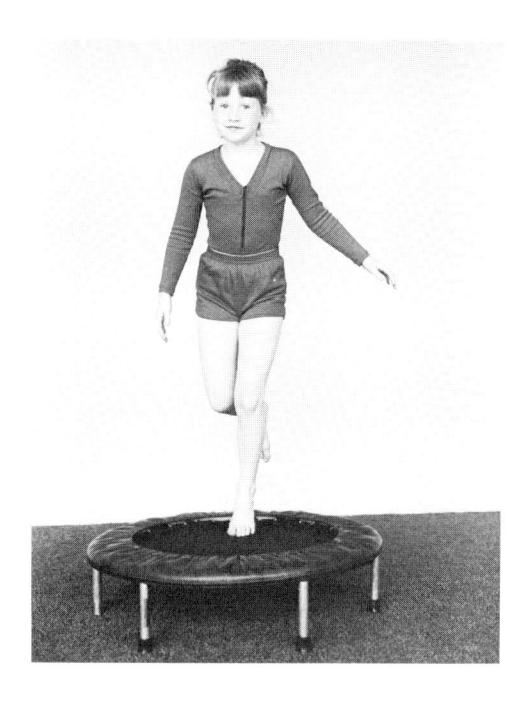

255. SIDE-TO-SIDE JUMPS

• *This is more difficult than it looks.*
• *Begin by jumping* both *feet from side to side and then from one foot to the other.*

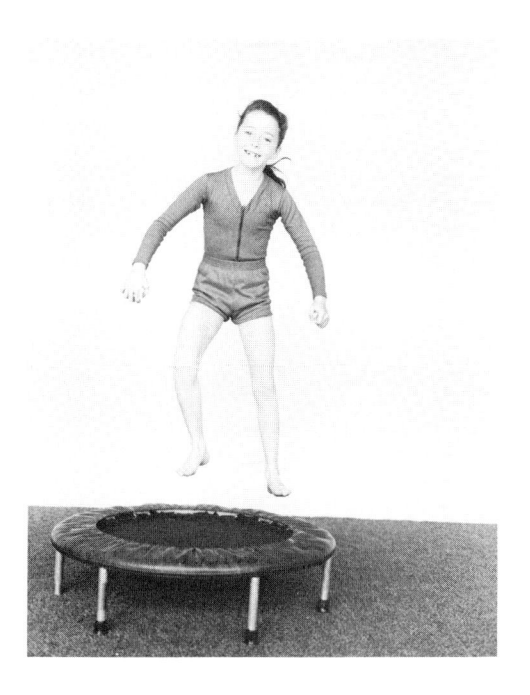

256. APART-TOGETHER JUMP

• *Jump both feet apart and then together on the next jump.*

• *As jumping improves, try to control the arms and point the toes.*

• *To make it more difficult, start with the feet together and do four jumps. On the fourth, spread the legs wide and land with them together. In time you will be able to spread on every second jump.*

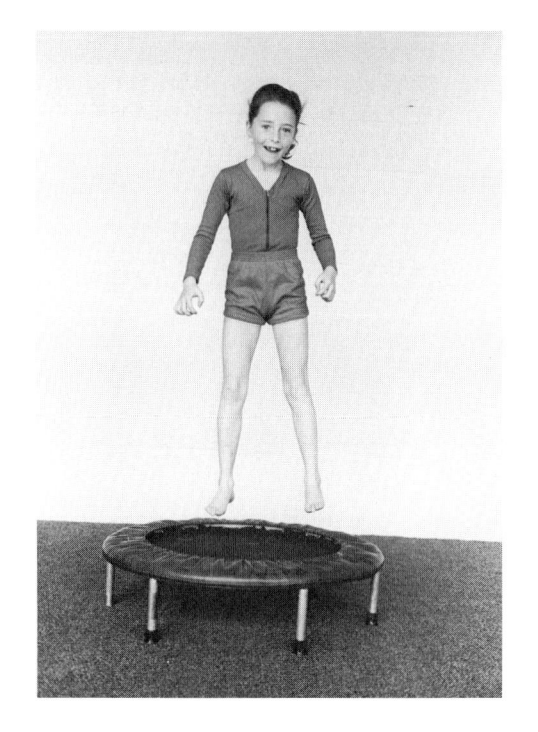

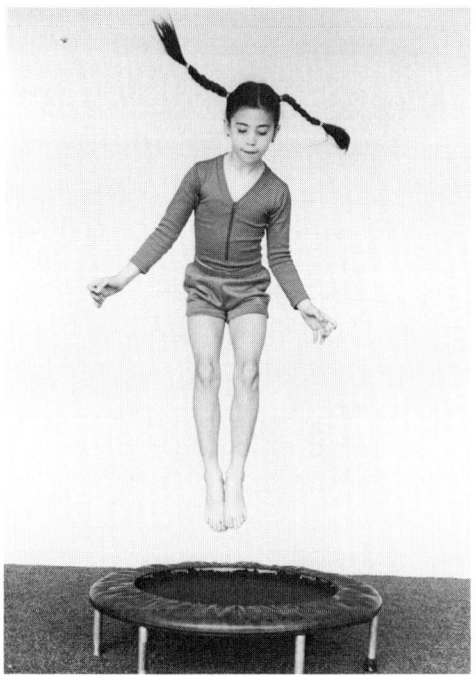

257. KNEE PULL-UPS
• Pull the knees high on every fourth jump, then every second, and finally every jump.

258. REBOUNDER JUMP ROPE
• Use your jump rope on the rebounder and see if you can double the overhead arcs of the rope with each jump.

259. JUMP SERIES

• Have the children design a Jump Series. Each one makes up a jump to be done to eight counts, for example:

Eight straight jumps
Eight apart-together for 8
Eight turning for 8 counts
Eight hip twists for 8
Eight pull-ups—use 2 counts for each which equals 4 pull-ups
Eight high knee lifts for eight
Eight goosestep kicks for 8

CHAPTER EIGHTEEN
DANCE

There are a thousand kinds of "dance," and they cover every variation, from the dancing fingers of an octogenarian tapping out the beat of a march to the wild gyrations of a bunch of kids at a prom. A tiny child "dances" when it bobs in front of the TV set, and the teenager "dances" in a similar sort of repetitive isolation to the stereo. The formal postures of ballet are dance, as is the freer movement of the "moderns." The Native American used dance to whip up his courage to fight, and much of the world's mating is preceded by dance. Dance is one of the most exciting and complete outlets for self-expression, and everybody should have the right to that outlet. As with every other form of creativity, the greater the "vocabulary" the more expression is possible, and random motions do not express very much. Before a child can *say* what he or she feels through dance, there must be a "bank account" of physical words to draw upon. Before "creative movement" can elicit more than mere release of tension, the body must be trained to do as it is told—it must be disciplined. Later, when the tools of the body (strength, flexibility, coordination, endurance, and *control*) have been developed, "creative movement" becomes art, with all the satisfactions attendant upon real art.

The tools of dance are also the tools of sport. When the body has control, it can do what the brain requires, and if it has endurance, the doing can go on for a long time. In terms of sport these qualities mean the difference between enjoying the whole day on the ski slopes and leaving at noon. They also mean the difference between playing the full game and subbing for the first quarter, riding a spirited horse or a hack, being in the tournament or watching, winning or losing.

When applied to dance, they mean the difference between really *dancing* and just moving oneself about. If you can get the ABC's presented here into the brain and muscles of your boy or girl, you will have given many basic words that make up the language of the body, the words with which they will be able to compose whatever their own creativity urges. To "feel" movement and not be able to dance it is like having the urge to write yet knowing no language; a terrible desire to sing but being mute; a longing to draw but being without hands.

When I began exercise classes for my own children, I told each to bring five friends to the Scout House in Harrison, New York, on Thursday at four and we'd *exercise*. I learned then about the tyranny of words. The three mothers who called that first evening to tell me they didn't want their daughters to *exercise*—they'd get *muscles*—knew nothing of either exercise or muscles. Had I not been a fast talker, three little girls would have missed out on a wonderful experience. I told the mothers that what I intended to teach was a form of dance. To be sure, it was dance, but had they known very much about real dance they would have known that *dance* is *exercise* and makes *muscles*. Of course if they had known anything about muscles they would also have known that they are terribly important and that anything that encourages them is helpful.

The next "word hurdle" appeared when boys started joining the group. The wild running and jumping, the exciting tumbling, and the simple equipment were complete joy, but what would have happened had I told *their* mothers I was teaching "dance"? The boys would not have been allowed to come. What, then, could I call what I was doing? I looked around for a word that could mean anything, everything, or virtually nothing, and came up with *conditioning*. For years hundreds of Westchester children learned to dance, to tumble, to ski, to climb, to create, and to perform—all under the ambiguous cover of *conditioning*. By the time the boys found out they were "dancing," they were so strong, so athletic, so well built, and so delighted with what they were doing that it didn't matter. If you can train your son in the skills contained in this book, it won't matter in the least if he can move like Gene Kelly or Fred Astaire. No one is going to challenge the star athlete; it wouldn't make sense. The sooner you start, the further you will get; but don't show him the pictures of Anne taking her first lesson in this chapter; he won't be able to imagine himself doing things demonstrated by a *girl*. *You* will have to learn the "steps" you intend to teach and then pass them on. Remember to use just a few minutes of these postures in each class. *They are for the practice of controlling form.* Little by little you will find the control extended to the exercises earlier in the book. Backs will straighten, legs extend fully, toes point, heads come up, hands relax—and movements will begin to look "finished."

MUSIC

If you have a trained ear, you will have no difficulty finding the music that goes with the action, but if you must start more or less from the beginning, look up records or tapes by Leroy Anderson. He isn't very pop, but then neither are Kabalevsky or Mozart. Both have written music that makes little hearts beat faster and toes point harder. The Gayne Ballet is especially exciting when it comes to floor progressions and the Russian Series. Try out various music on yourself. If *you* feel like dancing, so will the children.

CLOTHING

The same applies to "dance" as to "exercise": You want to be able to *see* what the body is doing. Also, you want the little dancers to *feel* like dancers. Today leotards are a part of every child's wardrobe; they even have tights for babies. Your dancers may want to wear tights with their leotards—fine, so long as they also wear ballet shoes. Tights with feet are arm breakers.

BALLET SHOES

Ballet shoes are to ballet what baseball shoes are to baseball, football shoes to football, tennis shoes to tennis, and golf shoes to golf. They are part of the act. They are, however, different in one respect: They are not really essential at the start, and even suggesting them for boys would be a bad idea. Wait until they are used to the whole idea before asking them to defend their new activity against the ignorance and prejudices of classmates and even uninformed adult relatives. If the floor you must work on is such that some form of protection is necessary, use the foot coverings worn by gymnasts. There is no stigma attached to them.

A MIRROR

If you can add a full-length mirror to your equipment, you will increase the speed with which good form becomes a part of each child ... and you. It is difficult to know what the body is doing when it isn't being watched by its owner. That's why posture is bad generally. People don't *know* what they look like, walk like, or dance like. In addition, there are small muscle spasms throughout the body that interfere with one or another muscle's proper function. You will read about that in the chapter on Myotherapy. For now just know that you need to *see*.

"I CAN'T DANCE ... I NEVER HAVE"

Well, if that's the case with *you*, it's time you started. Look first at the pictures of the teacher and take your cues from them. You needn't *look* like her, and your children needn't look like the little girl. Those are models; learn from them.

One thing more: There's no reason you can't go to dancing school *now*. One of the positive things to come out of the "fitness boom" is that people can go to classes and not feel out of place.

PREPARATION FOR DANCE

Ballet is certainly not the be-all and end-all of dance, but it is one of the best disciplines we have. There is only one way to do a plié and have it right. There are five foot positions, and they are either right or wrong. There are arm positions and ways in which leaps and turns are done. You have something to go by that doesn't change with the mood of the century. Those things are basic to ballet. They are like the multiplication tables: Three times three can only make nine, not anything else. If you go to art school anywhere, you will be taught the basics of three primary colors and you go on from there.

For many years now we have followed the progressive line. "Don't tamper with his or her creativity." Nonsense! The creativity comes *after* the discipline and the tools. Even Michelangelo went to school! So did Pavlova. Ballet *and* the preparation for ballet are both disciplines. The preparation makes the demanding work of ballet easier and gives the little dancer a passing acquaintance with the art. That prevents the destructive business of being the klutz in the class. Being the star doesn't guarantee a dancer (he or she may prefer the violin or painting in oils ten years down the line), but the *feel* of dance will be there.

The violin will sing with more understanding, the oils will have a wonderful rhythm, and the body will *know* things about itself that are denied the nondancer. Make no mistake, whatever the bent of the dancer later on in life, the little dancer keeps dancing, whirling, twirling, and floating in a lovely world no one who hasn't danced can enter. Dance was man's first art form and, like the song coming from a lovely throat, an art produced by the body, which is its own instrument. Whatever is learned young is retained. Let the children sing and dance. Give them those two incomparable gifts.

How often have you heard someone say to you, "Stand up"? How often have you wanted to say it to a little child. When you say it, the child will do her best to comply and will think she is succeeding. Some will push their shoulders back, some hike them up. Some poke their heads forward, and some who have had a little gymnastics training or have watched gymnasts on TV will arch into a swayback like this little girl. To begin with, there is nothing the matter with this little body except a bad habit, which can be trained out. She even has the strength required to stand the way her teacher stands, with a straight back. Her teacher, too, is a gymnast, but an aware one. If your little one has a swayback, do the posture exercises. Swaybacks on little children look cute. On adults they look awful and cause back pain. Children should be *able* to arch their backs, but have enough strength and discipline to do it only when a stunt calls for it, as in Back Bends or Walk-Overs.

Check to see that the child can carry the arms back and the chest up. If not, or if the head pokes forward, check his

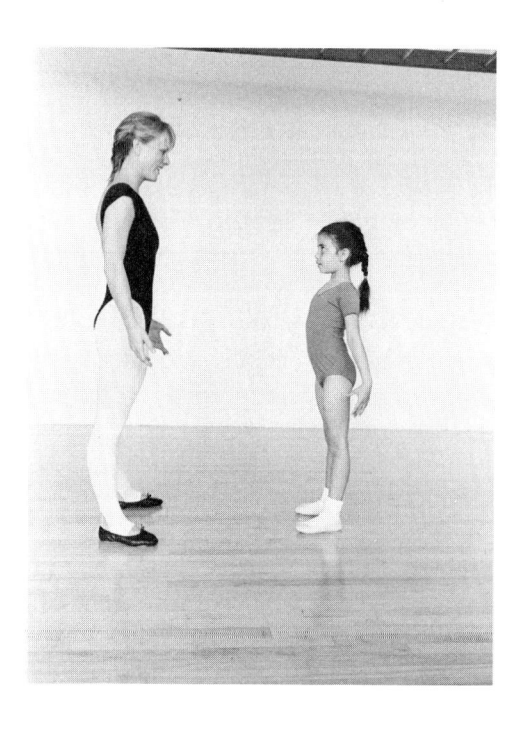

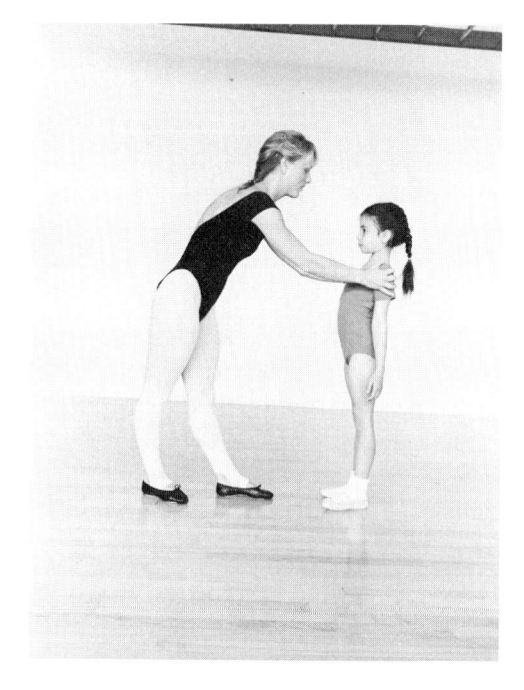

Dance

or her posture for round back. Foreshortened muscles in the chest may be pulling the shoulders, arms, and head forward.

Give the children the *feel* of standing straight. Begin your class with everyone trying to stand straight with backs straight and flat abdominal muscles, shoulders back, and heads on straight. *Watch!* If one has a high shoulder, a tipped head, pigeon toes, turned-out feet, a swayback, a round back, a flat back, or a protruding abdomen, note it and use the exercises for everyone to fix the one who needs help *and prevent those same posture anomalies from developing in the others.*

260. SHOULDER TWIST

• *Hold the shoulders back for your small student in the* stand-up *position.*

• *Twist first left and then right, urging her to feel when they are right. This is where your mirror will help.*

• *Step back and do sixteen shoulder twists facing each other so that she can copy you. If you are a beginner, too, and find the student doing better than you are doing, say so and copy her. Children don't worry about better or worse,* not unless you compare them with another child, *especially a sibling.*

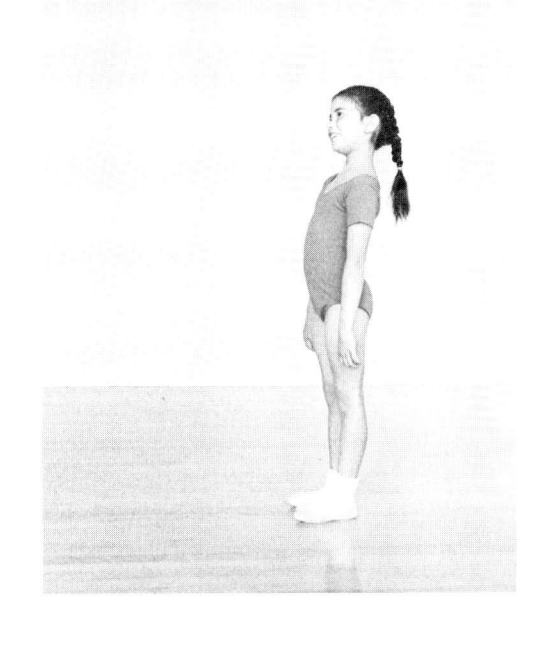

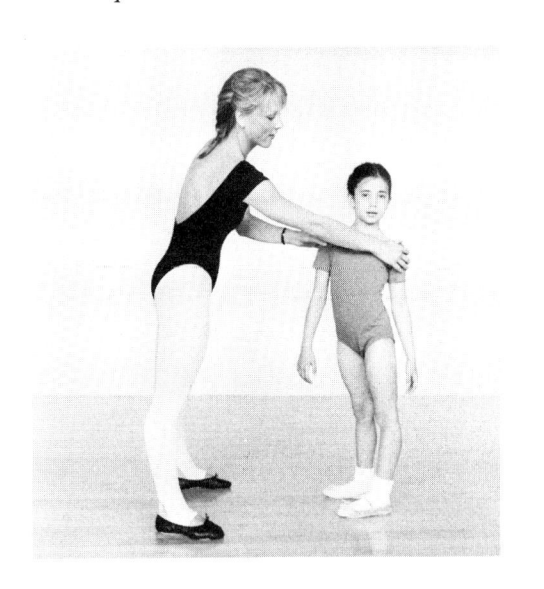

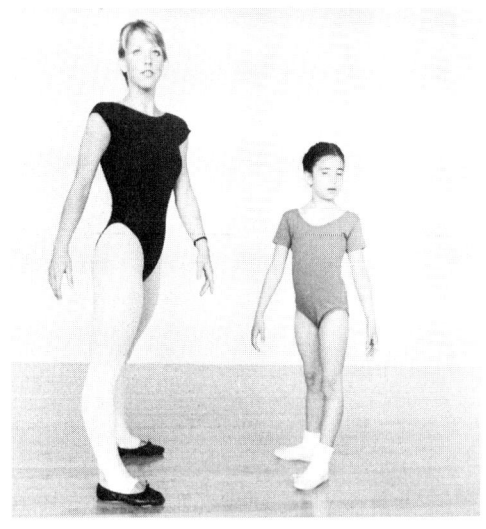

261. SHOULDER SHRUG

• *Many people* unconsciously *pull their shoulders up when* any *kind of stress. Learning to follow the teacher may be stressful for some. Do shoulder shrugs often.*
• *Pull the shoulders up to the ears and then press them down to make a very long neck. Hold the shoulders up for four counts and then down for four. Do eight.*

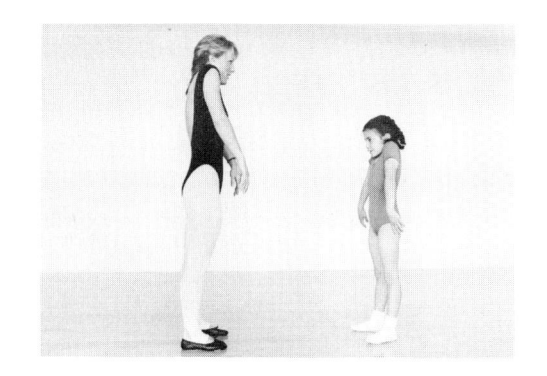

262. ALTERNATE SHOULDER SHRUG

• *Pull one shoulder up at a time* while you push the other down. *Everyone can pull* up. *Stress the press* down.

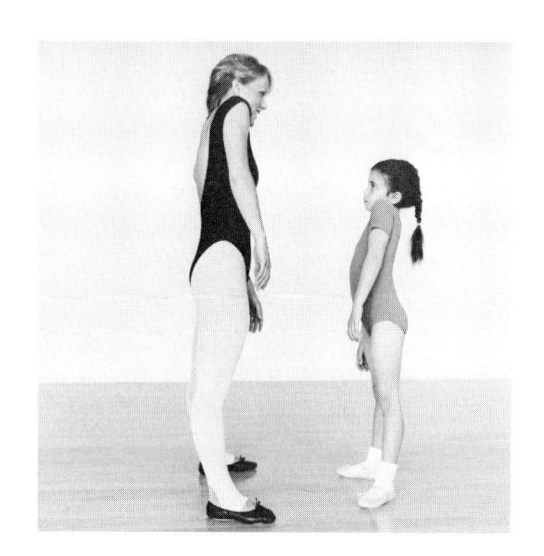

263. ROUND DOWN AND PULL UP

• *Start with the head and shoulders drooping. When this little girl was told to "droop," she rounded her back just fine and let her legs bend slightly, but she forgot to let go in her neck. That's the kind of thing you look for. Suggest that you both pretend to be very tired. The head will go down at once.*
• *From the droop, pull up into a straight stand.*
• *Shrug the shoulders hard and press the shoulders back as you lower them to a straight stand. Do four.*

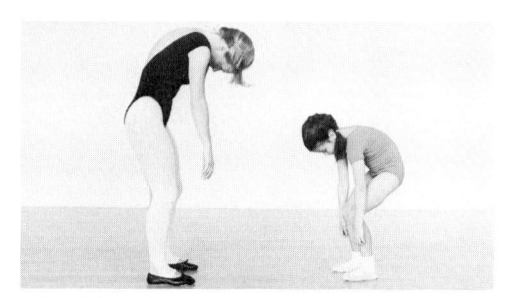

Dance

264. BACK STRETCH AND BEND

- *Start with the feet slightly apart and the knees straight.*
- *On* one, *lean down and grasp both ankles (if that is difficult, do exercise 6).*
- *On* two, *extend the arms backward and lift the head. The back should be flat and level.*
- *On* three, *bring both arms forward. It will be easier if you drop your head.*
- *On* four, *drop into a round-backed deep knee-bend. Grasp the ankles and repeat. Do four to slow music. If you are doing this exercise to music faster than you would like for this, just use several beats for each move.*

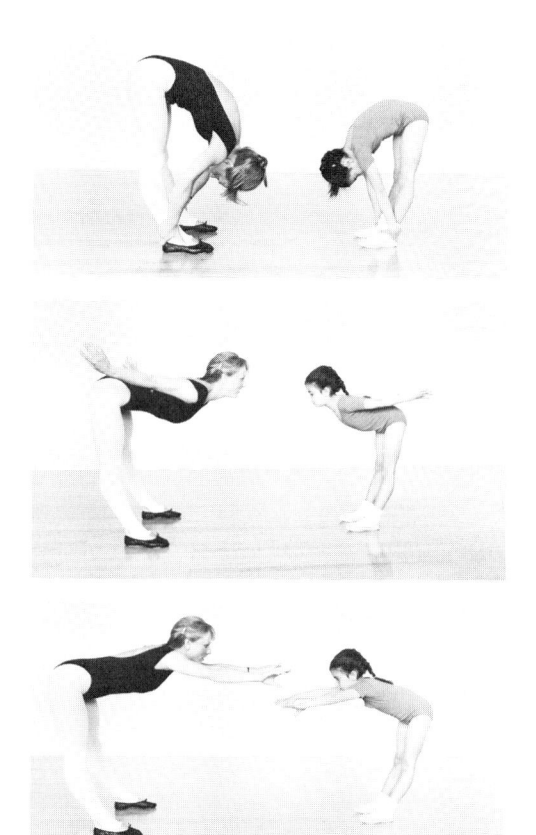

265. PULL-UP AND CIRCLE

- *After completing exercise 264, add the pull-up by slowly unrolling the back and straightening the knees.*

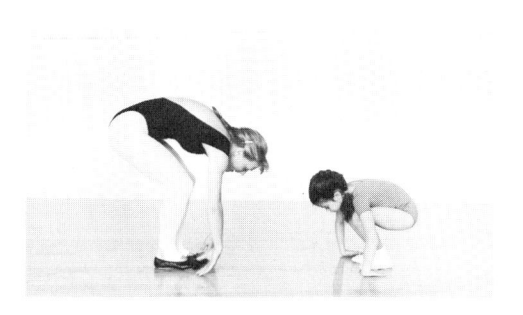

- *Twist the upper body as the arm circles overhead and the face is revealed.*
- *Stand straight, carrying the arm*

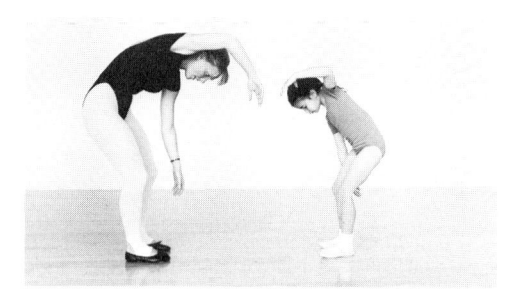

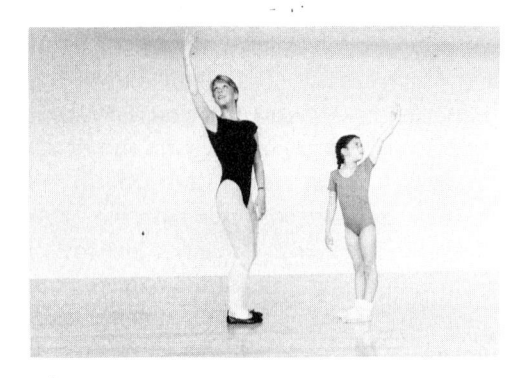

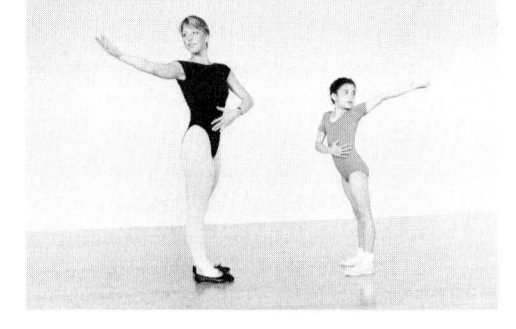

straight up and continuing the twist with the whole body.

- *The far arm is placed on the abdomen as the circling arm reaches back to the horizontal.*
- *Keeping the legs straight, arm out to the side and head up, bow low from the waist.*
- *Return to the standing position and drop again into the round-backed, bent-knee position. Repeat, using the other arm. Alternate for eight.*

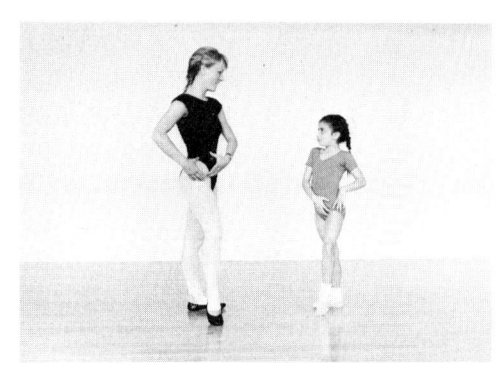

266. HIP ROTATION

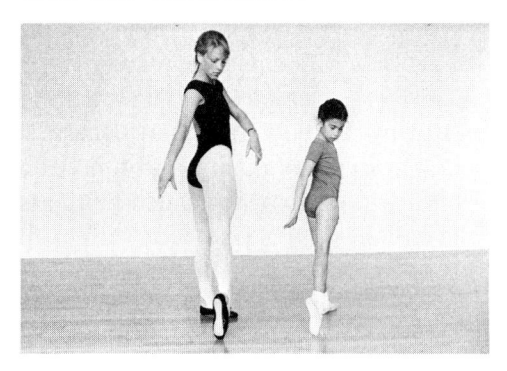

Control of the pelvis not only determines *how* the body will move, but also the effectiveness of both arms and legs.

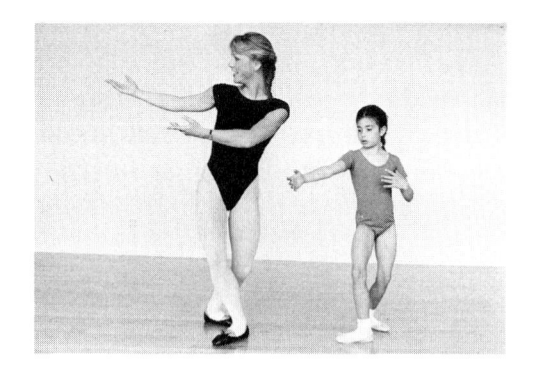

- *Place your hands at the very top of your thigh where the rotation can be felt as the leg turns in and out.*

Dance

- Turn the leg in as far as possible, touching only the toe of the rotating inward leg. At the same time lift the hip.

- Rotate the same leg outward, stepping down on the whole foot, which is turned out as far as possible. Bend both knees slightly.

267. LEG ROTATION ONLY

- Hold hands with your partner or hold on to the barre. Turn one bent leg in as far as possible, touching only with the toe.
- Turn the leg out while keeping the knee bent and touching only with the toe. Do eight to a side for a set. Do three sets.

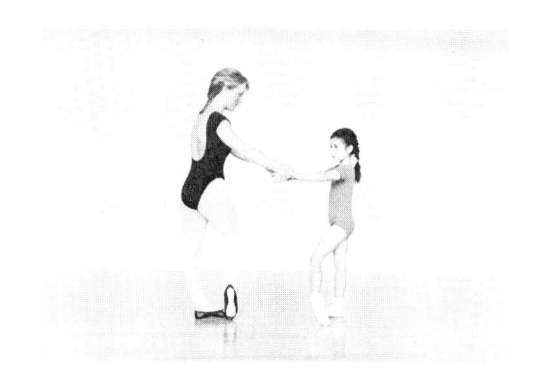

268. RAISED-LEG ROTATION

- Holding on to a person or to the barre, raise one leg and rotate the leg and hip inward, then outward. Do eight for a set. Do three sets.

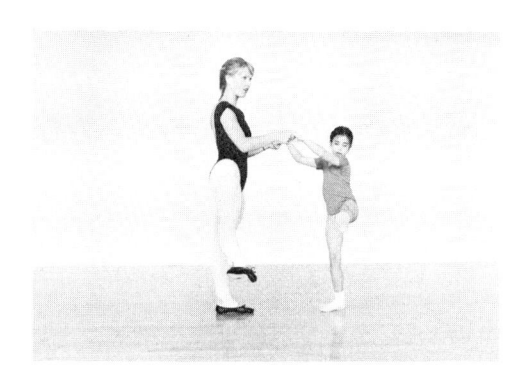

269. FLAT FOOT TO HALF TOE

Many older people lose the ability to go up onto a full half toe, in which the weight is supported by the toes and the ball of the foot. A well-developed foot can bend just behind the toes and the instep to make a straight line from bend to hip. This ability should be developed and protected with exercise.

- *Kneel down and place one foot in front of you with entire sole flat on the floor.*
- *Press down on the toes to keep them and the ball of the foot connected to the floor. Raise the heel. Repeat often enough to show the child what you mean by half toe.*

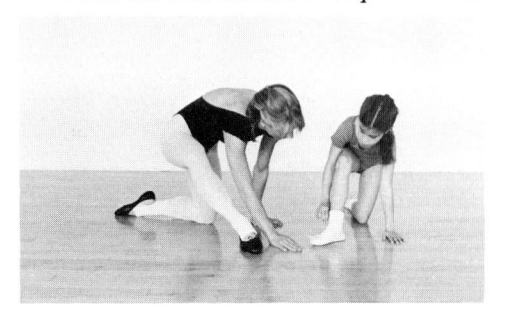

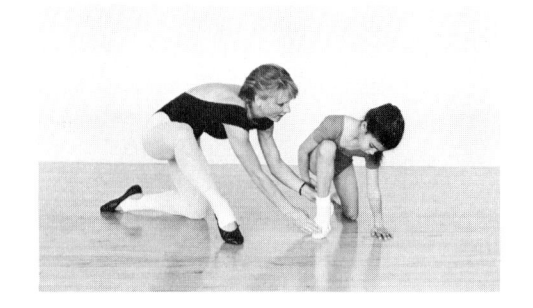

270. STANDING HALF TOE TO POINT

- *Stand on one leg and touch the point of the working leg to the floor.*
- *Use only enough weight to flatten the toes and touch. Alternate legs.*

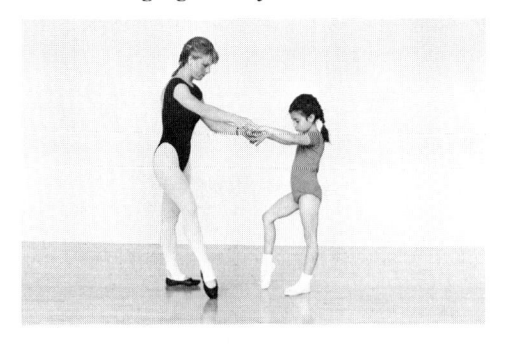

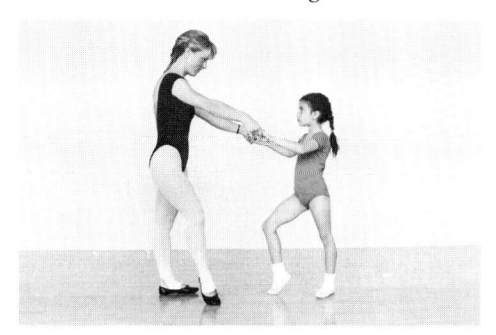

271. BENT-KNEE TOE RISE

- *Using partners or the barre for balance, start with the knees slightly bent and the heels flat. Rise to the half toe but do not let the head level change at all.* This will not only bend the foot, as in exercise 269, it will force the knees over the feet to further stretch the foot muscles. Do eight.

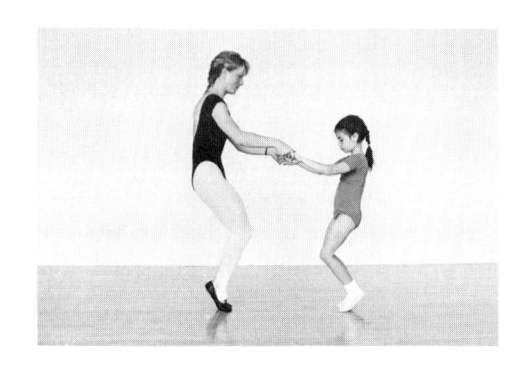

Dance

272. TURNOUT

Turnout is as important for ballet as a good shoulder is for a baseball pitcher. Turnout begins in the feet and ends in the pelvis. *A good foot turnout depends on the pelvic turnout.*

• *Stand with the feet facing forward as if ready for a march. Bend the knees slightly.*
• *Place both hands on the tops of your thighs with the fingers facing in.*
• *As you turn both feet outward to make a "fishtail,"* feel *the thighs turn outward.*
• *Press outward on the child's thighs, turning the knees outward. This will* feel *funny and look even funnier unless the pelvis is tilted under, which is harder to teach than you might think. Use pelvic tilts (exercises 19 and 38) for preparation.*

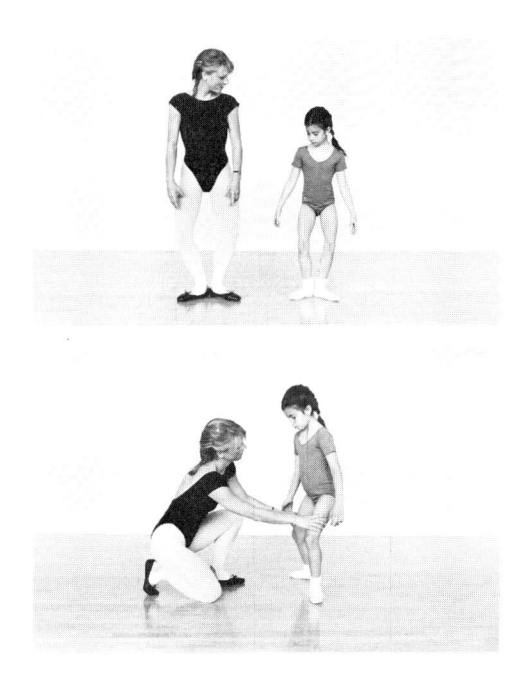

This is the point at which many ballet classes founder. The children are urged to "turn out," but no attention is paid to what the pelvis is doing. What it is often doing is poking out back to accentuate a swayback. From the start, *watch!* See that the pelvis is tucked under and use the Spine-Down Stretch (exercise 2) to strengthen the psoas.

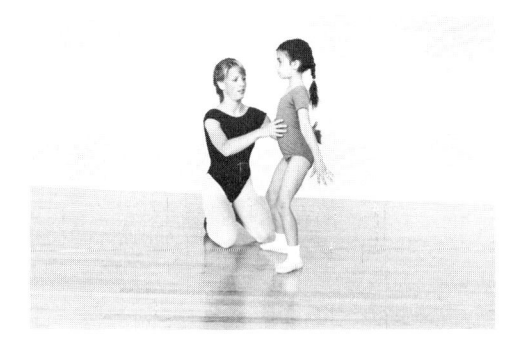

---

273. PLIÉ

When you were doing warm-ups right at the start of the program, you learned to cover your feet with your knees (see exercise 14). That is what you must do in pliés. If toes are sticking out to the outsides of your thighs, you are *pronating*. That really means using your feet and legs incorrectly, for whatever reason.

• *Place the heels together and bend the knees a little.*
• *Straighten both legs and tighten all the muscles in the legs, back, and abdomen. Do eight.*

274. PLIÉ, SIDE

• *Start as in Exercise 273.*
• *Take a step to one side and repeat eight pliés.*

275. PLIÉ, FRONT

• *Start as before and advance one foot about three inches forward.*
• *Repeat eight pliés in this position. Do not twist your hips to make the exercise easier.*

• *Return to the original position and advance the other foot. Repeat the eight pliés with the other foot.*
• *Be sure to keep the hips tucked under.*

276. HEEL-TO-INSTEP PLIÉ

• *With both feet turned out, place the heel of one foot against the instep of the other foot. Do eight pliés and change feet for eight more. While you are tucking the pelvis under and keeping the carriage straight, the knees may forget to cover the toes. This will put strain on the knee. When the legs are strong enough (and they will be if you use the exercises and floor progressions in the earlier part of the book), you will be ready to do the Grand Plié—safely.*

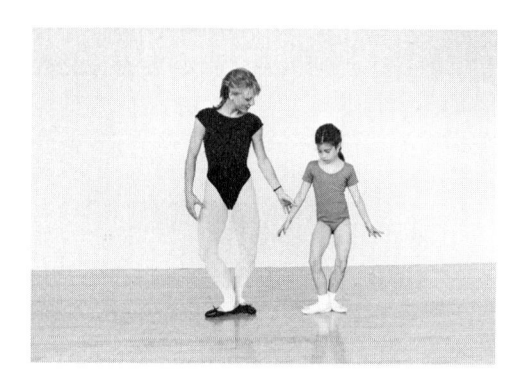

Dance

277. GRAND PLIÉ

- *Start with the feet in a "fishtail." Go into a slow half knee-bend. If that feels comfortable, continue into a full knee-bend with the knees well opened. Success will depend not only on leg strength but on crotch flexibility (see exercise 54).*
- *Start with four and work up to eight, to be done at the end of the foregoing plié series.*

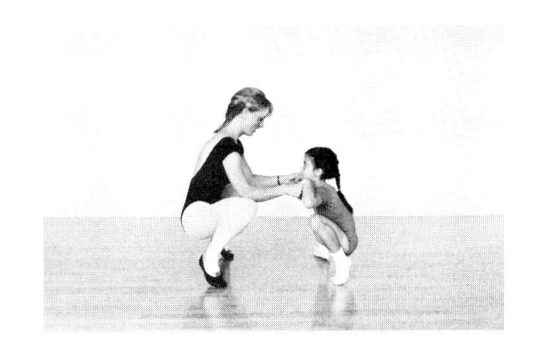

278. JUMPS

The opposite of down is up. As the legs strengthen with bends, they should find jumping easier and easier, higher and higher. Every sport demands different things of the body, and gymnastics demand that the jumps and takeoffs be done from the straight-forward foot. Dance demands the more graceful "fishtail." It is easier to provide both directions for young feet than for older ones.

- *Support the first jumps so that the little person feels what it is like to be up there and straight out.*
- *As soon as you can, after the pliés have trained the feet into the "fishtail turnout," work for pointed toes at the top of the jump, then "fishtail" pointed toes.*

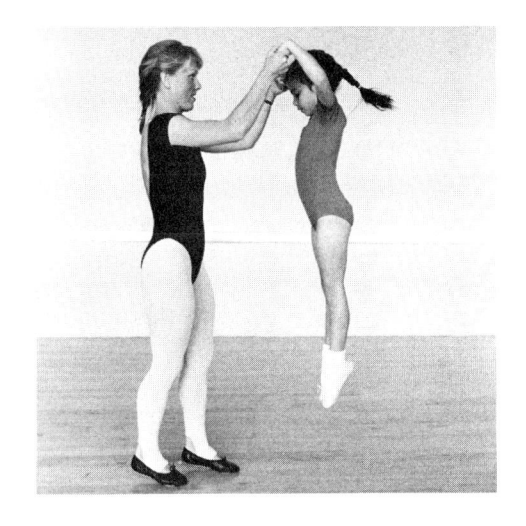

- *The landing should be soft, landing on the half toe and lowering to the heels without a jar. Try for relaxed shoulders and arms. Start with four.*

THE BARRE

We already have some familiarity with this piece of equipment, which also served as our pipe. It can be used as a barre by resting it on two sawhorses or two sets of stairs. You may prefer the doorway gym. It depends on the number of children you are working with.

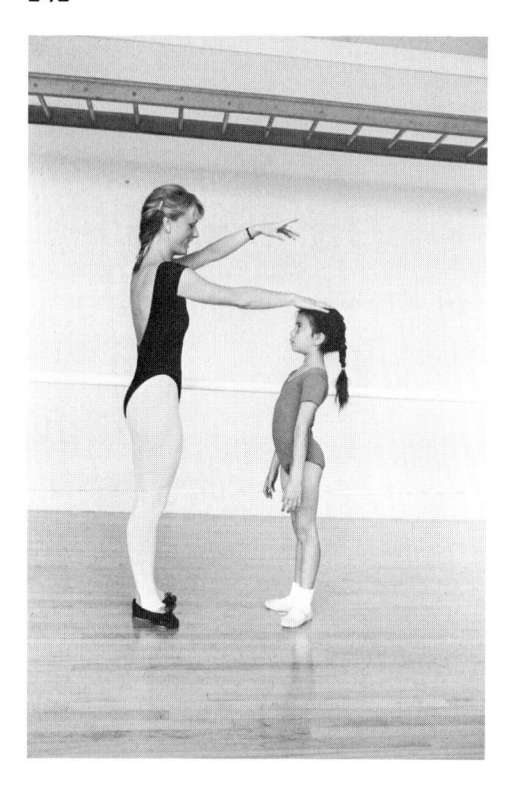

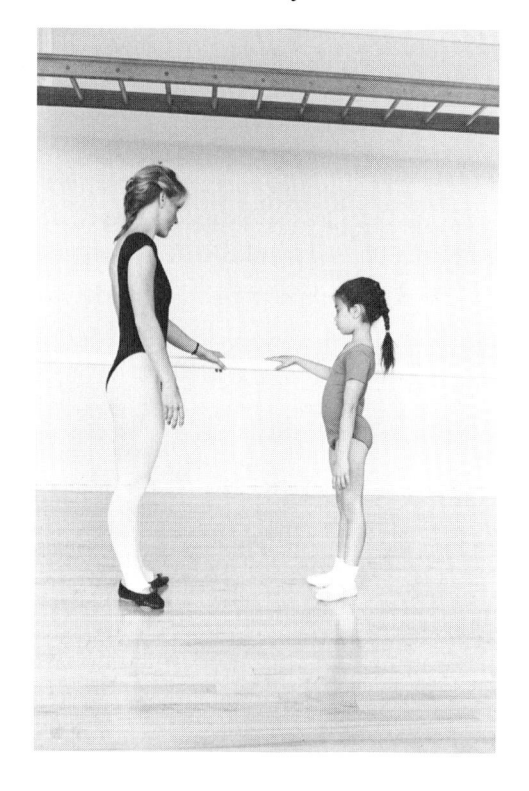

Barres are also easy to make of lighter pipes. Any good book on ballet should provide you with measurements. If you plan to go further than preparation for ballet, you will need a couple of good books, and I'd suggest a series of classes. You don't need to shine; just learn the basics.

Before you start with the barre, get across some helpful ideas to the children. Tell them to pretend there is a string running up through the body that comes out the top of the head like those on marionettes. While the barre is there to help with balance, it's really the string tied to the ceiling that keeps the child standing straight. They must *feel* and *think* tall . . . and they must do it all the time.

The barre is approached with a light touch, not a desperate clutch. The *legs* do the real supporting, and although the body is curved and seems to be both light and relaxed, it is covered with muscles that become as strong as steel bands. They don't *look* like steel bands; think of the beautiful little gymnasts. They don't *feel* like steel bands; a relaxed muscle is as soft as butter. They are responsible for the success of the child—with the help of the *watchful* teacher. A child who sags or leans at the barre is doing badly—and that is the teacher's fault.

Dance

279. ARM CIRCLE

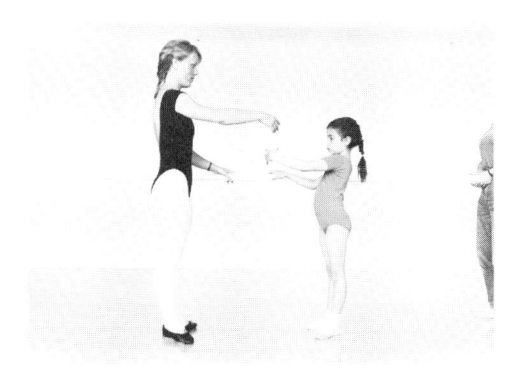

- *Start with the toes in the "fishtail," the body straight, and one hand resting* lightly *on the barre. The free hand is where the focus should be.*
- *Hold the arm out in front before you begin the exercise and pretend it is holding an orange.*
- *Turn the hand over and, without moving the fingers from the holding position, lower the arm to the side.*
- *With the hand* in that relaxed state, *bring it forward to barre level.*
- *Carry the arm up overhead and out to the side. As the hand reaches shoulder level, turn it palm down without tightening any of the fingers.*

Remember, every dancer carries the scars from the first teaching forever. If you put fancy hands to work, hands like those of the proverbial "lady" drinking tea with the "little finger well out," that dreadful affectation will last, at least in the mind, forever. Valuable energy will be spent undoing what should never have been taught in the first place.

- *Bring the hand to the side. Do dozens of such arm circles with both arms before going on to the next step.*

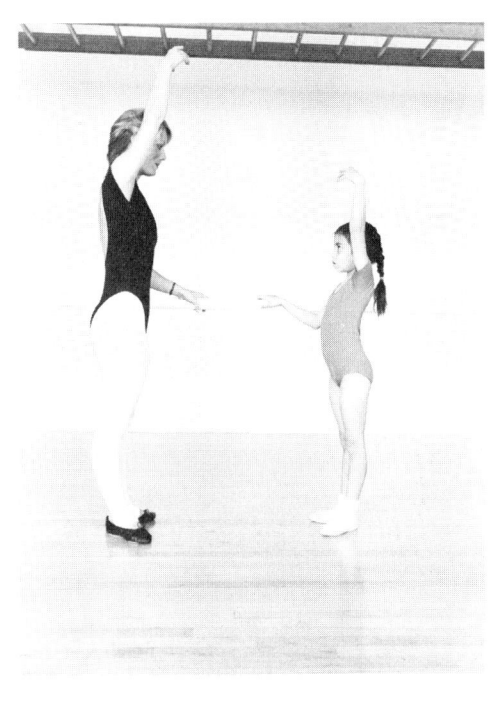

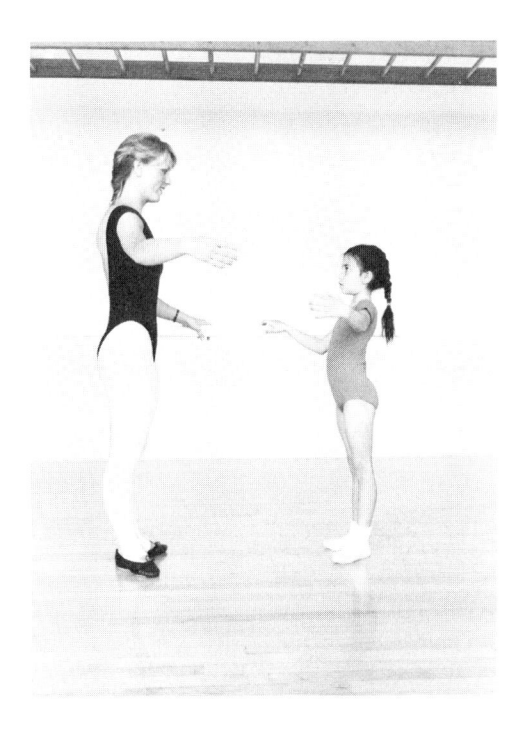

280. FORWARD POINT AND RETRACT

- *Check to see that the feet are "fishtailed" and, with one hand resting lightly on the barre, place the weight on the leg next to the barre.*

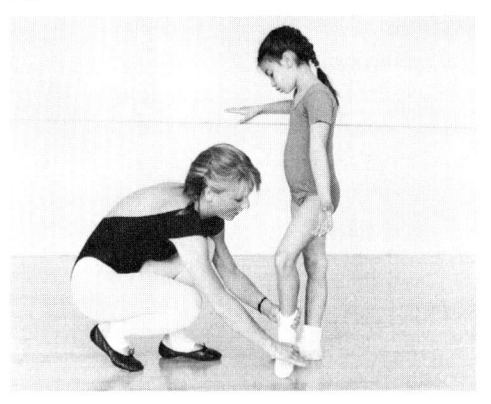

- *Brush the foot near the barre forward and point the toe hard.*
- *Return to the "fishtail." Do eight to a side and alternate for four sets.*

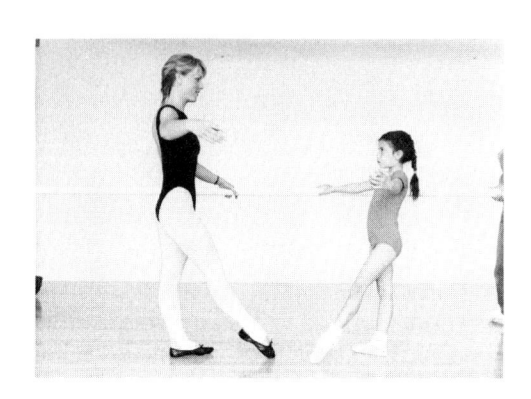

281. SIDE POINT AND RETRACT

Before you begin, be sure the little foot knows what you mean by "turn out," or "place your left heel at your right instep."

Sloppy performance is born with the help or laziness of the teacher. No foot, arm, hand, leg, head, tummy, or back should be allowed to get away with anything. It is at the beginning that good habits are born. If one of the children can't keep up, that child isn't ready. Don't overlook it—fix it. If you produce a few "stars" and a bunch of dancer-slobs, you will be known for the dancer-slobs. Sometimes it means telling a mother that this little one should stay with (or go into) exercise classes until ready for the more advanced work.

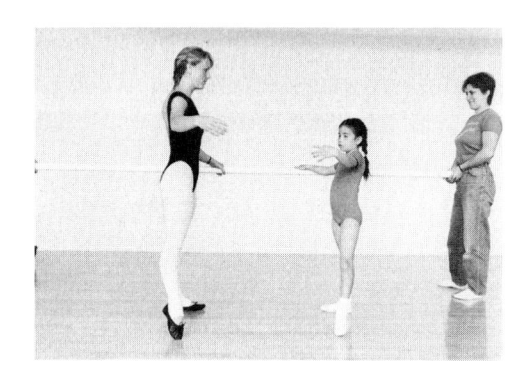

- *Do the same pointing as you did forward, but to the side. That doesn't mean almost to the side, it means to the exact angle.*
- *Turn and repeat with the other foot.*

282. BACK POINT AND RETRACT

• *Do the same to the back. Eight to a side equals one set. Do three. Be sure that the work is done to a beat. If it's too slow, it will be boring, and if it's too fast, it will be sloppy for a long time. These steps are like the notes of the pieces being learned by the young musician; make no mistakes as you play slowly and you will eventually increase speed.*

283. BENT-KNEE SIDE EXTENSION

• *Start in the "fishtail" position with the free arm out to the side.*
• *Bend the inside knee as you would in a plié and extend the outside foot to the side. Check for relaxed hand and arm, no swayback, and head up. Keep reminding the child to* stand tall.
• *Retract to "fishtail" and do eight to a side for a set. Do three.*

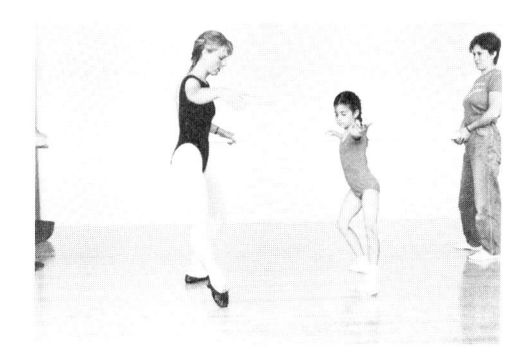

284. BENT-KNEE FORWARD EXTENSION

• *Do the exact same thing with the standing knee and extend the free leg forward. Keep the arm to the side. Do three sets.*

285. BENT-KNEE BACK EXTENSION

• *Do the same exercise to the back. Watch for the swayback. Do three sets.*

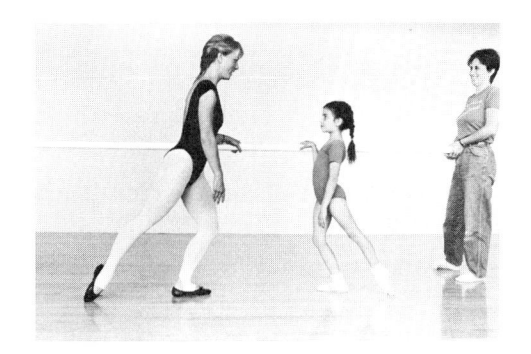

286. TOE-RISE EXTENSION

• *Just as you did jumps* up *after knee-bends* down, *do a toe rise from the "fishtail." Extend the foot away from the barre as far as you can with toe pointed* hard. *This will work the rising foot for strength and the extending ankle for flexibility.*
• *Do eight to a side for a set. Do three sets.*

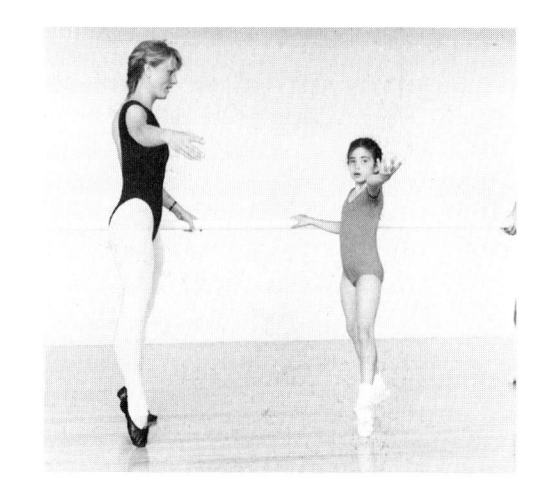

287. RAISED-KNEE EXTENSION

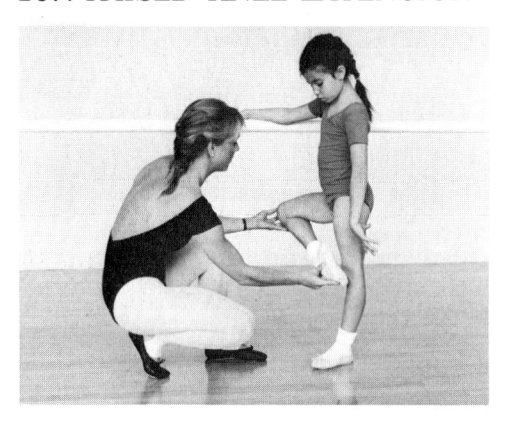

• Prepare by placing the foot where it should go. *The more you give children the feel of the foot or arm when they are where they are supposed to be, the better.*
• Lift the knee with the knee well turned out.
• Maintain the turnout as the leg is extended.
• Retract and replace the foot on the floor. Do eight with each leg for a set. Do three sets.

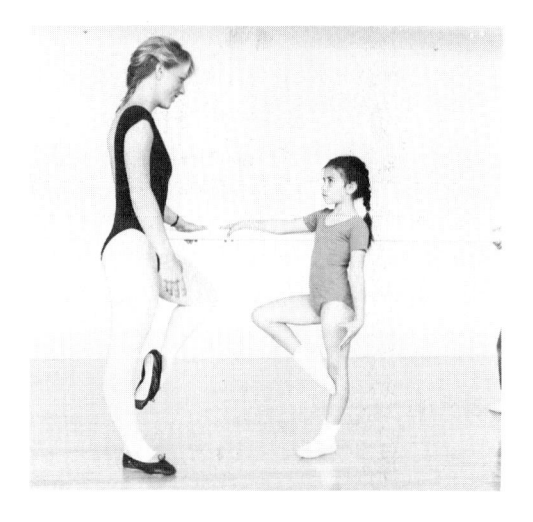

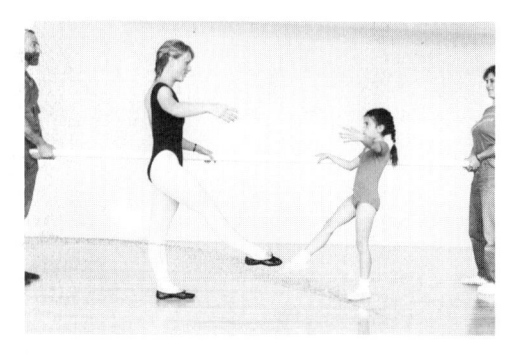

Dance

288. RAISED-SIDE EXTENSION

• *When you see a foot turned wrong, stop and fix it.*

• *Raise the free leg and bring the foot close to the standing leg, toe pointed and knee turned out.*

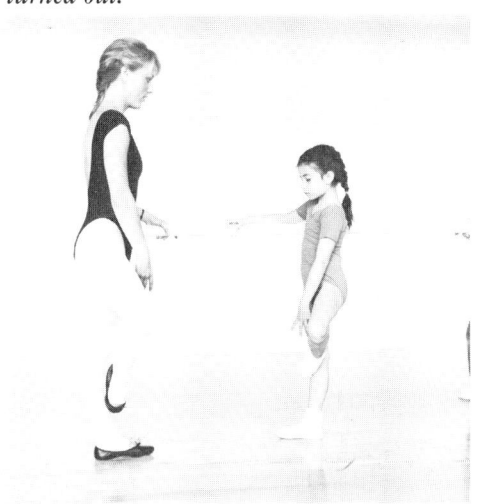

• *Holding that bent-knee position, extend, and retract the leg.*

• *Return to the starting position and do eight to each side for a set. Do three sets.*

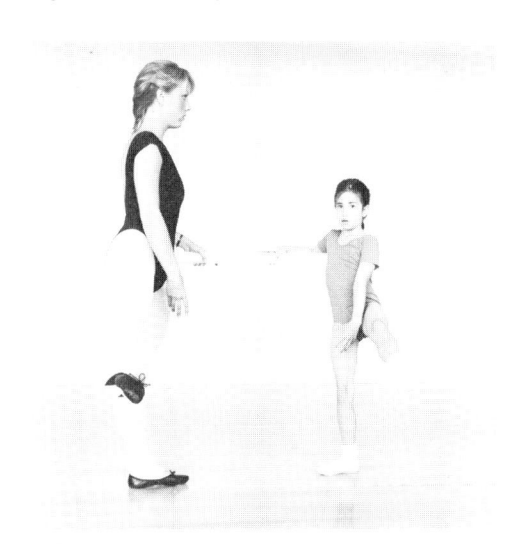

289. BACK EXTENSION WITH LIFT

You have already done two kinds of back extensions *often*. The leg should know how to move back correctly, and the foot knows about turnout. The next step should be taken in two phases. At each class, you should assist each child to lift the turned-out leg as high as possible. That is phase one. During that time nobody does phase two.

• *Phase two: Extend the leg* and *without assistance, lift no higher than 2 inches. Each week go a little higher, but not so high as to change the straight stance. If the leg height causes a forward lean,* it has gone too far for the condition of the body. *Use the exercises in this book to improve both the general condition of the children's bodies and also the specific needs.*

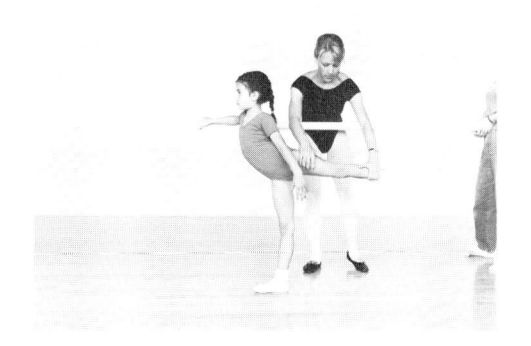

290. THE BOW

Finish the ballet practice session with the proper ending for a performance.

  • *Stand on the left leg, right foot pointed to the side and arms outstretched.*
  • *Draw the right foot in and place the full weight on it as you point the left foot to the side.*
  • *Finish by crossing the left foot behind the right and extending the left arm to the side and slightly back. The right hand, palm up, comes to the chest. Bend forward from the hips.*

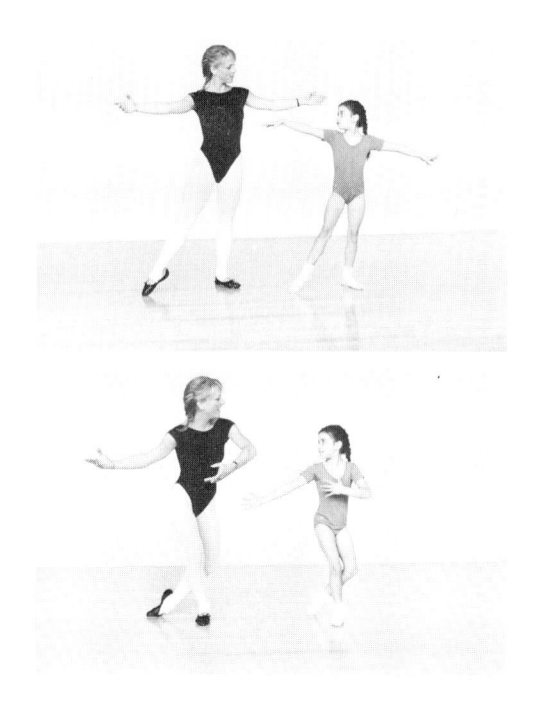

It doesn't matter whether your class is all girls, all boys, or a mix. It doesn't matter whether your class is made up of your own children only. *All* children deserve the joy of watching good ballet. There is a lot of the other kind around, and a lot of it is to be seen at local recitals. That's all right. Children love to watch each other. . . . but provide the real thing with either home video or a trip to the big city. If foreign dance companies come to perform, take the children to see them. Don't wonder if they are too young. If they are six, they're old enough.

CHAPTER NINETEEN
TENNIS

As in every other sport requiring skill—and they all do—tennis needs a foundation. The game does not begin on the court or with the purchase of equipment. *Long, long before the game comes the body.* It isn't just the tennis racket that makes the winning shot; it's the strong hand, firm wrist, well-developed arm, flexible shoulders and back, the powerful hips and legs, the stamina, and the self-discipline. *These are the things that can be developed years before the tennis bug bites.*

Awhile ago in Sydney, Australia, I spent a month working on some TV shows. Each morning on my way to the studio I passed young Australians going to school. Boys and girls alike, singly or in groups, they carried the inevitable book bag, but they also carried their tennis rackets—and fine, well-prepared bodies carried the whole business. Whatever other sport was a part of their school days, tennis would be a part of their lives. Always they would possess a release from the tensions of life, an outlet for the spirit of competition, a chance to get away from "daily" living, which does have an unpleasant way sometimes of seeming very "daily" indeed.

There is something else about tennis: like skiing, boating, hiking, cycling, and other similar activities, tennis is a sport for the individual sports person. Who is that person? He is the person who really doesn't get a big bang out of team sports like baseball, basketball, and football. It isn't that he is not athletic. He simply prefers a different sort of outlet. If you make a survey of your friends, you will find that doctors, physicists, and scientists in general come under the heading of individual sports type. Rarely do you find them out for the team, but the cliffs are covered with their ropes and pitons; the spring floods find them shooting rapids; they appear on the trails in summer; and they like tennis. The outgoing, gregarious salesman, company president, or insurance man usually has a major sports letter tucked away somewhere. This, incidentally, is one of the reasons why American doctors are at such a disadvantage when it comes to understanding physical fitness. Never avid athletes in schools that provided only the three bigs—baseball, basketball, and football—they missed out on close association with physical activities. If the drive is stifled owing to lack of opportunity, the skill is not developed when the body is at its young, learning best. If the body is not developed, the skill is limited, and when ability is poor, satisfaction is not sufficient to overcome inertia. The nonathlete does even less in college, and as work piles up, the postgraduate student finds other outlets. He arrives at full adulthood minus one of the most important assets for living—a good body and the means of keeping it in good condition.

The children of tennis players almost always play tennis. That is to be expected. But what of the others, the nonvarsity boys and the thousands of girls for whom the schools provide nothing at all? Perhaps tennis is the answer. You won't know unless you try, so try right—don't leave it to chance.

When you start your exercise and fitness program with your own children, with your friend's children, or as a teacher in school, think *sports*. *See* those little people in their parkas careening down the wintry slopes . . . perfectly. *See* them in their tennis whites out on sunlit courts putting in scorching serves and rallying happily with others just like them. *See* them on their horses, *see* them in their dance classes and on the stage as they present their art. *See* them *doing* what you feel is right for them to be doing. That's the beginning.

You need not be an ace tennis player to teach tennis the way you are going to teach it to young hopefuls because what you are really going to do is *prepare* their bodies for the sport. That last rarely "sells" a sport. There are, of course, children who can't wait to play. They are the ones with parents and older siblings who play. The instructor loves to see them coming, but they are the tip of the child-population iceberg. The ones underwater are the ones who know nothing of the game and don't care right now. They are the ones who will be given a racket in high school and told to get out there and learn . . . too late. Or they will meet a boy or a girl who plays and want to share . . . too late. Nobody wants to play with a dud, and the dud won't try to make up a foursome more than once.

It's so terribly embarrassing at a time when just about anything not absolutely perfect is embarrassing.

So how do we prepare little people for this wonderful pastime?

Ask yourself what really good tennis players have that tennis needs: speed; endurance; good knees so that they can get down for the low balls; a strong arm, wrist, hand, and shoulder. They need good peripheral vision and they need reflexes and courage for the net. Is your program going to give the children these things? Yes, especially if you pattern them exactly as I showed you how to do in tumbling.

The basics of tennis must be there before you need them.

1. YOU HAVE TO WATCH THE BALL. That means you have to be able to shift your eyes quickly from one object to another. So, for children you make a game of it.

291. EYE EXERCISES

Pick out four objects in the room (not too far apart) and give each a number. As you look at each one, say the number and the name, for example: "Table—one, picture—two, chair—three, lamp—four." Using a slow beat, look at each object in that sequence several times, at first naming them, then just saying the number in time to the music as you shift your eyes. Be sure you *center* your look on each object. After a bit, reverse your sequence so you start with the lamp and work backward to the table. Then skip every other one and jump from "one" to "three" to "two" to "four." Reverse that. When you can find each object with unwavering aim, use a faster beat. Use four different objects every day.

2. YOU HAVE TO BE ABLE TO KEEP A TIGHT GRIP ON THE RACKET. Put another way, it means being able to hold on tight.

- *Use the rope work starting on page 206.*
- *Make chinning part of every day and suggest to parents that they put a chinning bar in the bathroom doorway and that they stand by and* watch *as their children try to* improve. "Watch me, Mommy, watch me, Daddy" *will never again be the powerful trainer it is right now.*

3. YOU HAVE TO GET A "GROOVE" FOR LONG, SMOOTH STROKES.

The "groove" is the result of doing the same thing right, over and over, until there is no other way to do it.

THE FOREHAND

You will not need a tennis racket for this, although one could be used (with or without strings) for the older kids. For the little ones a Ping-Pong racket will do nicely. We use little paddles to which we attach long streamers to make arm exercises more fun. For "tennis" practice we fold up the streamers.

• *For the forehand (as well as every other stroke) you will need a strong wrist. For that you will need the weights on page 191 and the rope work on page 207.*
• *You will also need to be where the ball is, and that means speed. Practice the wind sprints on page 298.*

292. FOREHAND PATTERNING

• *You are going to stand in the middle of your room and pretend it is a tennis court. You* may *have trouble pretending, but the children will* see *a tennis court. They will also* see *a net, so in order to have them see it where it should be, you should run a piece of tape across part of the wall you face. Measure 35 inches from the floor for the correct height. Now you have a net to* think *the ball over. Don't treat this idea lightly. This is how Olympic athletes practice when they aren't in the gym:* They think themselves through their moves without a mistake. *comes to your* forehand. Watch! *The racket should move back and forth on a line somewhere between the waist and chest,* not in an arc, high at both ends and down in the center. Don't worry about affecting their swing later on. They will find their own best levels when they really play. What you are after here is swing and rhythm.
• *The music will be very important, and* a *slow* waltz seems to do the best job.
• *When you have shown the children what to do, start them swinging to the beat and then step back to correct.*

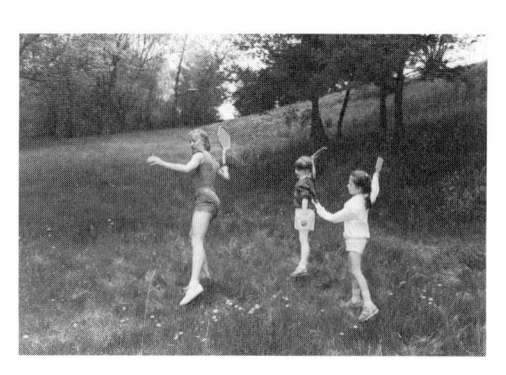

• *Stand with your left side toward the "net," your weight on your right foot, and your racket back, ready to take the ball as it*

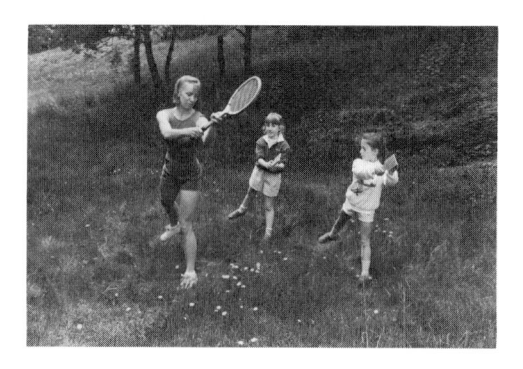

• *The stroke should end across the front of the body and, for the time being,* touch *the other hand,* but the back foot should not leave the ground. *(Both children have done so in this picture!) You want both feet grounded so that you can take off in any direction at a second's notice.*

• *When you have done several bars with the* forehand *move, go on to the backhand.*

To teach patterning for the forehand, you need to know something about it if you are not yourself a tennis player. Extremely important is the *preparation* for the stroke. The player shouldn't wait until he or she has run into position before getting the racket in motion for the swing. That's what the patterning does. It finds the place for the arm and the racket so that no thought is needed for the play. The mind says, "That thing is on my forehand side," and the patterned arm immediately pulls back at the right height. When that isn't patterned in, the player arrives at the spot and finds that the ball has also arrived. That leaves no time for a smooth swing. The result will be a hurried, jerky, incomplete stroke, with no power behind the ball.

Most people, when they begin the game, overrun the ball and end up with the racket handle in their ribs. It is far better to have run a little short and have to push your reach for the ball than to crowd it, have to change direction, strangle the swing, and cramp the stroke. One of the prime reasons for overrunning is not being sure of distance and speed. Use the running and wind sprints on page 248 and the floor progressions starting on page 107. The way to learn what your body can do is to train it.

THE BACKHAND

The backhand involves a conscious twist of the torso *before* the stroke. There is a twist in the forehand, too, but it comes *after* the ball has been hit and is just part of the follow-through. The exercise that loosens the waist muscles and permits an easy, full twist is the Waist Twist (exercise 9). It will also make the follow-through more fluid. If you happen to have a golfer in the house, it will do the same thing for both backswing and follow-through.

293. BACKHAND PATTERNING

• *Stand with your right side facing the "net."*
• *Pull the right arm across the body, ready to swing.*
• *The weight is on the left foot.*
• *Swing the weight onto the right foot as you carry the racket across on the same line as for the forehand.*
• *As soon as you have done these swings often enough to get a smooth rhythm and the racket on the desired line, add the head.*
• *As the racket swings back and the weight*

is transferred to the left foot, look over your right shoulder. *You want to know where the ball is coming from or you will overrun it.*

• *After you have added the head turn to the rhythm, keep using it when you practice.*

• *Remember, you are not playing tennis, you are preparing the body for the rhythm, the grooves, the power, and the flexibility tennis will require.*

• *The ability to turn the head freely is usually one of the pluses that come with youth—unless a whiplash accident* or an injury to the serving shoulder *puts a crimp in the right side of the neck. Many a backhand has become a liability due to inflexibility. If* you *are such a player, see the chapter on Myotherapy.*

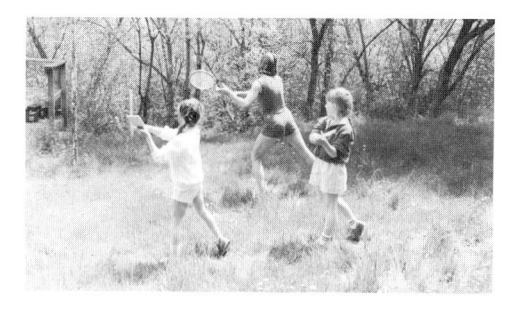

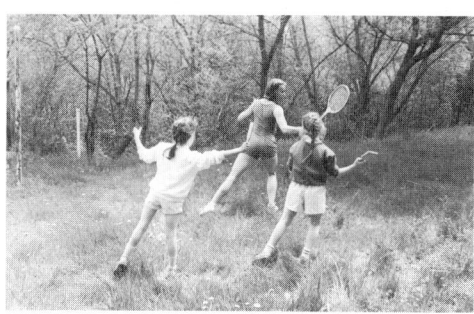

When a child learns to play an instrument, one of the first things a teacher impresses on that child is, "Move to the next note *fast and be ready for when the rhythm demands it. Don't take your time in between playing one note and the next.*" It's something like the army adage "Hurry up and wait." That's tennis, too. *Get there and be ready for anything.*

4. YOU MUST ALWAYS USE CORRECT FOOTWORK.

• *To pattern for either the forehand or the backhand, ask the children which foot should be somewhat ahead and which weighted in each instance.*

• *The answer for the right-handed player will be the left foot advanced and the left side toward the net. The exercises for the court are floor progressions, most particularly Side Skips (exercise 82).*

• *For the backhand, the right side is presented, so be sure to do many side skips to* both *sides.*

---

294. SIDE SLIDES

• *Stand with the right side facing the direction in which you intend to go. Step out right on the right foot and then* draw *the left after it until the feet are together.*

Tennis

• Repeat this action across the floor, doing it to both sides.

• After the form is learned, speed it up and you will have side slides. A side slide will permit you to close in on the ball and still keep the leading foot in front. There is nothing surer to lose the game than arriving at the right place at the right time but facing the ball straight on with two flat feet and your weight evenly plopped on both of them.

---

5. YOU HAVE TO HIT THROUGH THE BALL.

• *That means carrying the racket through the stroke* after *you have hit the ball. Why? Because the power you need must continue and not stop short. Most "backyard tennis" is made up of short pops that go nowhere because the players never learned to hit through* the ball. Tennis is like any other skill, made up of good habits carefully nurtured by a good instructor. A bad habit is like a missed stitch in an otherwise perfect sweater. It shows up all the time.

6. YOU HAVE TO BE ABLE TO FIND THE RIGHT LEVEL.

Tennis calls for action on many levels. Do your swings at knee level with the knees bent low enough so that the *stroke* is on that level and the racket doesn't scoop down while the arm and hand are up. This sort of action calls for excellent control of the knees. Do the Russian Series (pages 121–125).

7. YOUR WRIST SHOULD BE LOWER THAN THE HEAD OF THE RACKET.

When the children are doing well with their swings and the head of whatever they are using for a racket is held above their wrists, buy some lead wire. Wrapped around the racket (not the neck), it can be made to add a few ounces of weight at a time, and a few ounces is what you need, not pounds. That's where a lot of arm pain is developed. A racket that is too heavy for the arm wielding it will put *trigger points* into the arm, hand, shoulder, chest, and upper back muscles. As you will learn in the chapter on Myotherapy, trigger points are hypersensitive spots that get into muscles when the muscles are damaged, even a little. In tennis, injuries to little people can come back to plague the champion and lose him or her the match. No one will pin the shoulder pain on overwork of a given set of muscles at age nine.

8. YOU MUST WORK ON YOUR HANDS.

---

295. SHUFFLE PATTERN

• *In addition to hand strength and the ability to keep a tight hold on the racket, you need the ability to* shuffle *the racket quickly from the forehand to the backhand hold.*

- *Use a medium-slow beat for this exercise.*
- *Stand with your right foot facing the "net," your racket back and ready.*
- *Turn to the right so that your left foot takes a step forward and your right arm is drawn back, ready for a forehand stroke. In the middle of that turn you will have to rearrange the racket to accommodate the coming stroke.*
- *Each follow-through, however small, will give you the opportunity to do it. Do this across the room slowly and to the beat.*

---

9. YOU MUST DEVELOP YOUR FOOTWORK.

Feet not only get you to where the ball will be; they turn you in the necessary direction. Good footwork is as important to the tennis player as it is for the boxer and the dancer. The player with weak, inflexible feet is at a distinct disadvantage and will never reach full potential. That is true, too, for the person with the unattended long second toe. Read about that anomaly in the chapter on Myotherapy for yourself and then apply the principle to the children's feet. As long as they are barefoot, there is no need to worry, but once you put them into shoes (sneakers and ballet shoes are *shoes*, gymnastic slippers are not) you have a less than perfect foot.

All the floor progressions develop feet, as does ballet. In tennis you want to be able to get around with the feet apart a good deal of the time, so work particularly on Double Leg Jumps (exercise 73).

10. YOU NEED TO DEVELOP YOUR COURAGE.

Courage is not the same thing as lack of fear—that just might mean lack of good sense. Courage is what you have when you know full well what the dangers are but you feel sure you can keep your head and handle them. A preparation for courage is familiarization. If you have been exposed over and over again to a dragon who blows fire and smoke and yells at you—but never really hurts you—you lose the fear of him. You know he *could* step on you if you got in his way, but you are quite sure that you are faster than he is and you use your agility accordingly. When will your children (or you) be required to use *courage* in a tennis game? It will be at the net. So how do you develop this kind of courage?

DODGEBALL

Dodgeball is a game any age can play—and should. The game is usually played with two teams of twelve each. One team forms a circle, and the other goes inside that circle and tries to keep from being hit by a basketball that is thrown at them from the perimeter of the circle. As a conditioner, this game is a flop, be-

Tennis

cause the slower, less agile, and *less courageous* are hit at once and forced out of the game. They never get a chance to develop the very things they need—agility, reflexes, and courage. As those still in the center are narrowed down to the last few, the survivors are almost invariably those who *naturally* would be good at the net in tennis.

---

296. DODGEBALL FOR TENNIS

- *To make dodgeball work for our purpose, each person should go into the circle alone and the diameter of the circle should be made large enough to give the child a chance to get away from the ball in accordance with his or her ability. As the ability improves, the diameter can be reduced. Always remember that there are two kinds of fear. One kind gets the adrenaline flowing and makes miracles of performance happen. The other causes panic and often freezes the frightened person in the path of danger when getting out would mean taking a quick step left or right.*

297. SERVE PATTERN

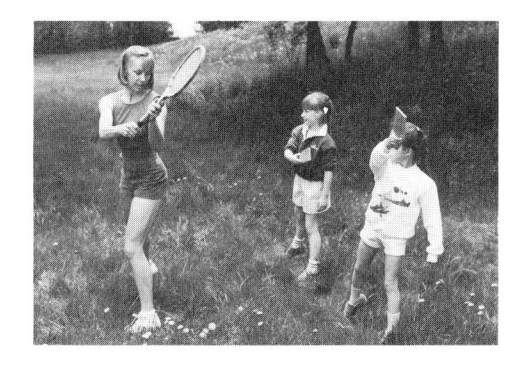

The serve is 50 percent of the game; the work done to pattern for it is important.

- *First, look down and see an imaginary line. It is the line you may not step over as you serve. Be sure the children "see" that line.*
- *Place the toes of the left foot just behind*

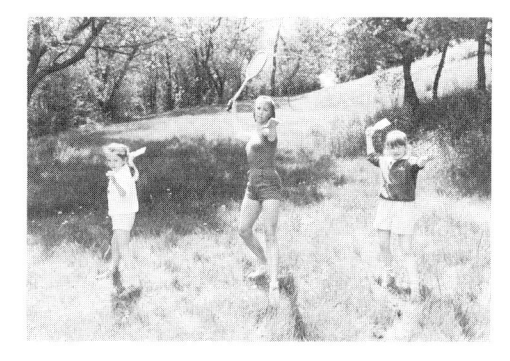

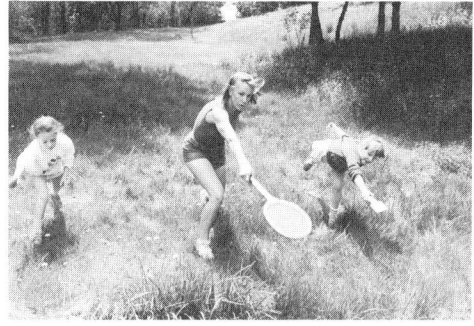

the line and thrust your racket out in front, one hand holding it and the other hand touching the neck as a steadier. That hand holds the imaginary ball. Make sure the children "see" and "feel" that ball.
- Drop both hands as you rock back onto the right foot.
- Do that about ten times, or until the swing is easy and rhythmical.
- Forget the racket hand and the racket for a while. With the left hand, toss the ball up a little in front of you and "see" it up there. Do that about ten times; then forget the left hand and the ball.
- Start from the beginning with the left foot on the imaginary line. The right hand, holding the racket, is out in front, balanced by the left.
- Now forget the left entirely and let the arms drop.
- That drop for the right hand is the start of a complete circle with the racket. Bring it down and at the same time shift your weight to the right foot in back.
- Carry your right arm down, back, and up. As the racket comes over and forward, follow through by taking the weight first on your left foot and then step forward onto your right as the racket comes down.
- Do many slow serves as if for a slow-motion camera. After a while you will hit a rhythm that works for you.
- The serve needs abdominal, arm, and chest flexibility. Do the Back Bends (exercise 111), then add Snap and Stretch (exercise 21).

Don't feel inadequate even if you have never held a racket in your hands. *You are not teaching tennis,* you are teaching the patterns that *prepare* for tennis and providing the necessary strength and flexibility. If you happen to have a twelve-year-old wonder tennis prodigy in class, let him or her demonstrate for you. The same exercises you are providing for the beginners will improve the hero's game as well.

THE SOUTHPAW

Left-handers in the past were often discouraged by both parents and coaches, who tried to make them over into right-handers. It never works, and besides, the lefty has some definite advantages. For one thing, southpaws are almost invariably excellent servers, and that's 50 percent of the game right there. Then, too, since most players are right-handed, they are used to playing with other right-handers. They are accustomed to the angles and the varying speeds that are achieved by such players, and their reflexes have been attuned to meet them. In effect they are playing against themselves. When the "lefty" presents them with a turned-around game, it often throws them off for several sets, and sometimes they never learn to "read" the other fellow at all.

There is one inherent weakness in the left-hander's game, and that is a cramped, slice backhand. This can be prevented with plenty of practice and *good coaching.* If your youngster is a southpaw, get him into the habit from the very beginning of almost turning his back to the net so that a full backswing is possible. If you work to music with racket but no ball hundreds and thousands of times, the groove will be worn into muscle and brain, and the stroke will be a plus rather than a minus.

GIRLS

Girls can play excellent tennis, but most do not. One of the reasons is early training, which counts as no amount of later coaching ever can. Most American girls get very little basic training. The swimmers do because they almost always come from swimming families and begin at birth. The skiers and skaters do, too, and for the same reason. The fact that little people cannot use a racket very well prevents early training with the sport itself. To get the most from a player of either sex, you must start early with exercise, equipment, and the outdoors.

If you must start now at whatever late date, you will get the best results with the "tomboys," who took from their environment whatever was available, like some little boys do. Dancers, too, if they have really been trained and not just provided with grace, make good players. Whatever the background of the little girl you want to teach, start now to build for the future. Along with the exercises and equipment presented here, get her going in track and field.

Make up a set of weight bags and teach her how to use them. Chase her up the climbing ropes until she is better at it than the boys. Girls are really tougher than boys, more flexible than boys—and they also have greater stamina than boys. With that in mind, pour on the coal and build a champion if you have champion material. If being a champion isn't in the cards, at least build a good player, one who will enjoy the game and give the other fellow a good game. You will find that when she grows up, she will understand that both her husband and her children need physical outlets as well—and she will provide them. If you accomplish that, you have done something for all of them, something that cannot be left in a will.

CHAPTER TWENTY
THE FAMILY—TOGETHER

It takes nine months to grow a baby, and during that time a lot of dreaming and planning goes on. The young people who were blessed with happy childhood years vow to provide the same for the child who is coming. Others, whose childhoods can best be described as nightmares, vow with equal strength that this time all will be different. Some carry their determination to make up for the lost years so far that the child is never permitted an unfulfilled wish.

When the baby arrives, there is rejoicing, a place is made somewhere in a family, and the child begins. From the very first moment things happen. *What you see* is a baby being bathed, dressed, fed, caressed, and cared for. *What you do not see* is a blueprint unfolding. Each new human slips into the world a complete entity with sealed directions for self-building, and no two are exactly alike. The influences of the first few hours, weeks, and months will show up in the personality and character of the adult twenty years later. The blueprints, plus the materials provided by the family, combine with the "feel" of that family to form the foundation. The height and width of the finished edifice cannot exceed the size and strength of the base.

Family life is a preparation for real

life, and the outside limit in years is about twelve. But no one had better count on that limit. By the time a baby has been in the world a few minutes, he knows competent hands from tense, nervous ones and will react accordingly. Watch a newcomer stop fussing when a grandmother who has already been trained by several babies plants him happily on an ample bosom and settles into a rocking chair for a peaceful half hour with the soap operas.

The baby who can scarcely walk already knows just how far he can push each of his parents. He already knows the going rate for a smile, a tear, a whimper, and a howl—and how to play one against the other. Long, long before he goes to school, the child knows the exact limits set by his own family. Rigid or not, exact limits are a help; they can be counted on as a constant, and they can be used like the North Star as a way of finding out where you are when traveling outside the family circle. At first the world is like a sea, and during preschool days the little mariner pokes around in bays and inlets well within sight of home and safety. Even if the rules change from day to day or mood to mood, he can still manage to reach his mooring. He's confused all right, but not lost. Then comes school and the world. He must sail out of sight of land. Imagine the terror that settles down on the ship without a compass.

A few years ago I did a study with some young parents to find out what they wanted for their children. I asked them to build a mental picture of what they thought their little one would look like at the age of sixteen. Then I asked them to imagine that for some unforeseen reason that boy or girl had to leave within hours for a distant part of the world and be on his own. Try it yourself with *each of your children*. Write down what you think each one will need to carry along as a part of the baggage, a part that cannot be lost or stolen.

Almost every parent started off with "health," which was both a sensible and an obvious start. Without health nobody gets far. Notice I said *health*—you can be handicapped and still be very healthy indeed. Lack of health means *sick,* and the sick feel too bad to set out into life.

Next in popularity was "purpose," something that interested, a *reason.* This seems to be in keeping with the wave of the future. My generation might have put "security" next, because they had had so little of it during the Depression years. Today young people are searching for a reason to be here at all, and this searching didn't strike the last few generations until they reached the late thirties. I think there must have been generations in which survival was a minute-to-minute thing, and few either had to wonder or had time to wonder.

The third on the list boiled down to "the tools for living." Education was one of those; a useful trade was another. "The looks to get a husband and the ability to keep him" was turned in by the mother of a pretty little girl baby, while another mother of a girl child hoped hers would "have the guts to go into a profession and make a go of it." This latter wish, too, is part of the times.

Every parent was concerned that the child be able to make a living. Most mentioned that good looks would be nice and that good sense would be even better. They all hoped for the child's self-confidence and the ability to get along with other people. Some of the men spoke (I think wistfully) about youth being a time for adventure, and two women hoped their daughters would want to be homemakers and have children. I think the rest just figured it would happen anyway and didn't mention it.

They all knew what they hoped their children would develop, but when I asked how they expected to get these things across in the next few years they admitted they hadn't given a whole lot of thought to that part of it. Have you?

Children learn by copying, not by doing what somebody says they *should* do. No baby was born speaking a language or with the ability to feed himself or change his own diapers. For a while somebody is going to have to help, but if the child is to be self-sufficient, that help has to stop the minute the child can help himself. Sometimes it's a lot easier (and quicker) to pick up the toys, tie the shoelace, clear the table, and sweep the kitchen yourself than to wait on two somewhat unsteady little legs, fumbling fingers, a daydreamer, or a master goldbrick. However, if you do it all yourself, you steal away three very important tools for a child's good life: a sense of worth, a sense of belonging, and a sense of responsibility. When you give in and do the things a child should be doing to maintain his *right* to a place in the family, you do an evil thing. You rob him of the security built on the ability to *strive*, to *do*, to *manage,* and to *succeed.* You also replace the parent he needs to respect with a servant who will be in no position to quit ten years from now when the young mistress or master makes exorbitant demands in keeping with an unrealistic self-image.

Children are the greatest tacticians in the world, and they constantly probe the opposition's lines. When you want a child to leave his play to do a job you know he can and should do, you become, for a while, the opposition. With unerring instinct he will find your weakness. Perhaps you are impatient, and if he delays long enough you will give up rather than insist. Perhaps you have a need for perfection, which he can twist to mean you do it better than he does. You do, of course, but if you aren't able to put his need for training ahead of your need for perfection, you'll be doing it better the rest of your life while he lolls in front of the TV set. Perhaps you aren't very observant and you don't even notice when you are being manipulated. Or perhaps you tell yourself that he's only a child and can't be expected to do this thing or that. Have you watched him when he was trying to get something he wanted or do something he wanted to do? He can manage just fine, and if you use that excuse for him, you will be finding ways to excuse him for the rest of his life. The teenagers today who have no respect for their parents *were robbed* of that ability to respect by those very same parents, who once thought their children *couldn't* when really they simply *wouldn't.*

So, first you set up the limits and provide the sense of security. Know and let it be known that you are a very nice person who will meet the child halfway. You

The Family—Together

will gladly *help* with socks and slithery shoelaces for a while, and you will praise lavishly for accomplishments. However, the accomplishments must be real (or you will turn loose an adult who believes life will reward him for doing nothing, and we all know it doesn't), and those accomplishments must come along quite regularly. Whenever you are tempted to overlook sloppy work, remember that the same brain and ability that moves mountains when he has something in mind for himself can be put to work for the family as well. If your child is to have the *security of belonging* to that family, let him earn it, and then he will know it is a fact.

If your whole family can work on a project that would provide pleasure for everyone when done and everyone can have some part in it, then the finished product *belongs to everyone.* If only the parents work while the young ones scamper around mostly getting underfoot and being told to "go somewhere else and play," the children are forced to become parasites. The parents will have the satisfaction of building something for the family, but the kids will have put in a day reinforcing the idea that whatever they demand is nothing more than their due and that while other people (parents) work, we (the children) get what we want *because that's the way it is.* Translated to later on, this means: Life owes me a living. Anyone who fosters that sort of erroneous thinking in a child destroys initiative and sets him up for quite a fall.

There are all sorts of possible family projects, but the most valuable are those that answer a real need. Children, like the elderly, who have much to give if only someone would need them, resent busywork. In America today chemistry has joined with the packaging industry to rob food of considerable value. If health is to be maintained, it has become a must for any family with a backyard to have a garden. A small plot coupled with a freezer and an old discarded refrigerator, which can be buried on its side and then covered with straw for the winter, can feed several families. The work of planting, weeding, picking, and helping with the storing (the things that used to go in root cellars do fine in the buried refrigerators) and freezing is anything but mere busywork. It means the difference between real food and a not very reasonable facsimile.

Children can learn a great deal about food, vitamins, minerals, and proper diet while caring for a garden. They are going to need that information if they and their children are to survive in the coming years, when feeding double the present population means even more chemicals and less true food. A wise mother comes to the plot equipped with a notebook, in which she meticulously notes what Mark planted, what's in Davy's and Jan's rows, and what Tari did to keep peace and harmony in the workforce. She and her oldest will team up to provide iced lemonade and certain other survival necessities that help promote a spirit of cooperation.

When it comes to harvesting, there is no need for hardship. Whoever is on picking duty just brings in four times as much as the family needs each day, and as it is prepared in the kitchen, the surplus is frozen right then and dropped into the freezer. One dinner's beans are on the table; three are put away against nongarden days. Carrots, beets, turnips, parsnips, and all such time-resistant vegetables, plus the fruit, go into the sunken "root cellar" that used to be Aunt Marjorie's refrigerator. When there is a big day of corn husking, that's the day there should also be one whale of a picnic with prizes for all, including Dad, who rented the Rototiller and got blisters preparing the plot. Corn that is cooked and frozen minutes after picking is something you can't buy in any supermarket.

Zucchini is an especially enthusiastic vegetable. Picked and sliced while the water is boiling, it makes a dish of indescribable delight. One summer we all learned something else. We had been away operating one clinic after another, and the zucchini were left to themselves in that lovely well-worked, highly fertile soil. After one ten-day absence we had Zeppelins in the zucchini patch. *What a waste*, we thought—but not for long. We peeled one and cut out the center, cut it up, and boiled it quickly in salted water. It was as good as the young ones, just different. Then followed Zucchini Day. We gathered in the whole armada and froze them in one morning. We are still having zucchini heated in a double boiler, covered with tasty tomato paste and Parmesan cheese—and it's spring. Incidentally, *never* throw the vegetable water away. It's loaded with the minerals your kids need. You need them too. Use it when you make soups or stew, or whenever it says, "Add water," on a can. Doctored with a few herbs and kept in the refrigerator, it can take the place of tea or coffee as a real pick-me-up and is just the base for one of those low-calorie bouillon cubes on a cold day.

There are some thoughts you need to give to the food you put on your table. For example, since much of it comes from far away and must be stored after it gets to your town, preservatives of all sorts are used. Preservatives aren't necessarily safe, and for the sake of your family you ought to read a couple of good books on nutrition. Unfortunately, medical doctors are still getting no or almost no training in nutrition. It is a science, however, that a lot of other people are beginning to study, and you can get good information either from the nutritionists or from their books.

Another thing, no matter what is done to the food you buy, no matter how it has been attacked by heat, strained through, added to, or subtracted from, it still comes beautifully packaged. Try to know what's inside and not be swayed by artistry in wrappings. There are, for example, only a few cents' worth of wheat in your dollar loaf of bread. As much as 50 percent of your hot dogs may be flavored, pink-colored fat. More than 80 percent of your "maple syrup" probably never got even close to a maple tree but came out of a cane field. Your peanut butter probably had a solid fat added to it, and smart bugs wouldn't be caught dead or alive in your dry cereals.

Chemicals are now added to food, and for your safety and the safety of your family you need to know what the different chemicals are and what they do *besides* dye, bleach, emulsify, preserve, flavor, buffer, acidify, alkalize, moisten, dry, neutralize, sweeten, condition, cure, hydrolize, hydrogenate, mature, and fortify. Then when you go to the market, don't just fill your basket with pretty pictures. *Read the labels.* Since you aren't supposed to read the labels because what you don't know won't hurt you much, take along a magnifying glass. You will soon learn which foods and brands to leave alone, even if the man on TV says it's just the thing you need for strength, energy, and go. Remember he is paid to say that while you are paying to feed your family. When you find that one brand of maple syrup is 83 percent sugar while a second brand is 50 percent sugar, and you just *must* have syrup or John's Sunday will be ruined, you at least have a choice. Nobody likes to be cheated, and when "all-meat franks" are all meat but largely fat at a time when uncolored fat costs about 49¢ and lean meat costs about $2.19, why are you paying $2.19 for a 49¢ commodity? To date, no law says what percentage of franks and luncheon meats can be fat, so until there is, you might do better with something else. Too expensive? Think over that price of useless and *dangerous* fat, and see if something else is really too expensive. It is of just such fat that heart attacks are made—and belly rolls.

One summer some people rented the house of a friend of mine, and I went by to help her straighten up after the folks went back to the city. They had left the kitchen shelves loaded with food they had not used, and as we emptied shelves, closets, and refrigerator, we were given a dramatic lesson in why America is fat and tired and has high dentist bills. There were five half-empty boxes of different kinds of sugar, all lacking in any nutritive value whatsoever, highly caloric and quite capable of using up stomach space that should have gone to food. I counted no fewer than *ten* opened jars of jam, jelly, marmalade, and preserves. These have about the same food value as sugar and the same calories. There were four boxes of cake mix and three packages of quick-mix sweet rolls. No nutriment there to speak of, but lots of no-nos. The pancake flour came in separate containers in which, by adding milk, you could shake up a batch in no time (at almost double the cost of the kind you mix in a bowl; this was in a kitchen with six bowls). There were puddings that could be made in the same way (same cost comparison), two bags of white flour, well bleached and therefore well gassed, and enough cookies, crackers, and fudge mix to give the entire family pimples for a year. At first I was aghast, and then my conscience gave me a good poke and reminded me that the reformed are apt to be more intolerant. I was only a few years away from my own garbage collection.

It was a brisk and colorful fall when my eleven-year-old daughter, Suzy, went off to the North Country School in Lake Placid, New York. She had been for her checkup and had "passed," whatever that meant. At least she was starting school without her usual miserable winter cold—that wouldn't show up until the snow came. Five cavities (the usual) had been filled. Since my experience with childhood dentistry had been similar, my only thought about that problem was: *That poor child, just like her mother.*

One week after the departure I received a letter from the school. Please, I was to send no food packages. The school believed in "natural food" (whatever that was). Store-bought candy, cookies, crackers, and cakes were not included in the students' diet. Their vegetables were home raised right there on the school grounds and were not sprayed with insecticides, nor was their fruit. Oranges for the school were sent up from a Florida grower who did not dye or treat his fruit. Beef was bought from farmers in the area who did not spray the feed or inject the animals with hormones or antibiotics. They raised their own chickens on the grounds and on safe feed. They also raised pigs, and those pigs were fed far better than most people. All the cereal the children ate was stone-ground every day from grain brought in from farms that were insecticide-free. Whatever was left over was made into the kind of bread that was once rightly called the staff of life. It had so much texture and taste that to butter or jam it would have been gilding the lily. There was no such thing as a peeled potato. They were cooked in their skins, and the skins were mashed right along with the insides. Thus no vitamins or minerals were lost. (Potatos with their skins are a great source of potassium, and potassium fights fatigue. Do you get tired?).

For snacks the children were given cookies made from that same freshly milled grain, fruit, juices, and raw vegetables. There wasn't a piece of candy or cake on the grounds except when a child had a birthday, and then everybody got a piece of cake, some ice cream, and a few pieces of chocolate—enough for a celebration, but hardly enough to compete with the table food.

The first week Suzy's letter was one long wail about her sweetless state. By the second week the wail had subsided to a whimper. The letter contained a tale about a teacher's hanging one of the juniors' baby teeth, lost in the normal way at age seven, in a glass of cola overnight and finding the enamel gone in the morning. The third week there was a request for work gloves, and the sweet crisis was past.

In the two years that Suzy spent at North Country School she gained three inches in height, but not a pound in weight. She did not have a single cold or cavity, and with her straight body, black hair, tanned skin, and almond eyes, she looked like everyone's dream of a light-footed Indian maid. The following fall she entered a boarding school near home where the food was plentiful and tasty but typical of most schools and colleges. The youngsters had access to food stores in the nearby village and a snack shop on the grounds. By Christmas she had gained ten pounds and had five cavities and a cold in her head.

One summer when I was visiting some children's hospitals in Switzerland, I had an opportunity to talk with the priest in charge. The question of the unfitness of Americans came up, and he allowed that, yes, it was strange that Americans with so much interest in sports should have such a poor record in fitness. He was very sorry for American children for many reasons. He had said all of this in French, at which I was terrible, and I thought I had misunderstood. I asked him to repeat, *mais lentement, s'il vous plait.* (I can say "Please go slowly," even in languages I don't speak or understand.) He took all the time in the world and even used a dictionary to explain that children in America seem to have a lot of "things" and many advantages, but miss out when it comes to the company of parents. Swiss children, on the other hand, have fewer material possessions and opportunities and also have to work hard at school and around the house, but when Sunday comes around (that's "family day"), they go off *together* to the lakes or the mountains for the entire day. On that day the two worlds of the children and grown-ups merge. They can both enjoy the same hours together if the grown-up has not lost touch with those things that mean much to children. It isn't how much time you spend with children, but what you do with them when you are together. If you can enter their world for even a little while, you can draw close. TV isn't their world; it's no world at all, just an escape. Children don't need escapes; they need reality—real sun, real rain, a chance to see things grow, a chance to feel heat and cold, wet and dry, a chance to share those realities with the people who are still most important in their lives. Fifteen minutes of "catch" with the kids in the evening will take the kinks out of your arm and out of your heart. It certainly need not be Little League for your children (only the best get to play as a rule, and it's anti-girl). Little League is very often another case in which parents *think* they go into the children's world, but far too often they insist that the children do it the adult way.

Of course you *could* take a walk.

What is a walk? A walk is going anywhere on two feet, and it's a great way to get healthy while you sneak a few valuable (much needed in today's world) lessons. "No, David, we can't go in there. See that No Trespassing sign? *No trespassing* means don't pass this gate or fence because the land there belongs to someone who bought it the way we bought our land and you bought your football. It *belongs* to somebody." Today there is a whole generation of young people who are convinced that the world and all that is in it should belong to them, whether they have earned it or not. This is not *their* crime; the dubious honor belongs to parents who have given children everything they ever wanted even before they got around to asking for it, and certainly before they had worked to earn it. With small children this results in waste. At the Institute we had a Lost and Found box, which literally overflowed with clothing, books, briefcases, glasses, jewelry, watches, and even money *that were never reclaimed.* Every bit of this loot had been provided by parents and would have to be replaced by parents. When these same careless children grow up, they have been *trained* to expect gifts and handouts. Habit is hard to break. Further, since nothing has any value that a young person can gauge, such as hours spent in hard work, vandalism isn't wrong— it's just adventure. Half the time when a young destroyer is picked up, Daddy pays the bill, which isn't all wrong, since he probably could have prevented the problem in the first place, but it doesn't help the youngster. He just wiggles out and goes on to bigger and better wrongs. There used to be a public-service plea on television that showed a set of car keys left in the lock, and the caption was "Don't help a good boy go wrong."

It isn't only the lessons of life that come out on walks. There is a world to be discovered: moss, fallen leaves, a baby oak that must be marked so that the brush cutter will avoid it, and small animals that come out if you rest awhile. Legs, hearts, and lungs grow stronger, eyes learn to see, and there is a sharing between the generations. Perhaps in the sharing the future gap will be less wide and less bitter.

There is also a sharing among siblings. At home, in the usual surroundings, little brothers and sisters can often be both boring and upsetting as favorite toys are sat on and smashed, favorite books lose their pages, and someone pours glue in the typewriter. For a long time little people are right out of savage land as they find new things to examine with newly developed finger muscles. In the woods, though, they can become what little brothers and sisters are "supposed" to be: inquisitive, busy with nature's toys, and attentive to what older siblings have to offer.

Cooperation begins early. It is big brother who baits hooks, fixes oarlocks, is trusted to take the kids down to the dock and bring them back. Little ones are often better behaved for big brother than they are for parents, but no *big brother* or *big sister* just happened, any more than responsible adults just happen. Both have to be trained, and if parents don't do it, life will, and often with an ax handle. It's hard work to develop a sense of responsibility in anyone. It takes time, patience, and a plan. Fun on Sundays isn't enough; the young human must understand seven days a week that if being older provides nice things like staying up later than the others, not having to wear somebody's worn-a-year ski jacket, and status (if you have to take him to task, *don't* do it in front of the others), it also demands responsibility. Youngsters sometimes feel put upon when they are asked to "help" and younger children are not. "You're the oldest" doesn't mean a whole lot when shouts of childish laughter come into the kitchen, the barn, or the garage where "the oldest" is working while others play. It's only fair that everyone works at the same time, and while it will take time to train each one at first, it pays off. If "oldest" does have to put in time when the others are at play, then it should be noted, praised, and appreciated aplenty. This applies to every age, including grown-ups. There is just too little real appreciation around. All the time you put in on the kids will come back to you. Count on it. True, it would take less time to do it yourself *for a while*, but one day you hear Jan answer the phone and say, "Just a minute, please, may I know who is calling?" Jan, seven, has copied David, who is eight, who has copied Tari, who is twelve; and next year Marky will copy Jan and you'll have complete phone coverage. It all began when you took the trouble to teach Tari and saw to it that she did it right.

If David sometimes seems to be doing nothing—you *know* there's no bait on that hook, or that he hasn't turned a page in half an hour, or that, like Snoopy, he is just lying on his back on top of the garage—be patient. Things move so fast that there must be time for consolidating gains. Dreaming is a part of childhood, just as it should be a part of adulthood. *Everything begins with a dream.* Lucky for the child if he can do his dreaming in clean air amid the peace that comes with the sound of water lapping against a boat. Many children must fight desperately for solitude, and some cannot find it anywhere anymore, nor can grown-ups. Pavements, buildings, machines, and noise crowd in on people to crush their spirits.

It is true that children are children such a little while. The same might be said of you. You will never be exactly this old again. Take a little time to dream. *Thoughts are things,* and if you don't dream them, they can never come to pass. Let children dream, too, but don't confuse dreaming with goldbricking. Even children must buy dream time with the responsibilities suited to their abilities.

The generation gap is not really a gap between generations at all. It is a gap between people. You will find that you are *really* not any closer to the lady down the street than you are to her children. You will find as much to disagree with when the garden club meets as you will at a teenage gathering if you really get down to cases. You'll just handle it a little better at the club because you are more used to those people—and *they* don't really change much.

It's a little difficult to get used to kids—they change so fast from week to week, and then, too, they hide it so well.

You change, too, *for them.* One minute you are way up there, and a little later your eyes meet. It would be a lot better if all of us were able to accept the fact that knowing other people is the only way to get on with them, and knowing people takes effort, even knowing one's own.

You have so much to offer your own right now, while you, too, are young and in a state of flux. And if they are not your very own children, that changes nothing. There are many adults who have much to bring to life. Every year I find more and more really interesting people coming to my five-day workshops to learn how to teach *real* exercise who say, "I want to work with kids." The "externs" at my clinics go into a happy dither when a child is brought into the clinic with scoliosis, "growing pains," a sprain or anything else. To begin with, they get well quickly, but also they are fun to work-play with. All of us are still children somewhere, and it often takes a child to help us find the child we once were. Instead of spending so much thought and worry on a "generation gap," we would all profit if we put the same energy to work for intergenerational communication. You will find that easiest if it can be done where the generations can and should be on fairly equal terms, doing things physical amid the gifts nature provides. Nothing good comes easy and the most valuable gift in life is time. You get back what you invest.

CHAPTER TWENTY-ONE
THE FATHERS

Fathers in America are in danger for their lives. They often have to work too hard, because every year it costs more and more to live in a country where fewer and fewer (let alone the best) things are free. Many leave home in the morning to travel miles on superhighways. There is no time for enjoying the morning.

Fathers are often caught in a trap. The young man fell into the job because it was the first thing that came along and it wouldn't hurt to try it for a few years until something better turned up. Then he married, and the children, not a different job, came along. Now, even if the new job is offered, he has a difficult choice to make. A man alone could take a chance, but what about the guy with a family? No, he guesses he'd best play it safe while the babies are little. Maybe later. But later there are doctor and dentist bills, Jeannie needs braces, and Tom shows real promise on that cornet. Then, too, they have a second mortgage. Perhaps when all the kids are in school and Dianne can get a part-time job . . . And so it goes. By the time the last one is in school and Dianne gets the part-time job, he's not the youngest fellow in the business and there are a couple of comers he'd better stay ahead of. If he should try a new job, would he do as well starting at the bottom as he is doing now in work that bores him but pays pretty well? Every day when the traffic backs up and the sameness of his days eats a little deeper into his soul, he wonders what he's doing there. This upsets his digestion and gives him a dull headache.

Fathers eat badly. They breakfast in a hurry and, if the family isn't considerate, amid a lot of *Sturm und Drang*. Of course if there is rioting at the breakfast table, he may have to accept some of the blame for permitting it in the first place, but no matter who is at fault, father will pay the price. He will either cut breakfast short or gulp it. Half the time he is served very little of value anyway. When he gets to the office he will have a quick cup of coffee (with sugar, cream, and caffeine).

Fathers lunch with associates to discuss a problem or with a client who has a problem, or they are the client with the problem. In any case the work goes to lunch with them and sits right there at the table. There's no relaxation, no peace, and when you are constantly jockeying for position, there isn't much letup. Father didn't do very well at breakfast, and his blood sugar level is way down. He feels hungry and tired. The waitress brings the menu and asks if anyone would like a cocktail. It will be fifteen minutes before they can get their lunch anyway in that crowd, so of course he has the cocktail. He may even have two. By the time lunch arrives, he is uncomfortably warm, the smoke from either his own or other people's cigarettes has got to him, and he feels as though his collar is too tight.

Back at the office the problems are piling up, and he can't get through one thing before another sets up a clamor. One phone call leads to another, and by four o'clock he has three calls to go and the mail is still untouched. By five he is worrying about the traffic gathering for the homeward surge. By five thirty he's in it. Driving through the poor visibility in spring and fall, and the ice and snow of winter's darkness, and the carbon monoxide of summer takes a toll, and he arrives home half dead. And what does he come home to?

Sometimes it's peaceful and a haven in a stormy sea. There really isn't a reason in the world why the house should rattle to the racket of childish games after six o'clock in the evening—not if the children have been outdoors all afternoon getting rid of their pent-up energies. By suppertime the children should have completed *their* day, and what is left of the day should belong to the hardworking parents. But such things as peaceful households don't just happen. Kids permitted to rule the roost all day are most certainly not going to give up that pleasure simply because the man who supports them has come home. If anything, since they, too, are probably tired, they will intensify the noise and demands. True, mother has been stuck with it all day, and father should share in the responsibility some time—and besides, when can they see him if not in the evening? None of that holds water. The kids were at school all day, and after school it is the mother's job to get them exercised as you would a racehorse. No exercise, a bad-tempered horse. As for *his* part of the responsibility—yes, but on weekends, not when he's done in. The American woman will probably be a widow for eight years if she and her husband are of the same age. If she would like to change that statistic, she'd best let him rest. As for when the children can see him—when they behave, he won't mind. If they don't, they don't want to see him; they just want to raise a ruckus, which they should be at liberty to do outside all afternoon, never at night and never when *he* comes home. Does it sound like the olden days when children were "seen but not heard"? It isn't really; that's what the misinterpreters of Freud would have you think. Actually, good children are a delight even when they can't (and shouldn't) contribute conversationally. They are lovely to look at, to hold, and to treasure. Monsters have none of the nice attributes, and all too often *we have made good kids into monsters by letting them run our lives and our homes.* That is what happened to many of the young people of today who want to rule the world before learning how to rule themselves. The trouble is that little monsters grow into big ones, and big ones can neither be sent to their rooms to think it over nor be developed into considerate human beings.

Constant irritation in the evening will send a father's blood pressure up, and probably before the evening is over, he will blow his stack. The kids will disappear howling, and his wife will sit mute with misery. By the time he is forty-five, he will have put up with 5,760 days of numbing effort and 7,300 nerve-shattering evenings. Somewhere between the ages of forty-five and sixty, millions of fathers die of heart attacks.

The preparations for peaceful evenings begin when children are born. Children are bright enough. If they know that it is their responsibility to keep the evenings pleasant—(and woe to him who breaks the peace, no allowances for age)—there will be peace. The home *is* the training ground for life, so ask yourself what would happen to father if he had a tantrum at a board meeting or in a client's office or in fact anywhere in the workaday world. Plenty, and all of it bad. Anger is often justified, but bad manners are something else again. So if you are fitting your children for life, and incidentally trying to make your own not only bearable but pleasant, you had better figure that there must be rules and see that they are obeyed.

Speaking of rules, father obeys the traffic rules, and if he doesn't, who is watching besides the police? Could it be the kids? Father pays the bills, and if he doesn't, the family won't eat. Father pays taxes, too, and if he doesn't, he could go to jail. Those are the rules. Evenings are for parents—that's the rule. Evenings are not for parents to do homework. Kids can do their own homework if the right to a TV program is the price. Evenings are not for reading endless boring stories—one is enough, and even that one ought to happen *after* all the rules have been obeyed. Evenings are for parents, not for bathtub battles, tyranny at the table or endless delays, seven glasses of water and twenty-three good-night kisses. If you are trapped in that sort of mess, don't blame the kids. *You* permitted it, but *you* can correct it. It will take about a week of constant effort, and even then be on the alert for sporadic forays for roughly two months. That ought to take care of it if you are consistent, and do be consistent with the rules or it may be you in five years who can't understand when it all went wrong. It goes wrong at the beginning.

Fathers do like to be with their children when they are rested and can enjoy them. It pays to gather one or another up when you have to run an errand—not two, just one. Just as two puppies will tussle and roughhouse when they are together, children keep up a kind of teasing static. One lone puppy or one lone child is easier to get close to, and you can ask and get both help and camaraderie from so little a person as a seven-year-old.

Anyone can learn almost anything, from sewing to Sanskrit, if the interest is high enough and the source is at hand. If you are a father and are given the opportunity to share time with a small son or daughter, you are a walking treasure chest. The things you have done in your life are more exciting than the best stories ever written, because *you* did them. Tell. The dreams you had and have are the most exciting dreams in the world, and never mind if you didn't fulfill them, children can't tell fact from fiction, which sometimes saves their sanity when bad things happen. Your dreams may still come true, because *you* dream them.

My walks with my father never led to real things. Life robbed us. But I bought the woods he intended one day to buy. I put the apples out for the deer as he would have. I don't chase the beavers away because he taught me about them. I can read the tracks in my pasture and my father's Indian ancestors, who are also mine, allow me to know of their presence here where the Stockbridge Indians once roamed. So did his dreams come true? Did he give me imperishable gifts? My father knew Indian lore and he gave that to me, too. He skinned eels and wrapped them first in leaves and then clay and baked them in the fire where the corn, similarly wrapped, was steaming. He broiled venison on two sticks: one held the venison chunk and the other, bacon that dripped fat onto the venison. My father never got lost in the woods, nor do I; I know how to mark my going with the landmarks that will bring me home. I can build a good lean-to and sleep warm under branches and leaves. I can make a fire even in the rain, and probably most important, when I leave a campsite, there is only bent grass to show I have been there. Bent grass will stand straight soon enough—*and I never walked with my father after I was six years old.* On my sixth birthday I was sent away to an orphanage where things happened that I can hardly talk about even today—but only a part of me was there where those things went on. The rest was with my father in the woods where he had taught me to whistle and chew birch bark, look at the North Star . . . and dream.

Who, then, are the fathers? They are gods come to earth for a little while to teach little mortals about hopes and dreams and impossible adventures that may or may not be true, but that put the North Star within reach. Fathers have a message to impart to sons and daughters that no one else can give. What message? Only the children will remember, for gods forget their golden messages even as they give them. The one I got from the god who was in my life for a little while is, "Remember, there's always a way it can be done. If it doesn't work one way, don't waste time on that way or you'll get stuck. Walk away and find another way. It is there, somewhere." That has been the North Star for me all my life.

If you are a father, or if you know one, know, too, how short immortality lasts . . . and how very long—if you handle it right.

Time is the most valuable thing parents have to give, but that works both ways.

Now that my daughters are grown and off living their own lives in other places, I can always call them back by remembering my daughter Petie hiking along the Tuckerman Ravine Trail on Mount Washington on Columbus Day. She wore little leather britches and an Alpine cap we'd brought her from a trip to the Tyrol. Her boots were authentic, too, and so were her muscles as she struggled along under her pack. I can hear Suzy as she clung to a cliff up in the Shawangunks saying happily, "A little bootht, pleath." She had lost all fear of heights long before she lost her lisp. I can remember sand castles and rowboats, a slide down a Maine waterfall with Petie, and losing Suzy in a sleeping bag when she slept on a downslope. There were skiing days and horseback rides, cooking over campfires and sleeping under stars. Every moment spent doing things to remember was an investment. Don't wait "until they are old enough to go along" or until they "get sense." They are old enough now, even if they have to go in a pack on your back—and their *senses* are alive—*now*.

Take pictures of them doing any and every thing. One day you will be the next best thing to a father, and that will be a grandfather. Grandfathers are special, too. They can tell you what your mother or your father did when they were your age, which of course is the most important age at the time. Those pictures will be your chapter headings, and who knows, maybe you will still have messages to impart.

CHAPTER TWENTY-TWO
THE MOTHERS

Who are the mothers? The mothers are the women who have had the babies in the first place, and they are the women (with or without babies of their own) who influence children along the way. They come in all sizes and with every attribute, but just as no one of them is either both fat *and* thin, tall *and* short, or old *and* young, no one of them has *all* the attributes that go to make up mothers. There is no such thing as a *typical* mother. There are only mothers. True, women are forced from time to time into playing the motherhood role expected of the times, but behind their eyes you see someone quite different, no matter what they do, wear, or say.

Mothers have the same credits and debits in their various makeups as anybody else. Some are quiet, gentle, and shy. Others are vivacious, gregarious, and fun. There are the serious, the intellectual, the driving, the phlegmatic, the confident, and the unsure—just like anybody else. When they have children or work with children, they bring these things with them.

There is no *typical* child, and the several children in any one family can be as different from one another as the wild flowers in a field. What will serve one perfectly could be all wrong for another. They, too, have different attributes, and according to one's philosophy one can think that the matching of parents to children is a matter of either luck or plan. If you think it's luck, then do the best you can with it; if you think there is a plan, then you have to do better than that. You have to give each child what that child was sent to find with you.

For starters, have you ever looked into a child's eyes and said silently, *Who are you anyway?* That can be disturbing enough if you look into the mirror and ask yourself the same thing. You may get the feeling that something inside of you answers: *Well, at last you have got around to it.* You won't get any world-shaking answers from the eyes in the mirror, but you may suddenly realize that there is someone there you haven't met before, someone you should know quite well but have not taken the time to look up. Children's eyes have no shields yet; you can learn a lot from them.

Whatever you believe about life, if you look around you and see what some people build with their lives, you cannot help but know that they didn't start the day before yesterday to do those things—they started as children, or before. If the blueprints that come with the baby tell him how to put himself together, when to be born, how to breathe, suck, excrete, grow, add size, heal himself, *and think*, would it be too far out to believe that the blueprint also may contain sealed orders that tell him *what job he has been sent to do?* If that is permissible, could it not also be possible that you were selected to help prepare that person? If so, you were not selected because you were a *typical* anything, but because something in you has value for the particular children in your house, not the same thing in you for each one, and certainly more for some than for others, but something of value, and yours to give. Whatever it is—and it could be anything from providing a listening ear to placing firm hands on the reins of a wild stallion—do it the best way *you* can, not the way somebody says you should do it. Whether you are a parent or a teacher, *you* have value, and what's most important, *you have it right there.*

While those things haven't changed much if at all with the changes in the world, other things have. My mother's time was so like her mother's time that they are almost indistinguishable except for the unrest that came with World War I. It was followed by the first stirrings of women's lib. True, the revolution was only surface and was confined to shortened skirts, wild music, shorter haircuts, high heels, cigarettes and cocktails, necking, and advanced education for a few. Most mothers did what their mothers had done and had the same attitudes their mothers had held. Father was the breadwinner and mother kept house, raised the kids, got the meals on the table, sewed on buttons, and often made the family's clothes, the curtains, and sewed for the Women's Guild. Baths were on Saturday, church on Sunday, and Monday was washday.

Except for a few precarious islands here and there, those days are gone forever. World War II told the world of men that women could do men's work and often better than men could do it. That was welcome news when the war plants had to be filled, but shock set in when the war was over and women refused to go back to the old subservience. They had tasted a new kind of life and found it good. There was no turning back. What women had been told all their lives—that they *had* to depend on their husbands and that husbands were the only way out of their parents' homes— had been proven wrong. It slowly dawned that the major obstructions were gone and not everyone was glad, nor did everyone know what to do with their freedom. They still don't. The atomic bomb blew up more than two cities in Japan, and nothing will ever be the same—for anyone, but most of all for the mothers.

Today most mothers have either part-time or full-time jobs. Some fall into the category called single parents. Divorce started that category, but its numbers have been swelled by women who have elected to become mothers without marrying or who were caught in the riptides caused by the "Sexual Revolution," another phenomenon of our times. Those are usually the very young mothers who, dabbling in sex without proper education, found themselves having babies while still little more than babies themselves.

Today *mother* doesn't mean the lady who sits at home and "does" for everyone else. Today mother can be a high-powered editor, a secretary, a medical technician, a waitress, a teacher, a surgeon, an electrician, or a firefighter. She can be thirteen or forty plus, or anything in between. She can have a helpful husband who will pick up the kids at the day care center, do the shopping, and get supper on . . . or come home in the same car pool from the same job, sit down, put his feet up, and read the paper. She can go to work on the 7:15 out of Rye, New York, while her husband gets the kids off to school, cleans the house, and writes a column for the local newspaper. On the other hand, she can start at six to feed the baby, get herself and the children dressed and fed, the baby off to day care, the children to school, and herself to the job—all by 9:00 A.M. She can put in anything from a few hours to a full day with all the attendant worries of keeping the job, advancing in the job, taking care of emergencies, making ends meet while worrying over what the children are learning at school besides the three Rs. She also has to worry about the three Rs, since school isn't what it used to be either.

Once, the only jobs open to women were teaching, nursing, and clerical work. Now the sky's the limit for those willing to pay the price. The superior teachers have become the superior workers in the women's workforce. Inferior education is one of the results. Of course there are still good teachers, there are just fewer *really good* teachers and there are more children. Of course there are still homes where discipline, manners, and preparation for higher education are taught, only there are fewer such homes—but more children. It is a time of flux, just like a growing business that has too much business to be handled by the present staff but not enough money to hire additional staff. So the existing staff is asked to put in more hours and work harder and harder—until . . .

Until what? Until we Americans (especially American women) rearrange things. We can and we will, and there will be men to help us in time. Some are in place already, as those with helpful husbands will tell you. Some see the handwriting on the wall, as those who have instituted pregnancy leave, day nurseries at the workplace, and alternative work schedules will tell you. It all takes time. My mother, who had been accepted at Hunter College, wasn't allowed by her parents to go. She was a girl, and what did girls need with college? I didn't have the money to go straight to college from high school, and when I tried to enroll at Sarah Lawrence when I had enough money, I was told I was too old—at thirty! Today we would both be welcome.

When my mother was a mother, we had maids. Maids went out with World War II. When I was a mother, there was just the beginning of nursery schools, and day care centers were for "poor" people who "had" to work. When I was a mother, there were *some* children called latchkey children because they went home to empty houses while their mothers worked in the war factories. What we see now are thousands of children coming home to empty houses. Incidentally, the latchkey children I had in my ski club, Scout groups, and exercise classes were every bit as cared for (sometimes better cared for) than the children with stay-at-home mothers. The latchkey kids were often more responsible than the others, too, and happier as well.

What we have to accept is the fact that most mothers are probably going to have to work or will *want* to work. What has to be done for both them and the country is a different kind of help for children. It has all been done in one place or another—successfully. There *are* day care centers that are well staffed and that *do care for children.* There really are nursery schools that care properly for children. There are even schools that educate children and some that have found ways to educate, exercise, nutritionally feed, bathe, and interest children *all day.* It takes intelligence. We have intelligence. It takes selling. We can sell. It takes dedication. Lots of mothers are dedicated, and so are fathers. None of it is impossible. America has been a leader in the world for a long time. It is time it took seriously the needs of two of its most important groups—the children and the mothers.

This is a book about fitness, and we cannot overlook the role played by the mothers when it comes to that important facet of life. Today's young mothers are victims of a paradox, several paradoxes. We are considered one of the most "sports-minded" nations in the world, yet our children are the weakest in the world and growing weaker with each generation. The last naturally fit generation of Americans is now over fifty years old. They are the last of us to have walked to and from school and been able to run home for a hot lunch at noon. They are the last who as a generation played freely outdoors and had nothing indoors to keep them there. Today's mother entered America at the time of the school bus, the TV, and the start of danger in the streets. There has been no *real* physical education since the early 1930s. So they have had no *real* training, ever. Of course there are those who were sent to dancing school, riding school, the Turnverein, or Sokol. Of course there are those whose parents played tennis, sailed boats, skied, and hiked. That means they did it, too, and that their children will. But that's not a generation, that's an elite few.

The next paradox for the mothers came with the so-called fitness boom. They and several millions more were sold on "fitness," but they didn't know how to get it. They signed up for whatever was available—jogging on the road, "aerobic dance," spas, and weight machines. With untrained bodies and no education, they became the victims of America's purveyors of nothing for something—advertisers. Sadly, they didn't get just "nothing" for their time and money: those mothers got shin-splints, calf strains, injured knees and backs—and there is more waiting for them when they reach fifty, which will not be the magic age it was and is for their parents. They didn't make the good bodies when they were little that guarantee continued fitness after fifty.

So in the land of million-dollar sports salaries, millions of sports fans, and billions spent on health, our mothers and their children are not only deprived, they are in grave danger. What can be done about it? Plenty, and the answer is right here in your hands. If you are concerned enough about your children to read this book, then you must be aware that *you* are one of the answers. And to be an answer, you have to be in shape. How? By doing *yourself* what you are reading up on for the children.

Who are the *mothers? Women* are the *mothers*—and no one can replace them. Women shouldn't be asked to do it all, however, and more important, they should know *they can't do it all, no matter how hard they try.* There is another generation that *could* try, it is the after-fifty crowd. Recently my book *Bonnie Prudden's After Fifty Fitness Guide* (see Sources) came out. It told that generation how basically fit they are and how to reclaim the bodies they had when they were younger. In the last chapter, "What Shall We Do When We Grow Up?" it told them to get busy with exciting *new* things. You and your children and your needs are exactly what those people need. *They* remember the games your children were never taught. *They* know how to take a walk in the woods. *They* can make kites and tell stories. People over fifty are like people under fifty, all different. Look around for some of them to help with your problems. You have a need for *good* day care, *good* nursery schools, *decent* education, after-school centers that provide things of value, jobs that allow for changes in schedules and emergencies. They could help you get them. Meet with them, talk to them. Remind them that *their chances for doing something of value will never be better.* And for my part, I will tell them about you, our most valuable national asset—*our mothers.*

CHAPTER TWENTY-THREE
A UNION FOR PARENTS

It was pouring rain when I answered the doorbell. There, sopping wet and carrying a bag of tools, was a skinny little kid who said his name was Wayne and he'd come to fix the tractor. I thought the father of the boy was probably waiting out by the garage, so I went to let him in. There was no father waiting when I opened the door. Wayne explained that *he* was the mechanic and could I please tell him what symptoms the tractor had. I could, and he fixed it.

Wayne liked tractors. He knew more about the one we had than the grown-up mechanic in our area—and, I suspect, more than his dad, an engineer at General Electric, who had taken on the tractor franchise in preparation for retirement. Wayne said he had been "watching and helping for years," and as the saying goes, he had watched real good. Not only could he take care of machines, but with those machines he could mow in one afternoon after school the same area two grown men had tended for one full day once a week. It is an age of machines. Those who understand them are well ahead, and the earlier the better.

Watching Wayne ride his steadily diminishing circle around the lawn, I wondered at all the changes. What became of chores? What became of waiting and saving for the things we wanted as kids—things that compounded in value in the waiting and dreaming? What sort of sinister star did we hitch our wagons to when we decided to give kids the things *we* didn't have? Well, what didn't we have?

We didn't have ice cream every day or pizzas on demand or potato chips or unlimited allowances or a free pass to perpetual entertainment. We didn't have permission—or worse, encouragement—to date seven nights a week. And we couldn't get the car either. We may have thought our parents were pretty mean sometimes, but we never suffered from the numbing conviction that these people in charge of our lives were so square that we, their children, could con them into or out of anything and everything.

We never had to wonder what to do with free time; there wasn't enough to wonder about. If we did have a chance to go out, we didn't have to wonder where the limits were; we knew that, too. We didn't have pot and we didn't have pills and we didn't have to keep up with the kids who did. We didn't have to decide at fourteen whether or not sex was love and love meant sex. We did know where babies came from, but we didn't have to decide at fifteen whether we'd have the baby or abort it.

True, not *all* the kids smoke pot, share crack, or order sex with the hamburgers at the diner. But it would be as foolish to pretend there are only a very few who do as to commit suicide over the ones you know who do. The way it looks from here is that the kids are getting a lot of things we didn't have and that we would rather they didn't have. What to do about it? Form a union.

The union I'm suggesting is serious business, and before any good can come of it, parents will have to come to an agreement *with themselves*. First ask yourself a question: *Do the children who eat at my table, wear the clothes I buy, and share the roof I built have the right to tell me where to get off?* Put that way, most people would say certainly not, but then someone injects a confuser: No, but they have a right to their opinions. Right, and if they express themselves considerately, you will consider those opinions, provided there is plenty of experience behind them and you can see that the opinions have merit and are not just "self-expression." There's the confuser. It came from those "woollies" who said children would be warped if they were not allowed to "express themselves." It's hard to say how many well-meaning parents fell for that one, but we do have some very odd young people around today who have been raised on "self-expression."

Next question: *Do my children have the right to waste their time while I am paying for their education?* Young people have the right to question. They have always questioned, and occasionally some of them have set out to make changes. But making changes takes time, effort, determination, and knowledge. Time is not a week, a month, or a single year. Effort is not breaking all the windows in the chemistry lab and joining six of your friends to beat up a teacher. Determination is not getting rid of the principal, and knowledge is not knowing how to tie dynamite together, fuse it, and blow up a dormitory. Those are not yet your children, but they are the upperclassmen, the ones the juniors try to copy—*if they have no firm convictions*. They get convictions from you. What *are* yours?

Do your children have the right to disturb your life with strife and discord right now while you are supposed to be enjoying the things you have worked for? And finally, *do those little kids who inhabit your house have the right to tell you that what you happen to want out of life is wrong?* No, indeed they don't. Their turn will come, and when it does, you can be as sure as you are of taxes that they won't ask you how *they* should live. If they are wiser than many in our generation have been, they will see to it that their children wait their turn. They are not overly endowed with either patience or understanding.

Many of you who have children under twelve are saying that these things don't apply to you: *Your* family works on the principle that love and security will bind you together. But what do you mean by love? What do you mean by security? Love isn't giving in to kids; love is helping them to grow. Security isn't protecting them from life and their own wrongdoing, whether that wrongdoing is skipping school or skipping down the aisle of a department store with a schoolbag full of stolen articles. Security is giving them an honest map they can follow when you aren't there.

On top of all the confusions that beset the American parent, the most damaging one is guilt, and I really don't know *where* we got that one. We have been so worried about a kind of ersatz equality—"Timmy has to have a bicycle; *all* the other boys have bikes and he'll feel deprived"—that the real inequalities have been overlooked for many years. When we fell into that trap, the kids had us. They didn't know how come they were so lucky, but they didn't waste any time cashing in. "Emily has Adidas. *All* the kids have Adidas. Why can't I have Adidas?" "The Morrises have a new car. *All* the kids' parents have new cars. Why do we have an old beat-up rattletrap?" "*All* the other kids are going. Why can't *I* go?" This might not have gained so much momentum if *all* the kids' parents met at church, the club, the PTA, the Y, the community center, or even the store, but they don't anymore. Groups are fragmented, and opportunity for unity has been almost nonexistent—up to now.

The parents who form the union to save the family will have to get together, really get together. They will have to meet at one another's houses, in apartments, in school auditoriums, and in churches. They will have to decide what *they* think is good for children, what should be allowed—and they will have to stick to it. No kid should get away with "*All* the kids are—why can't I?" because now you know that *all* the kids are saying exactly that to *their* parents, and by *all* the kids, they also mean yours. At each meeting there should be a collection of the things that the children are saying *all* the kids can do this week, and if possible a list of kids who come under the blanket of *all*. You will be amazed at how often your name is given—amazed and after a while good and burned.

Then measures will have to be taken.

There will always be a few children who wander as they please, and you won't find their parents in the union if you could find them at all, but those children would rather belong somewhere than wander, especially if someone cared whether they showed up or not. It will be a lot less expensive for the union to provide gyms, pools, and personnel than to set up places for the treatment of addicts age twelve. It will be a more permanent arrangement, too, because too few addicts of any age ever get permanently cured.

Our union will have to go into the schoolroom, too. Once upon a time if a youngster misbehaved in school, it was taken care of in school. The youngster prayed quietly that no note would go home, because whatever happened in school would go double when mother or father got wind of it. It is true that there were some pretty mean and horrid teachers, but they were nowhere near as damaging as the helpless and frustrated teacher of today, who is forced, by interfering parents and school administrators who refuse to back them up, to take whatever the bully boys dish out. *Your* children watch these teachers, whom they must respect if they are to learn. *Your* children watch Artie get away with murder in class. *Your* children cannot learn because Artie is disrupting the class, nor can they respect the teacher who can't handle Artie, who is no bigger than they are. The teacher *could* handle Artie, but parents in general won't let him. The price for such misplaced protection of dear little Artie? Chaos.

This goes a step further. Children are copycats, and Artie is now the hero. If he gets away with it, why not try the same thing? It works in school, so why not try it at home? Then, when in shock and confusion you don't handle the first attack, you damage and ultimately destroy the only solid thing in life for most little children—their respect for you, their belief and faith in you. As for you, you become that most ridiculous and pitiful of creatures, the giant brought low by pygmies.

Discipline is something we cannot raise children without, and by discipline I don't mean beating them to a pulp. You are not only big enough to do it if you had to; you are also bright enough so that you don't have to lift a finger. Our children today are addicted to a number of things, and probably the most prevalent is TV. The day the school bus came in, afterschool discipline went out, so you must entice the teachers into your union. They won't be long in coming when they learn that you intend to back them up. If Tommy is obstreperous in class, he is a boulder on the tracks of learning for the others. He is also a trouble to himself. If Tommy's parents knew just how big a trouble he is to himself, they, too, might be willing to help. In school the teacher has no weapon as strong as the TV set. If Tommy is denied TV time until he has proved himself in class, chances are he'll quiet down. But what if Tommy's parents are indifferent? There is always group pressure, and that is the most powerful of all. If Tommy upsets the class and all the other parents turn off the TV, you can be darned sure that the class will turn Tommy off posthaste.

Responsibility brings us back to Wayne. Wayne *wants* something, just as every kid should be allowed to want something. If you fall all over yourself trying to find out what your child wants so that you can buy it for him before he can ask for it, you steal from him. You steal wanting. It's important to want, to plan, to dream. If you, in your desire to *give* (which is actually as much fun as wanting), overgratify the child's desire, you interrupt the natural scheme of things. First, there is the dream, and as it takes shape, the feeling of need arises. It could be for anything at all—a dress, a bike, a room of one's own, a trip, music lessons, an education, anything. Next comes the scheming, the working, the saving, and the satisfaction of nearing a goal. To realize his dream, Wayne does gardening. He learned how from his father, and it is his father who is wise enough to help him dream and help him grow while he works to acquire. How much better than saying, "You want that? Here, go buy it."

How about your son or daughter? Do you help him to grow, achieve, and acquire by honest effort? If you have a garden, ask yourself who does the hard, hot jobs. It's no real chore for an eleven-year-old boy to drive around five acres of lawn on a high-powered tractor. That's the icing on the cake.

It's something else to weed the beds and push a power mower through the trees. Do you pay your Lilliputian help for doing the easy jobs while you do the tough ones yourself? Is that the way life really is? When you make it easy for your child, are you doing him any favors?

Then there is the matter of sticking to your job and doing it as well as you can. Do you? Where did you learn that valuable trait? Edging with a hand tool separated the men-to-be from the spoiled kids in one short Saturday morning.

When kids lack the ability to stay with it over the long pull and take hapless refuge from life in drugs and dropping out, more than likely someone forgot to teach them how to keep going when it would have been easier to stop. Everywhere we hear that young people are "copping out" because they don't like life as they see it. That's a reason? If you don't like what you see, change it. All you need is the will to stay with it, and that can be developed in an eleven-year-old child if somebody wants to.

Who bought the tools? Who bought his bike, her skis, their snorkel and fins? You did. When was the last time you could find your scissors? Who had the cards last? Who dropped the portable radio? Who left the saw in the rain? Who let the light burn out in the basement? Have you, by any unhappy chance, given anyone the idea that there will always be another to replace it?

We have made great strides in convenience. The laundry does itself while you do the shopping. You can put together a meal in half an hour from what are called convenience foods. You have a convenient garage next to the house or a part of the house or downstairs in the basement, and your car is conveniently ready at any time of the day or night. The shopping center is conveniently located, as are the medical center, the dentist's office, and the church. The one thing in our lives that is just as inconvenient (if not more so) as for our grandparents is the raising of children. There is no easy way to raise children. They usually arrive at an inconvenient time. They teethe most inconveniently when you have people in for dinner. They have inconvenient chicken pox for Christmas and inconvenient measles for Easter. They fall most inconveniently from trees and inconveniently are rushed to the emergency rooms with assorted cuts and gashes. They have inconenient stomachaches and inconvenient moods—but you love them. You love them and you want to enjoy their short stay; you want to give them the tools for life and send them on their way. Really, not since one child in four died before the age of two has the raising of children been quite so difficult, so uncertain, or such a challenge. Try to remember that when you form your union. Tell your friends and their friends that they won't be able to do much for the children after the age of twelve if they have not already done it before. For once, be stronger than the kids who rule by numbers. Alone, they don't stand a chance of outwitting you, nor can their numbers prevail if you will take the time to gather numbers of your own. Everyone today is frightened for children. Everyone is saying, "But what can *I* alone do?" The answer is form a union to save the children—not around the world, *right here*.

TWENTY-FOUR
BACKYARD TRACK MEET

To have a backyard track meet, you need one or more children *and you.* It is quite possible for children to mark off and set up an area of sorts without any help, but the excitement is then dependent on the attention span of children, which is notably short. If you want to get even a fraction of the potential offered by such activity, it will take the help and interest of an adult. A few materials and direction when it comes to setting it up will produce an excellent track and field area, but the main and most important ingredients are time, interest, and encouragement.

Whether you are an old track star yourself, an elementary school teacher, or a parent whose only connection with sports is Saturday afternoon on TV, you can do a tremendous job, and you don't need experts for your team. Quite different from so many activities available for children today, there doesn't have to be a winning team. Ellen, who falls over her own feet, has only to run a little faster next month and she "wins." Tom, who can't see to field a ball, may turn out to be a wonder with the shot put, which requires his strength rather than his eyesight. Mel, who has energy to burn and hostilities to match, can receive a workout and even be rewarded in the distance run, while Bill, who is too short even to make a team, can vault like a bird and will beat his own records with clocklike regularity. But you and they will never know about this progress unless you keep accurate records. If possible, you should invest in an inexpensive stopwatch to go with your "coach's" clipboard and pencil.

To make a very efficient track area, you will need a few supplies, most of which can be purchased at the local lumberyard. The few necessary tools can be found in any home or school tool drawer and the garden section in the garage.

TRACK MEET EQUIPMENT

- *One bamboo pole 8 feet long and strong enough to support the weight of a child using it for vaulting.*
- *One bamboo pole approximately 7 feet long to be used as a bar for jumping and also as a javelin.*
- *Two or three garbage pails full of sawdust for the jumping pits.*
- *Six pieces of 1-inch-by-3-inch boards 3 feet long for hurdles.*
- *Six pieces of the same stock, but 2 feet long.*
- *Six pieces of the same stock, but 1 foot long.*
- *Six pieces of lathe 6 inches long.*
- *One board 4 inches wide and 5 feet long for a takeoff board.*
- *A small supply of 1½-inch nails for the hurdles.*
- *About forty 3-inch nails for the jumping and vaulting standards.*
- *Two 8-foot lengths of 2-by-4 lumber.*
- *A folding ruler or yardstick.*

In addition you will need a rake to smooth the pits, a shovel to dig them, a hammer, some adhesive tape for the vaulting pole, a few feet of very heavy cord to make the javelin grip, a wheel from an old wagon or baby buggy to be used as a discus, and a smooth, round stone about 4 inches in diameter for the shot put.

As each piece of equipment or area is completed, take time to test each youngster for that "event" and keep score in a notebook.

You can use one side of your newly plowed garden, or if you want to keep practice going all summer, you can prepare a separate jumping patch. Dig a hole 5 feet square and about 6 inches deep. When it is clear of all loose dirt and debris, check carefully for small, potentially bruising stones. Fill the hole with the sawdust. Have the children take turns jumping into the pit so that they will become familiar with the feel of landing 6 inches below the apparent surface.

When the pit is finished, go to work on the two standards that will support the bar. Lay the 2-by-2s side by side so that you will be able to match the bar-supporting nails evenly. Start 4½ feet from one end of each and sink one of the 3-inch nails ½ inch into the lumber. Make the intervals 2 inches apart.

When the standards are ready, dig a 1½-foot hole for each one about 6 feet apart on either side of the jumping pit and be sure the slimmer bamboo pole will make the span. Be sure also before you fill in the holes that the nails are even so that the bar is level. The standards should be right at the edge of the pit on the side of the approach. *See that the nails face the pit.* Tamp in the earth firmly, measure up from the ground to the first set of nails and ink in the distance. Continue right up the standard, inking in feet and inches; this will be very important when the youngsters start practicing alone.

High Jumps The trials can be held for all the children at the same time. Just be sure that the starting height is low enough for even the littlest and least able youngster. Don't groan when Willie crashes at 2 feet 3 inches; just remind him that if he works hard, he can improve most of all.

During the trials give no instructions other than to start each child from a distance of at least 30 feet from the bar. You may also tell them that while speed is not essential, an even, running step will help. Set up your trials a little like the old game of "High Water, Low Water." All the children take a jump at the lowest level, and when all have finished, raise the bar one nail and everyone jumps again. Enter the last height that each child jumped successfully, and that becomes the starting mark for that child. *From that moment on, no child sits and watches.* Each one knows where to set the bar, and the height is determined by who is jumping, not the chance to jump determined by the height of the bar.

When you start your track and field workouts, be sure that all the children do *warm-up exercises* first, even before running, which is all too often considered warm-up enough. While warming up may not seem essential for very young children, it is important to ingrain the habit while they are little; then it will become part of them and will always assure a wider margin of safety as well as better performance.

---

298. HIGH JUMP

• *Start by putting the emphasis on* lift *right from the outset. Remind the youngster that running speed is not nearly as important as a steady running rhythm, and then the* lift. *Watch to see that the speed, whatever it is, does not slow during the last three steps before takeoff. If anything, it should increase.*

- *The jumper should "gather in" before the spring, and this is done by pushing the shoulders down a little and lowering the hips by running so low that the feet barely skim the ground.*
- *The body is crouched low as the takeoff foot hits the ground, heel first.*
- *The direction of the jump is forward and never to the side, even though the bar is to the side.*
- *The kick upward with the lead leg is vigorous, and thought should be concentrated on getting lift.*

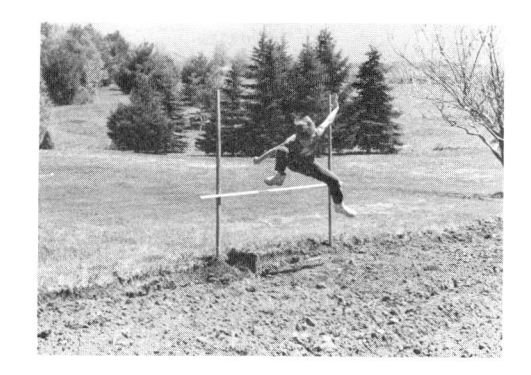

To improve the legs for jumping, do the floor progressions (pages 107–120) and the Russian Series (pages 121–127).

Broad Jumps There are two kinds of broad jump, and both should be used if there is space for both. One is the *standing* and the other is the *running* broad jump. Clear a jumping pit by softening up the earth (dig it up, don't just scratch the surface with a rake) in an area 5 feet wide and at least 5 feet longer than your best jumper can cover. The runway should be about 100 feet and as smooth as good care can manage. At the end of the runway at the edge of the pit, sink your 5-foot plank into the earth flush with the running surface. That is to be the takeoff line. Rake the earth smooth in the pit and start your first runner.

299. RUNNING BROAD JUMP

The youngster runs as fast as possible down the runway from whatever point permits him to build up maximum speed yet leaves him room enough to keep up that top speed for at least eight strides and still have space for four "floaters." These are steps that sail along on the buildup and don't require him to push hard. When each child finds his own best starting point (they will all be different), that is the practice point. In this way the fumbling and shortened strides will be eliminated. As a child grows in height, strength, and skill, the starting point will change, but at least he will adjust the change to performance rather than trying to adjust himself to a uniform (for everybody) starting line.

Measure the jump from the board to that part of the body that touches the ground nearest the board. Since this puts a very severe penalty on falling backward or lagging with one foot, insist that a *controlled* jump that nets a pretty good score *every time* is better than the occasional all-out stretch that makes tremendous distance and then ends in a fall back onto hands or seat.

310. STANDING BROAD JUMP

Use the same jumping pit and takeoff board. Stand with both feet behind the edge of the board, knees flexed and feet apart. Crouch slightly with arms back. On the jump, swing the arms forward hard and lift the chest. Distance is measured the same way as for the running broad jump, and the penalties for falling backward are as severe. Three tries for a score.

Jumping will be improved by running (see page 298) and by the Russian Series (pages 121–127). Do all the floor progressions as well (pages 107–120).

311. HURDLES

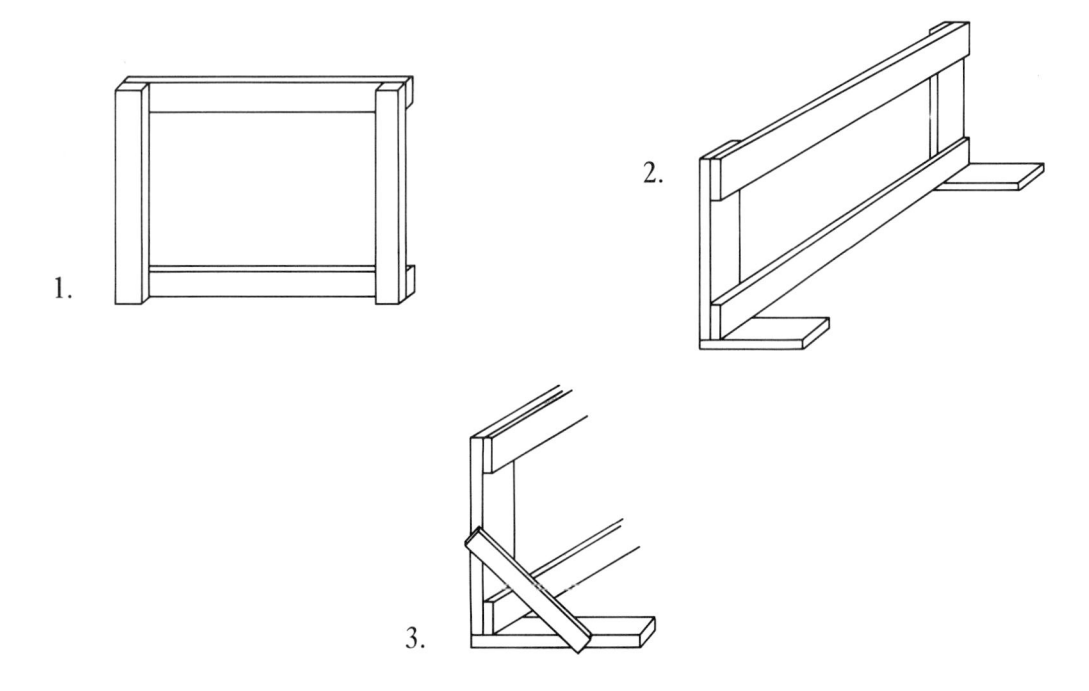

Lay two of your 3-foot boards parallel to each other about 2 feet apart. Then lay two of the 2-foot boards over each end to form a rectangle. Nail the 2-footers to the 3-footers and repeat this twice more to give you the start of three hurdles. Next, you will need a base or stand in the form of two feet nailed to the bottom of the rectangle. Nail one of the 1-foot boards to each of the two corners that will make the bottom of the hurdle. It should look like an L.

Next, nail one of the 6-inch lathes from the upright board to the "foot" at an angle on each side. This will give you a sturdy base that will keep the hurdle upright unless hit by a leg or foot, at which point it will fall forward with the stride.

The placement of the hurdles should not be a haphazard business. They should be far enough apart to permit three full strides between one hurdle and the next. This will mean dividing your runners into groups; however, the division should not be made by age or sex, but rather according to running speed and skill. The beginner always finds that three strides will never get him there if the hurdles have been set for practiced runners. Start with the hurdles six feet apart and then adjust for the groups, allowing greater distance for fast runners, less for the slow.

The object is to get over the hurdles safely without loss of speed in taking off, clearing, or landing. The body should move in a straight line rather than in waves like a horse going over a jump. It is impossible to do a good job of hurdling at slow speeds, so the preparation for this event should include a great deal of running to build up leg strength and speed.

The Takeoff
 Take off in full stride.
• *The lead leg exaggerates the knee lift of a normal stride and then reaches forward with a relaxed knee.*
• *The back leg exaggerates the forward push of a normal stride as* the body leans forward.

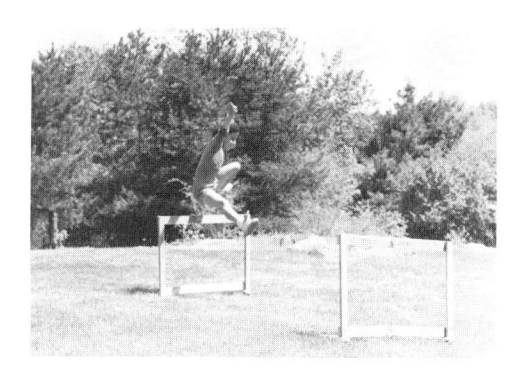

The Clearance
The back leg is *whipped* to the side with the knee bent. The runner should try to get it up to hip level.

The Landing
 Land on the ball of the foot of the lead leg.
• *As the back leg comes around over the hurdle, the foot swings down* but the knee stays up.
• *The front leg resumes the normal running stride.*
• *The back leg stretches out to the full-stride length as the body straightens up from the forward lean.*

Be sure the runner takes off quite far from the hurdle—this keeps the action flat rather than undulating. The hurdler should *drive forward* both during the run and when going over the hurdle. To keep up the speed, recover the back leg at hip height and then strike out hard. Getting a full stride on the first step off the hurdle is essential, and if the knee is not held up at hip level, the stride will shorten. This makes the flexibility exercises for hips and crotch a must, especially for boys, who are notoriously inflexible unless trained.

Let the children run the hurdles several times before you tell them anything about form; then when you do, they will have had enough experience with the feeling of hurdling to understand. Don't make the mistake of thinking they are too young to learn proper form. That's when it is best learned and creates a firm base for improvement.

JAVELIN

The javelin throw involves *all* the big muscles and not just the arm. It requires considerable timing and agility as well as speed. It is also a sport that should be practiced with care and attention as to where it is thrown. Javelins were once weapons of war, and they retain the ability to put both enemies and friends out of business.

302. JAVELIN

To improve the strength of the arms, chest, and shoulders, do push-ups, pull-ups, and the weight-training section (pages 189–196). To ensure shoulder flexibility, do exercises 18 and 21.

The Grip

Find the center balance point of the slimmer bamboo pole and wind the heavy cord around it to make a firm 5-inch-long hand grip. Lay the javelin *diagonally* across the palm so that it crosses from the base of the first finger to the outside heel of the hand. Place the first finger on the shaft *behind* the cord. The rest of the hand rests *on* the cord. Don't grip too hard; a tight hold will interfere with the throw. The grip

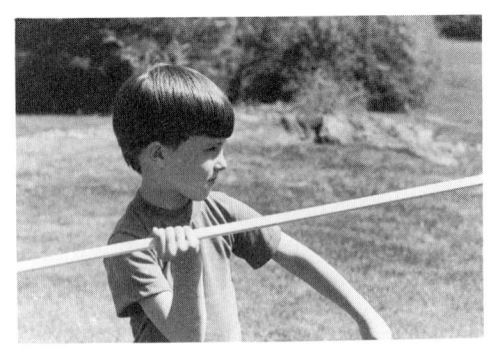

Backyard Track Meets

should place the shaft in the direct line of the throw and must control the javelin from every angle. If the point rises above the head too soon the pressure of air will cause a poor throw.

The Run

Use the same runway as for the running broad jump and the takeoff board as the foul line. The run can be as long as 60 feet and should provide maximum momentum so that the javelin already has speed from the body and is not totally dependent on muscle for distance.

During the run the javelin is carried toward the line parallel with the ground and at the level of the chest. As the line is reached, the javelin is drawn back *but with the tip still low.* If at the last second it is too high, the javelin will rise at too steep an angle and lose distance as the air is attacked by the entire shaft rather than the tip. At release the shaft should pass as close as six inches to the thrower's head and the head should turn slightly away. Be sure to throw so that the elbow precedes the hand. As in tennis, follow through.

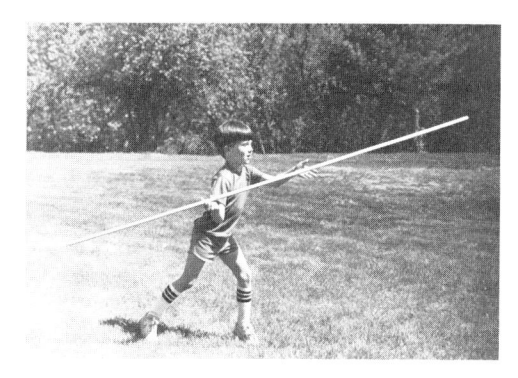

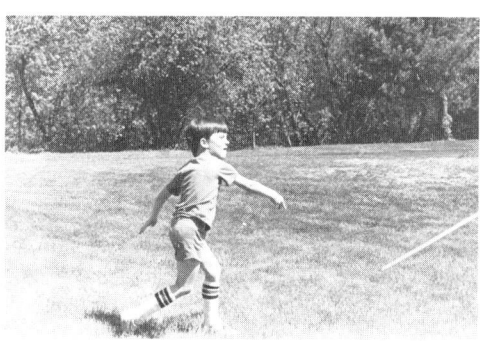

DISCUS

The discus, too, depends on the coordination of many muscles rather than just the arm and shoulder, and the same exercises and weights suggested for the javelin will serve as well for the discus.

To mark the circle needed for the throw, tie two pointed sticks to each end of 3½ feet of cord. Hold one stick point in the ground of what will become the discus and shot-put circle, then mark the circle with the sharpened end of the other stick.

Lay the discus in the palm of the hand with the first joints of the fingers curling around the rim. The thumb, which helps control the discus, lies flat against its surface. Some throwers bend the wrist outward in what is called a talon grip, but most coaches prefer the flat grip, which is considered more natural and normal.

303. DISCUS

To improve, train with weights and do exercises for shoulder flexibility.

• *Start in the center of the circle, placing the right foot near the rear of the circle on an imaginary line that bisects the circle and points in the direction of the intended throw. The left foot is on the same imaginary line about 2 feet from the right foot. The legs are slightly bent and the body erect.*
• *Take several preliminary swings to loosen shoulders (which have already been warmed up) and set up a rhythm, rocking the body weight forward and backward from one foot to the other.*
• *Spin the body into a turn to the left with the weight on the ball of the left foot, body slightly forward. Complete the turn by hopping from the left foot to the throwing position, the right foot landing slightly before the left.*
• *The discus should spin off the hand at shoulder level, like the last skater in "Snap the Whip" who has let go at the height of the snap.*
• *At the finish both feet will again be on the imaginary line, the right slightly past the center of the circle and the left approximately a foot from the edge of the circle.*

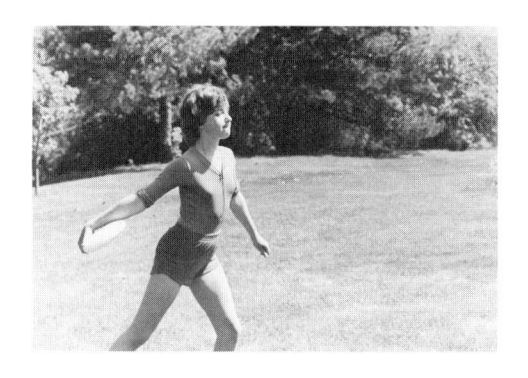

SHOT PUT

The same circle can be used for the shot put, but there must be a firm edge at the throwing side. A pole will work, but a line of heavy stones following the curve of the circle would be much better. *Do not let the youngsters throw heavy stones.* The one in the picture, brought in by my team, is far too large. Most boys would not be able even to get out from under it. Find a smooth rounded or oval stone that will fit easily in a small hand.

314. SHOT PUT

The Hold
• *Place the "shot" low in the hand rather than at the base of the fingers.*

• *Stand at the back of the circle with the left side facing the direction of the throw. The*

Backyard Track Meets

body should be erect and the weight over the right foot.

- *The shoulders are* level, *and the shot is held at the shoulder against the base of the neck. The right elbow points toward the ground at a 45-degree angle. The forearm is squarely in line with the intended "put." Look straight ahead, not in the direction the shot will go.*

The Hop

- *Bend the right leg slightly and then drive across the circle in the direction of the "put." Present the left side to the direction of the "put," but do not turn the head to the left.*
- *Keep the shot at the neck during the hop. Most beginners start to pull the arm back in readiness for the throw—don't.*
- *Start the push against the shot before launching.*
- *Launch as you turn and finish with the right side toward the "put."*

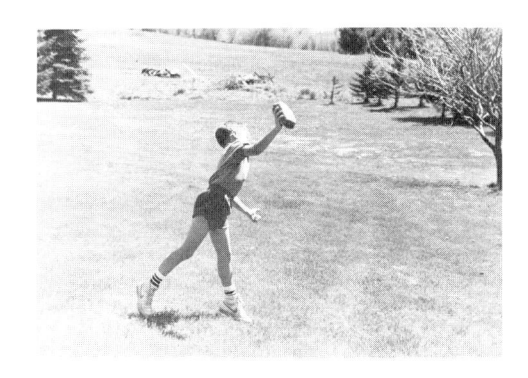

Try to remember that the arm "punches" the shot and the power comes from the upper arm. The lower arm is the last force to hit the shot, and the line between the elbow and the shot should correspond with the line of force. *There should be no whip.*

POLE VAULT

Every kid in the crowd will want to try his or her hand at the pole vault the minute you have standards, pole, and bar. It looks like fun, and it is fun. It is also quite difficult and demands speed, strength, agility, and coordination. Those with training in gymnastics and tumbling will do better than those without such disciplines, but it will also take training in running plus arm and hand strength (weight training and pull-ups).

305. POLE VAULT

The Grip

Tape the grip with friction or adhesive tape. The position of the right hand on the pole determines the grip height, and for the beginner it should be rather low. It might be best to alternate black friction tape with white adhesive tape every 6 inches for a good spread. Let each child use the band that suits him or her best. As strength and skill improve, children should move on to higher grips.

The Pole Carry

The pole is carried parallel with the ground, the front end slightly higher than the rear. It is held close to the body at hip level with the backs of the hands facing up. The pole tip faces directly forward. The left hand (if the vaulter is right-handed) crosses the body and is almost parallel with the ground. The right arm is extended back and is slightly bent.

The Run

The greater the speed, the more power will be available for the *lift*, but the speed must be controlled. A wild run means a wild placement of the pole, and from that moment on it's all downhill in a tangle. Grown-up vaulters use a run of about 100 feet; youngsters should try for 50 or 60 so that stride can be lengthened and rhythm established.

The Advance and Shift

At approximately two strides before reaching the takeoff point, the pole is *advanced* toward that point and the right hand and pole start to move upward. As the pole nears the point, the left hand slides up until it is close to the right. *The right hand stays at the same point from the start of the run to that second when the vaulter leaves the pole.*

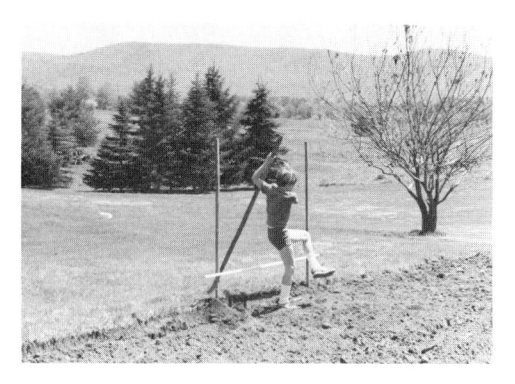

The Takeoff

At the second of *takeoff* both arms are above the head and slightly bent to absorb the shock when the body takes off the ground. Takeoff is made from the left foot as the right leg continues forward and *up*. The youngster should try to think of that right-leg lift as another high, knee-lifted running step.

The Swing

If you were holding on to a rope tied to a branch over a brook and you wanted to get over to the other side, the effort you would make to accomplish that act would be a "swing." In the pole vault the swing is *up* rather than across. Just before the "swing" the youngster should be running fast. The pole point goes down into the ground, and as it takes hold, he should *pull up* with an all-out effort (for preparation do chin-ups, push-ups, and the weight training as well as apparatus). The "swing" itself is an easy, relaxed move upward between the vigorous run and the vigorous pull-up.

The Pull-up

The pull-up is that all-out action as

the pole nears the vertical. Most beginners vaulting over fairly low bars don't see the necessity to *pull up*, since their *swing* usually permits them to clear the bar quite easily. However, as the bar rises, they will either have to *pull up* or hit the bar. Then they get the idea. The ability to chin oneself several times makes all the difference.

As the vaulter's hips get close to shoulder height, the pull-up is made and the body *turns*. The practiced vaulter does what amounts to a handstand (exercise 108) *on the pole* with his back to the runway. Not all the children will have the sort of determined, unflappable personalities that do well in vaulting, and not all of them will get high enough to do a handstand on the pole, but all should be taught the handstands that would make such a feat possible.

The Push-off or Fly-away

While it takes a lot of practice to get to the handstand-on-the-pole stage, the form for the fly-away should be worked on from the start. At the top of the pull-up (no matter what height) the vaulter pushes his body over the top of the bar and, when the push is almost completed, lets his legs fall. This acts a little like a seesaw and lifts the upper part of the body clear. At the second the pole is released to fall back on the runway, the backs of the hands are brought together so that the arms also stay clear.

The Landing

It is true that no fall ever hurt anyone, but the sudden stop is another story. Needless to say, as the youngsters practice, the bar must be kept low enough to assure control. As height is *slowly* attained, the ability to fall correctly is also attained (see chapter 12, "Tumbling"). Watch to see that the pit is big enough and the sawdust bed soft enough.

Constantly remind the young athletes that running and gymnastics play a tremendous part in the preparation for all track and field events. Push them to weight work, rain or shine. To prevent either injury or discouragement, vaulting should come after considerable time has been spent with tumbling, running, rope work, and weights.

The secret to a successful track team is the coach, and you are the coach. The slightest improvement should be important, and records should be kept from week to week and season to season. What is learned this season "cooks" in the subconscious and is ready to be brought forth *next* season. So if today's workout was disappointing, remind the child that good things are happening even when they don't show. What will keep him working, of course, is you.

CHAPTER TWENTY-FIVE
RUNNING

Once upon a time running was a way of getting away from danger, catching up to one's dinner, or covering long distances in a hurry. Now it is an activity children don't get much chance at and men over thirty do to prevent heart attacks. Running can tell you a great deal about your condition and the condition of the children. If one hundred of them were running around and around in a gym, you would soon see that no two of them run exactly alike. Some would be running flat-footed, usually with their toes in a ten-past-ten position. Some would be skimming along on their toes, busily setting themselves up for leg cramps. There would be stiff-legged runners who are so lacking in any feeling about their own bodies, they don't even know their knees are not bending. You would see finger flappers, arm pumpers, neck stretchers, and many other varieties of mismovers. There will also be a *few* boys and girls who run easily, naturally, and well.

Before you start to train young runners, check their times over a predetermined distance. Don't tell them anything about form, just let them run as they will. You will find that the ones who run well (they look it) will have the faster times; the ones who run poorly will be slow. Those who run poorly but have fairly good times would probably be able to do twice as well if they ran properly. Assure *all* of them that you don't care a hoot who has the fastest time. You care about improvement, and *all* of them are going to improve.

Look over the slow ones first. Try to spot the obvious faults. Do they plunk down in a flat-footed way? Are they flat-footed? If so, suggest the foot exercises on page 82 and check for the long second toe (page 435). Are their shoulders stiff? Suggest exercises 18 and 21. Are their arms awkward in the swing and do they swing at all? Are the fingers stiff, and is tension showing in stretched necks or facial expressions? Do they swing the feet out in back from side to side in what is erroneously called "the typical girl's run"? Do they pronate or roll over on the inside edges of their feet? Just what do they do that you can spot and identify? Put it down in your record book and then *correct one thing at a time for each child.* If you tell Mario, who slops along, to lift his knees, and Andre hears it (Andre's are high enough), you'll mess up Andre. Each may have a different quirk, and it is always better to treat each runner individually.

After you have watched your little (or large) group run and have written down in your book what you think is wrong, check with the tests (pages 12–17) to see if they tie together. The "round back" will probably run with the neck stretched and shoulders stiff. The child with anxiety often tenses when running (he tenses during everything else, too). The "swayback" leaves his seat out back and sometimes turns the toes out, too. The "flat foot" usually turns out as well. The "weak abdominal" may flip the feet from side to side in back. The "inflexible" will have a shortened stride. The "pronated ankles" and "wobbly knees" probably have the long second toe.

When you have tied in your standing postures with the tests for function, add the times. Set out a dash area of 50 yards. If possible, make it a permanent fixture, such as to a tree and back, around the house, to the corner or the telephone pole. Make it close enough so that you can say, "Go try the run and I'll time you." Kids need all the encouragement you can give them today: Running is not something they do naturally in outdoor play or to school because they are late. As you gradually correct their various problems and build both strength and flexibility, good running form will develop. Times will improve until even the slowest and most unaware youngster who hasn't the slightest idea about *how* he runs will appreciate that at least he is running *faster.*

Self-competition is good for everyone. Besides, it's fun to be able to chart improvement. Test your group and assure your young aspirants that they will do better with practice. Any practice at all will prove you to be right and may lead to more practice. The more improvement, the more you can appreciate and praise. The more of that, the more practice there is going to be.

Check for the following faults and list whatever you see on the child's test card:

Too stiff
Swayback
Round back
Flat back

Individual Track Chart

Date	Name	Dash	B. Jump	R. B. Jump	Jav.	Dis.	Hurd.	Shot	Vault

Stiff shoulders
Forward head
Grimaces
Breathless
Clenched fists
Stiff arms
Stiff hands
Flat-foot run
Pumping arms
Tiptoe run
Pigeon toes
Short stride
Toes turned out
Feet flipping back and sideways
Poor rhythm
Stiff legs
Wobbly knees
No speed
Tires easily

Watch for anything else that strikes you. Your eye will become the keener for a little practice in just looking.

The whole body should be relaxed because any tension will interfere with good performance. Explain that stiff arms and hands should be loose. Be sure you have spent some time on warm-ups before the run, and for the stiff-shouldered people do the shrugs on page 74. Tell the grimacers to practice "Indian face." A calm face often leads to a calm body, just as whistling when you are scared can make you feel a bit braver. The running itself will help to work out tension.

Teach the ones with stiff hands and clenched fists to run with the hands half open and the thumbs facing upward. If they run with palms down, the deltoids at the tops of the upper arms rotate, which tightens and destroys the free swing of both arms and shoulders.

The child who lands heavily on his heels may have flat feet now and will probably end up with a headache later in the day. This, as well as his running so badly nobody wants him on the team, will probably give him a very good reason (to him) for never running at all. Flat feet can be made to work as well as normal feet if the anterior tibialis is strengthened (see exercise 78). Also do all the foot exercises (pages 81–85).

When the foot pronates or turns either in or out, be sure to check for the long second toe and encourage the use of the little pad that puts the foot on a firm base (see page 436). If foot and leg strength are then improved, running may become such a pleasure that it will be a hobby for life. This will further protect the legs and especially the knees when the child goes out for football or basketball. When running, the feet should not turn in any direction other than straight ahead.

When watching arms, you will see

everything from the extreme pump, which can bang up to bloody a nose, to no motion at all. Ideally the arms, too, should be relaxed and coordinate rhythmically with the legs. The hands drop back as far as the hip pocket and swing forward as far as the center of the chest. Motion starts in the shoulders. There is little play in the elbows and none to speak of in wrists, hands, or fingers.

You will find that as you are able to correct one fault, others simply disappear. When the feet start to track forward and abdominals are strengthened, the arms will stop their wild flailing. When fists relax, shoulders will follow suit. This in turn will permit a straighter carriage, which will increase speed and make the whole business easier.

RECOVERY

Leg action is less complicated than you might think. Start looking at what is called *recovery*. It begins with the kick-up behind. Most youngsters kick up naturally, but whoever doesn't will find maintaining the run for any length of time virtually impossible. Recovery is completed by bringing the leg forward and *keeping the knee bent* as the leg moves under the body. At that point the heel almost touches the buttocks. Then the knee leads the leg forward and, when the thigh is well to the front, unhinges so that the foot reaches ahead.

If balance and rhythm are good, the fewer steps taken in any given "pace," the longer the "pace" can be maintained. A long, fluid stride is always more efficient than frantic churning, but for the long stretch one needs back and hamstring flexibility. If you spot churning and short steps, refer to test 6 (page 17) and use the corrective exercise (page 30).

THE STEP-DOWN OR REACH

The most important movement for stride length is to bring each thigh well forward before extending the lower leg. This keeps the foot in the air for a longer time, giving more distance. *It stays in the air as long as the driving foot pushes the body forward.*

The two most likely errors are failure to complete the *recovery* and failure to *reach*. In the first instance the kick-up behind is accomplished all right, but then the leg is just dropped to the ground without bringing the knee through. This cuts short the push of the driving foot. The second is failure to kick up behind. The leg is swung through as though a wedge of wood were stuck in each knee joint. The child who does this has not run very much because he simply couldn't. He can't improve because he avoids running whenever possible. The instructions that help him kick up behind will change all that, *and possibly his personality as well.*

Running as self-competition and as an exercise in form should come first. Only *after* the children can really run correctly should races be permitted.

Begin your competition with warm-ups for everyone. Children should be fully aware by this time that warming up will improve performance.

THE RACE

THE START

A good start gets you away fast with no wasted motion. Every runner eventually develops a style all his own, but the initial teaching should give each a good foundation on which to build. Insist on the following:

1. Place the left foot back of the starting line (the right if you are left-handed and left-footed).
2. Place the fingers behind the starting line squarely under the shoulders.
3. Kneel on the right knee with the left knee beside the right foot so that you will know where to dig the holes that will give the feet purchase.
4. Dig a hole for the toes of each foot.
5. Take the *marks position.*
6. Look where you will go, and relax.

GET SET

1. Rock *up* out of the kneeling position.
2. Rest all possible weight on the fingers and front foot.
3. Rock forward as far as possible without falling or losing control of the position.

GO!

Drive hard with the front leg. The rear foot is brought through low, just missing the ground. The body also starts low and straightens up gradually. If the runner does not have complete control of the start, he may stagger forward, losing speed as he struggles to recover. If he stands erect too fast, he loses the forward drive from his first effort.

Here are some starting faults that are easy to spot:

- The arms are spread too wide. They should be just under the shoulders.
- The hips are too high and the head is too low. The line of the back should be close to level.
- The weight is too far back, which will cause a slow takeoff.
- There is a tendency to stand up at the starting signal. Instead, stay low and recover gradually.
- Arms may just hang after takeoff. They should whip into action as quickly as the legs.
- After the race, *walk* your runners so that muscles can cool off.

Running for distance, especially comparatively long distances, provides an excellent opportunity for general conditioning. This is not true of dashes or any sort of all-out effort in sports. As in most of the games we play, we must *be* in shape to do well. Therein lies the tragedy of American physical education, which gave up *training* in the thirties and provided *games*. Later we will take a look at cross-country running, which, because it works for aerobic improvement, can also help with speed.

When any form of exercise is used, the body adapts in many ways, but most of the important adaptations come only after the activity has gone on for a long time. One of the best-known signs of such adaptation is the *second wind*. The misery that may precede the second wind is a sign that the body is getting these arrangements under way. When you feel the blessed recession of misery and a kind of shift into high, you know that all the body functions relating to energy production have been stepped up. You are indeed traveling along in top gear.

One cannot get to this delightful level with vigorous but short bursts of action because the body under such muscular stress manufactures fatigue products such as lactic acid so fast that they cannot be carried away quickly enough. They accumulate with such rapidity that the bloodstream is loaded with them and the muscles cannot respond properly to voluntary nerve stimulation. When that happens, the individual must stop his activity even though *his capacity for action in all other respects* has hardly been touched. His body is still full of strength, but the muscles simply cannot respond. In a swimming race it may become almost impossible to lift an arm out of the water.

OXYGEN DEBT

In any dash, oxygen is burned at a much faster rate than it can be replaced right then and there, and the body goes into what is called *oxygen debt*. This is comparable to taking a trip and finding out that it is costing more than you happen to have with you. There isn't time to stop off and get a job to replenish your cash—the trip is too short and the purpose too urgent. So you wire your brother and borrow. You would then be in what might be called a *money debt*. You will pay it back as soon as you can stop traveling and work a little. In oxygen debt you use all of the oxygen you had available in your body before the start of the dash, borrowing from your tissues to keep you going and promising to pay back with a lot of fast panting as soon as your quick trip is over. You can't replenish your supply en route because no matter how fast you breathe during the dash, the oxygen cannot be absorbed in time to do you much good. Instead of stimulating the circulation and exercising it, the dash uses up whatever oxygen was available and, like the quick, expensive trip, leaves the swimmer or runner owing his body a debt of oxygen he will have to repay. Sometimes being in oxygen debt is quite as uncomfortable as being in financial debt. One more thought: Can you imagine what sort of shape the man or woman is in who goes into oxygen debt from a single flight of stairs or a quick twenty-foot dash to the bus?

It should be your aim to get the youngsters to use *all* the functions of exercise and thus improve those functions. Fast running prevents sufficient use to produce maximum benefit. A few factors of exercise are quickly forced to the limit, and that in turn forces all the others to cease functioning. With this in mind, use dashes and relays (children love them) as icing on the cake. In distance running the runner puts out more *total effort*, and this sometimes leads parents and teachers to feel that younger children should confine their running to short stretches. This is a mistake. Adults *and children* should run for distance. It is just a matter of building their bodies to adapt, and this should always be done in stages. At the Institute, we started three-year-olds on mile runs. It took nineteen turns around the track to clock a mile, so the first week the little people ran once around the track and then went on to other things. Each week one more turn around was added until first we had quarter-milers (with quarter-mile pins). In time we exchanged the quarter-mile pins for half-mile pins, and still later for mile pins. This was only the beginning. They wanted to "run a million miles," which meant keeping track of the miles run. The trouble was that we didn't have enough teachers for the job, and the "threes" couldn't count for themselves and still remember which round they were on. So we gave each group two baskets, one containing nineteen small stones and one empty. Each trip around the track they transferred one stone from the full to the empty basket. At the conclusion they carried their baskets into the office and their miles were recorded in their notebooks. At the end of the season we had seven three-year-old *one-hundred-mile runners.*

Their bodies had adapted to the demands being made upon them. Hearts were stronger, and so were their determination, confidence, and pride. Since every part of their bodies had approached fatigue at an even rate, they had been able to work each part to the fullest and thus build the whole. No one overworked section called a halt before the job was done.

---

306. CROSS-COUNTRY RUNNING

Now comes the pièce de résistance, the cross-country run. The cross-country run is *it* when it comes to *overall* training, but it contributes a lot more than that. In the 1970s, when the so-called fitness boom came on the scene, jogging was the "in" thing. If you jogged, you could wear really snappy outfits; at a party you could mention that you had jogged your usual five miles that morning. Other people took note of you. People who had never run to the corner in their entire lives bought jogging shoes, shorts, and headbands. Without a thought in the world as to training or safety, or the future, off they went down the road, smug, self-satisfied—and later on they would add, sad.

Jogging on the road became the rage, and clubs soon formed. People began to take themselves and their jogging very seriously and filled their own and each others heads with words such as *high, hitting the wall, peaking,* and so on. Unless you could *talk* about your jogging with the right vocabulary, you were definitely not with it. Those were the years when *you know*, and *like* were also "in," and a morning greeting from one sweating jogger to another went something like this, "Like, howfarjoorun?" Second sweater checks his watch and answers, "Since early, like, you know, sisaclock." People weren't important to most runners; times and miles were. Panting and a stone face showed you were really putting out. But, like most fads, jogging-for-everybody began to lose followers. Why? *Injuries*. People had paid all kinds of attention to the shoes they were wearing but none to the surface they were running on. Anyone who knows anything about expensive horses would never run a horse on macadam or cement; it would ruin those valuable legs. But people . . . people's legs are unimportant. They are not noticed until they begin to hurt, and it wasn't very long before that began to happen to thousands and thousands of joggers. One year, at the height of the craze, there were thirty million *registered* runners.

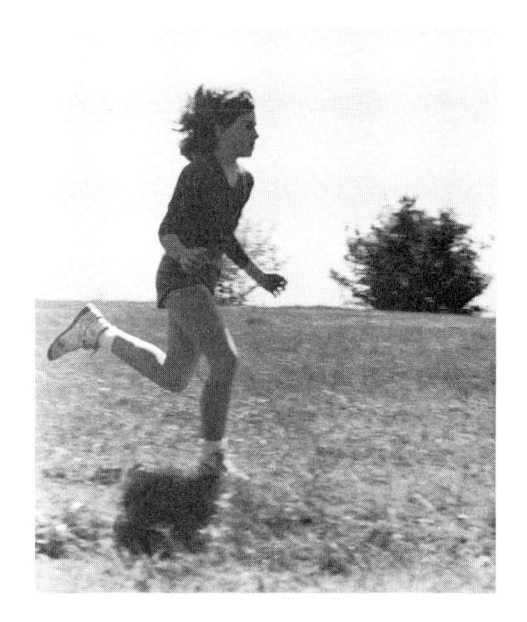

Within five years fifteen million of them had quit running due to injuries to feet, legs, knees, backs, and groins. Then the conversations began to go, "Jog?" "Used to, but I pulled a muscle in (almost anywhere) and had to give it up." "What do you do instead?" "Nothing much, everything seems to hurt."

If you are that ex-jogger, refer to the chapter on Myotherapy and get rid of that pain, but *never* go back to jogging on the road. Take up cross-country running and really get yourself in shape. Take the kids along and, incidentally, teach them how to do Myotherapy on you as well as each other. Then if you *should* pull a muscle or step in a hole and sprain an ankle, you will be painless in a couple of hours and back running in one or two days.

Before you start your cross-country or distance running, measure out the course. Have a definite starting place and mark the route to be taken with wands, blazes on trees, or colored ties on branches. A quarter mile is 1,320 feet. Borrow the longest tape measure you can find and ask a friend's help. Don't guess; measure. You can put encouragements along the way in the form of stakes with numbers for tenths of a mile. Another possibility is to push a bike with a speedometer over the course distance.

If you are just starting, use a walk/run combination in which you walk seventy-five steps, counting only the right-foot step. Then run for twenty-five. In a few days start adding steps to your run while keeping the walk at seventy-five. When walk and run are equal, start subtracting from your walk steps. Soon you will be tireless the whole way.

When your runners can keep up a good pace over a mile course, institute *wind sprints*, in which they trot at a comfortable pace for a while, then take off for an all-out dash for a *short distance*, then drop back to the ground-covering trot.

Remind your young athletes that running is required training for all track and field events and that the more they do, the better their skill will be in all other sports as well. For yourself, know that their bodies are improving day by day and that they will have at least one sport for all their lives. Know one other thing: While *they* are getting into shape, so are *you*.

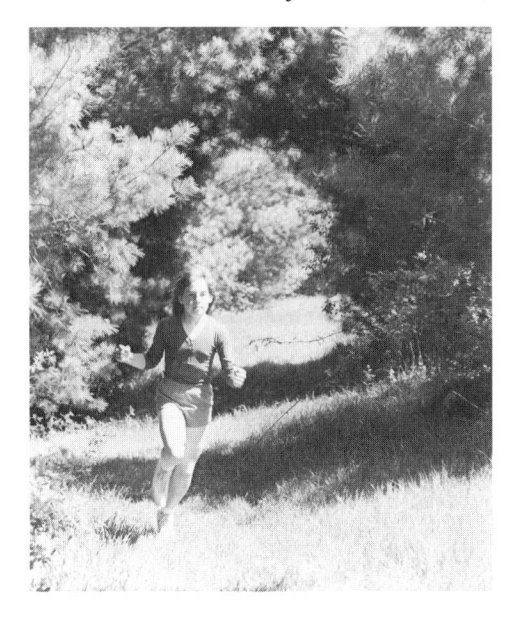

CHAPTER TWENTY-SIX
SWIMMING

For a long time there have been wise and enterprising mothers and teachers who exposed newborns to warm water in the "total dunk" form. In the early days, American whalers returned to New England with fabulous tales of the islands, not the least of which was seeing a new baby *swim* away from the mother who had just birthed it. Probably no one believed the tales. In those days Americans were not overly concerned with bathing to begin with, and for a Puritan offspring to dive into the icy waters off Maine and New Hampshire with a newly emerged babe in arms was inconceivable. *We* couldn't imagine such a thing, but a Tahitian mother couldn't imagine any better way for a baby to greet the world than in the arms of the sea goddess.

Those Americans who did understand the value of water can't claim first dibs on the idea either. Russia, the land of ice, snow, and steam baths, was way ahead of us. We are now beginning to consider the needs of the baby at birth, and in a few places—mostly birthing centers, which are themselves very new—we are beginning to turn the lights and noise down and to give the baby to its mother *before* assaulting it with Phisohex and shiny, cold instruments. In Russia they are even birthing babies under water. Babies love warm water, are totally at home in it, and don't have to learn to swim; they are born knowing how.

About twenty-five years ago, roughly five years after we discovered the sad facts about American *un*fitness, I was giving a seminar in Detroit's Northeastern YMCA. "You ought to have a Baby-Swim-and-Gym Class here" I said to the young, vigorous, open-minded general secretary. "How would we go about that?" he wanted to know. "Easy, we get a mother who isn't afraid of the water, a teacher who isn't afraid of the water, *any* good teacher of anything will do, the baby, and the Detroit press." "Done," he said. "My assistant's wife is both a swimmer and a new mother, and the baby is calm and delightful, like her parents. Jane, my fiancée, can teach anything, and I've got an in with the paper."

On Thursday I spent half an hour with the three soon-to-be-famous members of the new group. They learned about hugging in the water, listening to the heart pump while warm arm skin was pressed all around the baby's back and bikini-revealed midriff pressed against the front. Mother-smell went into the little nose that rested against shoulder skin. In short, we had reproduced the womb feelings of just a few short weeks before. "Lovely," said the mother, "Um, lovely," thought the baby. "What a shot!" said the photographer the next day.

"What's going on?" asked the reporter as mother and baby quietly slipped beneath the surface for a few seconds (which, she said later, felt like an hour). What was going on was "Old Home Week." Within minutes teacher and mother were playing "Pass the Baby" on top of the water and then the same game *under* the water. Before a half hour had passed, the mother and baby were *swimming* together under water. How was that possible? Simple, if you know some facts:

• Babies are born with reflexes that protect them in a water environment. The first reflex shuts off the trachea, the pipe to the lungs. If that reflex weren't there, how do you suppose the baby could keep from inhaling the amniotic fluid in the *womb?*

• The baby has swimming reflexes that go into action when the baby is face down in warm water. Froglike kicks are a part of every healthy new baby's repertoire, like sucking and swallowing. He or she also makes propelling arm motions, which, like the grip reflex, will get lost through disuse or be reinforced by the opportunity to continue swimming.

• Babies are like seals. When their faces go under water, a whole survival system goes into effect. All blood flow to peripheral areas—the arms, legs, kidneys, and digestive system—is slowed drastically. The blood not needed for immediate survival is rerouted to the heart and brain. This enables seals to stay at good fishing depths for a long time. This allows the baby to be safe under water for a much longer time than the mother, who has lost that ability through disuse. We all have many survival aids, which we lose either because they aren't that useful anymore or because we don't know we have them and know nothing of their value. We know much less about ourselves at the age of twelve than Navaho children know when they reach that age. A Masai, too, could give us lessons. What is more important, we can learn from our own babies if we will *watch*.

The session with the reporter and photographer was a huge success. The reporter was a swimmer from way back and a woman. The photographer was an artist. The spread came out over the weekend, and the Y's new Baby-Gym-and-Swim program was full before Tuesday.

From there it spread to other YMCAs, and then some YWCAs picked it up. Then the "scairdy cats" got into the act. They fall into the crowd I have labeled "perennially menopausal," but they aren't all female, and those that are are rarely mothers. In this case neither sex is comfortable in the water. A few doctors have been talked into that group, but they usually want their names in the paper. Call your own doctor and ask his or her opinion. If he or she is athletic or a swimmer, you'll probably get the "all-systems-go" sign. Best of all, use your own common sense. One "good" reason for keeping a baby out of Gym-and-Swim is a series of earaches. If your child gets earaches, wait awhile. Most of the other reasons cited—infectious diseases, meningitis, and a host of other "itises" you have never heard of—belong to the warner only and are a sign of neurosis. In the many years since that first baby-swim class we have never had one complaint other than earache, which often seems to run in families.

Why get the baby into the water? Several reasons. Swimming is like language: The earlier you learn it, the better you do it. Children under the age of three are the most vulnerable group when it comes to drowning. They are also the easiest to teach how to swim.

According to the National Safety Council, drownings were the third leading cause of accidental death in the United States in recent years. That figure is rising steadily as we increase our leisure time and as more and more families build backyard swimming pools.

Over 60 percent of those drowned were young people under the age of twenty-five, and the greatest number of drownings was suffered by fifteen-to-nineteen-year-olds. Most of the casualties were boys, and two-thirds of them didn't know how to swim. Imagine. That is the age of the young people planning to have babies in the next ten years. Do you think learning to swim is going to be high on their list of things to do? Not likely.

Over the years, the Joint Committee of Physical Fitness, Recreation and Sports Medicine has made numerous suggestions as to what we ought to do to prevent children's deaths by drowning. One was putting fences around water hazards. While about 40 percent of the drownings occurred when people were swimming or playing in the water, it seems that *only 5 percent happen in pools* that might conceivably be fenced. Seventeen percent happened while people were boating, and 39 percent were due to falls from shores, docks, bridges, and so on. It is virtually impossible to fence a shoreline. Here again we should say that it is impossible to protect a child from the perils of the world. We can't protect an adult either. We can, however, *prepare* people of almost any age to meet those perils. Learning to swim is the best way to prepare against drowning.

Babies don't have to be taught to swim, they come with the knowledge already built in. All they need is the opportunity; an ideal environment; *warm,* clean water; and a parent with patience and stability. If you are a parent or teacher embarking on this, I have made a film and a tape and written a book that will help (see Sources).

Children have to learn, if they have let their swimming license lapse by not swimming as babies. Given a shallow pool and some friends and an adult who likes to play in water, the whole neighborhood will swim by the end of the first summer the pool goes in. Children who have never had a lesson will busy themselves hunting for pennies or poker chips in the bottom of the pool—if they are wearing a mask. The way to use new equipment is to present it in a known environment. The following exercises and equipment are a small sample of what we have used and what we have done.

Before you start your swim program, give everyone the test for vital capacity (page 36). It will improve during the program, and you should be able to point it out. Long before the swimming season, *your* swim season should begin. Robert Kiphuth of Yale used to start his team out on the gym floor weeks before they were allowed to get their feet wet. He set the style for preswim exercise. You have probably heard that swimming is an all-around exercise; it isn't. You will need to strengthen the swimmer's body and try for the kind of flexibility enjoyed by fish. If you are in the market for a swim team, here's the way to start.

307. WARM-UPS WITH FINS

Whether you intend to go into the water in a little while or merely use this as a preseason workout, *warm-ups are essential.* If you do them with fins or flippers on your hands, you add resistance to your effort—a kind of full-range weight program.

• *With legs straight and apart, do a regular overarm stroke to a steady rhythm just as you learned back in the warm-ups section (exercise 8). Swim forward for eight; eight left; then eight right. That makes up a set. Do three sets to brisk music, wearing fins on* hands. *The weight of the fins will hurry your strength along, as will their resistance to the air through which they pass. Keep in*

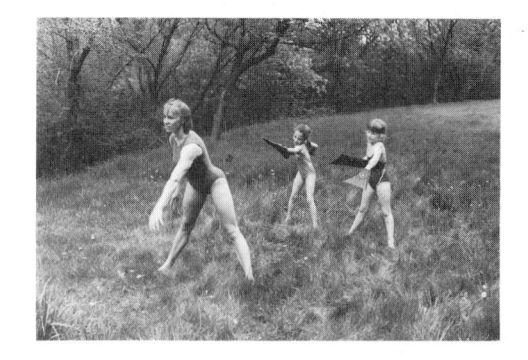

Swimming

mind that children love equipment and that there are dozens of pieces of equipment with which you can "swim." Frisbees, like fins, can be used beneath or above water, and both can be used in the same exercise if you stand in water.

308. WAIST TWIST UP AND DOWN

A limber waist is needed in most sports, but is not developed by all of them, biking and swimming, for example. That means that calisthenics must make up the difference.

• *The arms will soon tire with resistance exercise, so avoid flooding the muscles with fatigue products, which curtail activity and also cause stiffness and pain. Spread the legs wide for balance.*

• *Bend your arms at shoulder level and twist the upper body right and left for two sets of eight. Let the weight of the fins carry you around as far as possible. That extra weight will pull the body farther than mere arm swings like those in the warm-ups section (exercise 9) could do. Do sixteen twists* up *and then add sixteen* down.

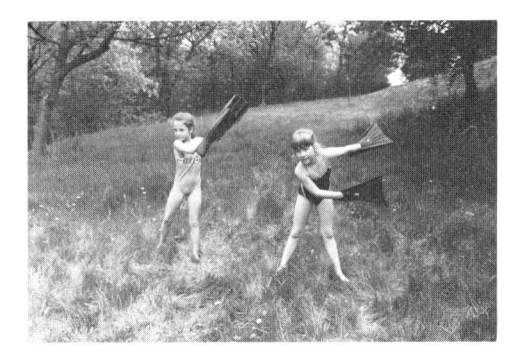

• *Bend forward from the hips and continue the twist exercise, but with the upper body parallel with the floor.*

• *You have done sixteen* up *and sixteen* down *to make up a set. Do two sets. Before you start the next exercise, which calls for arm and waist strength, do the Shoulder Shrug (exercise 13). Let your arms dangle at your sides.*

309. OVERHEAD REACH

• *Place the left hand on the left thigh and the right straight overhead. Slide the hand down the leg, which will bring the other hand across to the same side and put considerable pull on all the side muscles.*

• *Bounce the fin downward four times and then four times to the opposite side. Repeat the set three times.*

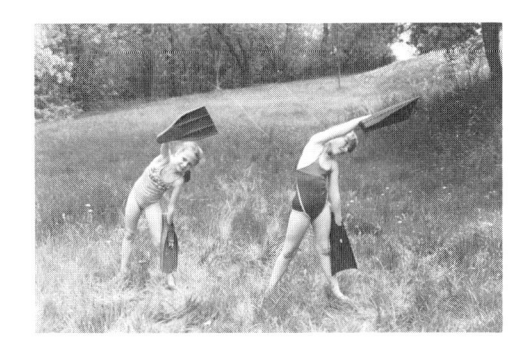

310. THE BIKE

• *Sit down on the edge of the pool or the floor of your practice room and put your fins on your feet. Lean back on your elbows and do the "bicycle" movement about twenty-four times straight ahead.*

• *As the legs improve, lean on your right hip and both elbows and do twelve.*

• *Then lean on your left hip and both elbows for twelve.*

• *Much later, go back to the first leg position, straight ahead.*

• *Lift both legs and arms for twelve.*

At the finish of the warm-ups your muscles will be warmer and more flexible. (If you are wondering what quality goes best in the water, it is flexibility.) To improve your body for swimming, do the flexibility series starting on page 97 at least once every day. Warm-ups plus flexibility exercises will prepare you for a swim class or competition—they get muscles ready and step up circulation. This means that your tissues will have an excellent oxygen supply *before* you go into oxygen debt. (Read the information about oxygen debt on page 303.)

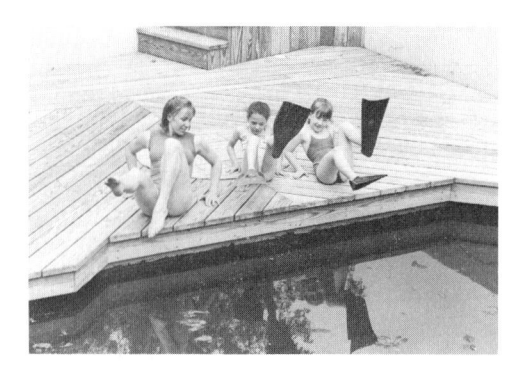

TOWEL EXERCISES

There is one piece of equipment every swimmer has handy—a towel. Whenever you are just resting or "hacking around," *use* it.

311. TOWEL SHOULDER-STRETCH

For smooth swimming action and long reach, you need shoulder flexibility.

• *Hold on to both ends of your towel and, keeping both arms straight, start with the towel in front of your thighs.*

• *Pull outward as you lift the towel slowly overhead and backward down to rest on your*

Swimming

seat. Let's hope you have the pectoralis flexibility to do this without bending either arm.
• If you cannot manage it, get a larger towel. As stretch improves, shorten your grip on the towel. Do eight forward to back and then eight back to front.

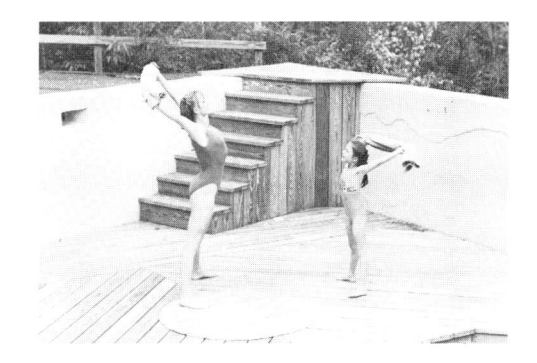

312. TOWEL FORWARD-PULL

• Put the towel across your back and hold the two ends in front.
• Push forward with both hands as hard as possible as you count slowly to eight. This will strengthen your hands (which swimming doesn't) and your arms, chest, shoulders, and upper back. The abdominals too. It is called an isometric exercise, that is, contraction occurs but doesn't result in movement. Do eight.

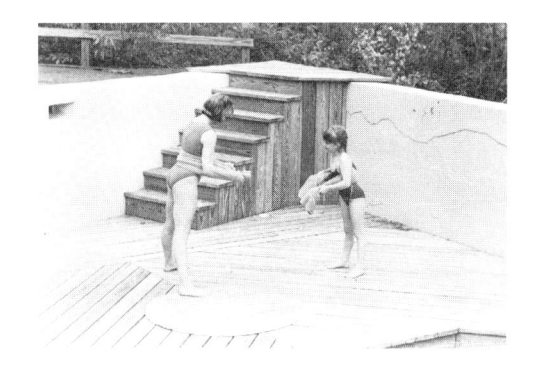

313. TOWEL LEG-FLEXIBILITY, PULL-OUT

• With feet well apart and legs held straight, grasp the two ends of the towel.
• Lean forward from the hips as you pull outward with both arms and bounce the upper body downward eight times. Keep the knees straight. Be sure to maintain the outward pressure on the towel ends. This is a combination of isometric (arms) and isotonic (hamstrings) exercise. That means keeping your mind on two things at once. (In isotonic exercise, movement does occur in the working muscle.) Do eight.

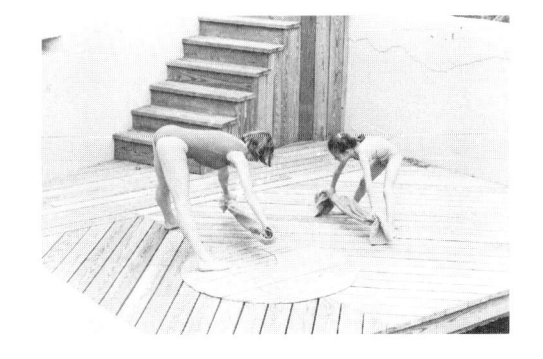

314. TOWEL, NECK PULL

- *To work the triceps in the arms, the hands, neck, and chest muscles, sling the towel around your neck and pull both ends forward with both hands.*
- *Hold the pressure for eight slow seconds and do eight. (This is another isometric exercise.)*

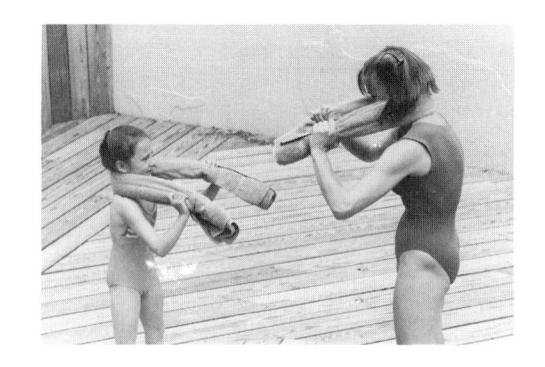

315. TOWEL, LEG PULL

- *To strengthen hands, wrists, arms, shoulders, back, and thighs, sit down and put one foot in the "sling" made by both hands pulling on both ends of the towel. Hold for a slow count of eight. Do eight with each leg.*

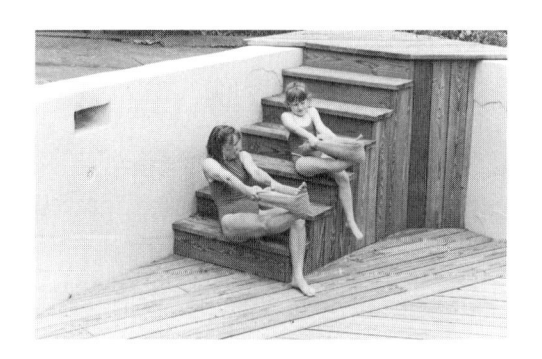

316. TOWEL LEG-PULL, BALANCE

- *To add balance to the exercise, stand up and balance on one foot as you do the towel exercise with your other foot in the sling.*

Hold for eight slow counts and relax. Do eight with each leg in the sling.

PARALLEL BARS IN YOUR BACKYARD

More and more people are adding pools to their backyards. If you are planning such a valuable addition to your life, take a look at the leftover space and think of an inexpensive, permanent piece of equipment—parallel bars.

The parallel bars most of us know are found in gyms and used during gymnastics competitions. Very few American students ever get a chance at them today and only those over fifty ever had any training on them. Fortunately, one doesn't need special training to use the ones shown here and they do give enormous returns for the investment. They can be used by anyone over five or six and even the littlest members can be helped to tight-rope walk on them and hang on them. Anyone knowing anything about children knows they love to show off and while showing off, will outdo themselves. If the bars are near the pool, where the whole family gathers, there will always be a ready audience.

Use two 24-foot lengths of two-inch conduit. Twelve feet of each piece becomes the bar part, leaving six feet at each end as supports both above and below ground. A hydraulic press (plumbers and electricians have them) can bend the corners for you. A two foot hole is dug at each end and the four ends placed 22 inches apart. Then concrete is poured around them.

317. STRAIGHT HANG AND TUCK

• *Take the straight-hang position by placing the hands on the bars and jumping up to hold in a straight-arm support.*

• *The body should be kept straight and the toes pointed. If any part of the child's body seems to be straining, it is. Strength is the needed ingredient. If the body is lacking that strength, the child will still try to perform by substitution. That means pulling into play muscles not meant to do that kind of work. If some of the smaller children strain, hold them back and keep them on weight training and tumbling.*

• *The* tuck *part of the exercise employs abdominals and the quadriceps. Draw the knees up to the chest, taking two counts.*

• *Lower the legs to full hang in two counts.*

• *Do four tucks and then jump off to rest the arms before trying again.*

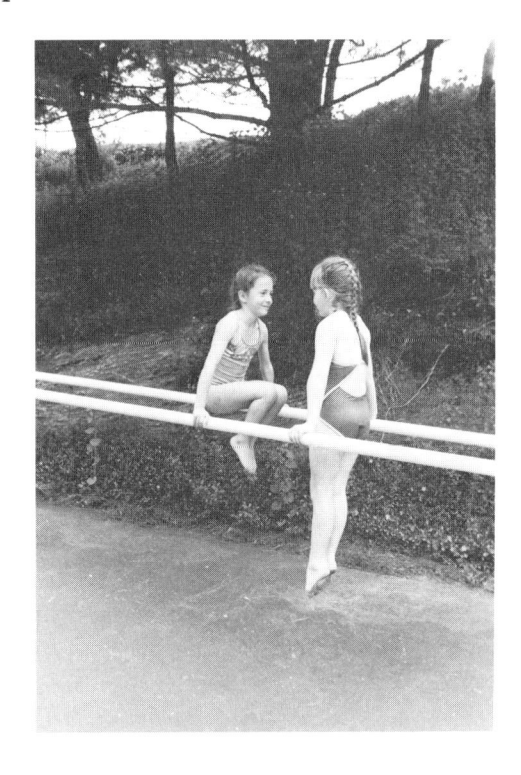

318. TUCK AND SPREAD

• Start by jumping up to a Straight Hang (see exercise 317).
• Tuck as in the foregoing exercise.

• Lower the legs into a spread-leg hold. Repeat four times and dismount to rest.

319. LEG EXTENSIONS TO SCISSORS

• Start with the Straight Hang (see exercise 317) and then raise one straight leg while the other hangs straight down.
• Lower that leg and raise the other. Lower the second leg.
• Raise one leg in front and one back as far as you can manage.
• Next, Scissor the legs past each other eight times. Dismount.

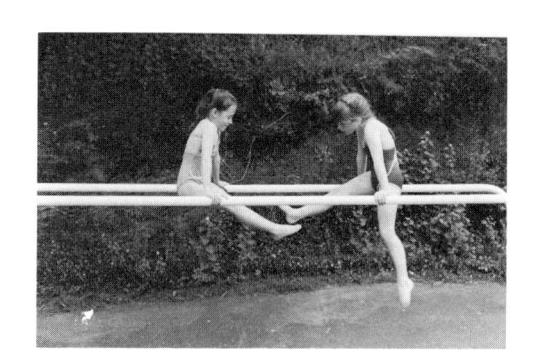

320. UPPER-BACK BOB

This exercise has many facets and should be done in increments well learned before the next is attempted. By this time it is assumed that much time has been spent with weights, tumbling, and the special exercises aimed at abdominal, groin, and back strengthening.

• Lay a pillow over one bar and jump up into a Straight Hang (see exercise 317) supported on the one bar, hands on either side of the pillow. This will bring the groin against the pillow-covered bar.
• Keep the legs straight and, with the entire body held stiff, tip the torso forward. The calves of the straight legs will come up against the underside of the other bar to act as an anchor. (Spotter: Be on hand the first few times and check to see that the pillow that is protecting the symphysis pubis, the pelvic bone in the front of the groin area, is in place. Thigh muscles not the bone, should take the weight.)

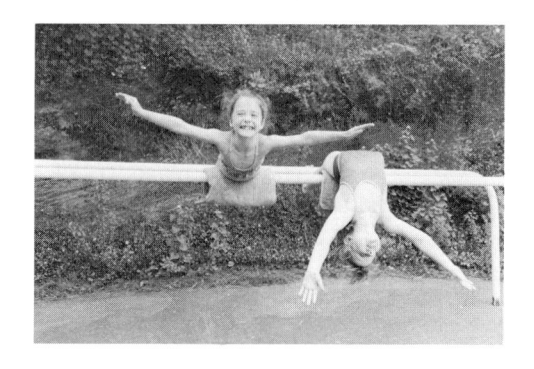

Swimming

• *Allow the upper body to droop forward and down, totally relaxed.*
• *Raise the upper body and head, leaving the arms in a droop. Do three and dismount by placing the hands on the bar and letting the lower body drop into a straight hang.*

321. HORIZONTAL ABDOMINAL HOLD

• *This calls for good spotting. Sit on the pillow so that your legs are hanging down between the bars.*
• *Slide back so that the bar is directly under the crease between leg and buttock. The legs can then be raised up to rest against the underside of the bar.*
• *Reach forward with both arms, round the back, and drop the head.*
• *Roll slowly back, as you did in the first abdominal exercises (pages 25–26).*
• *When the body is horizontal and supported by the legs,* hold *for a slow count of five. This is resistance against gravity. (Spotter: Stand at the head to support the upper body if needed.) Do three.*
• *On the next set of abdominal exercises on the bar, sit up with arms folded across the chest just as you did in the beginning (see exercises on pages 25–26).*
• *When there is sufficient strength, sit up with arms behind the neck.*

322. ABDOMINAL STRETCH

• *From the Horizontal Abdominal Hold (exercise 321), allow the upper body to drop down as you did on the equipment earlier. Preparation for this includes exercises for the abdominals. (Spotter: Don't allow this as a solo until the Horzonital Abdominal Hold is easy.)*
• *Fold the arms across the chest and sit up. Do three.*
• *When the child is big enough to reach the floor with the hands, dismount via a back walkover.*
• *See exercise 320.*

323. LEG BOB

• *Walk around the bar on the outside to where the pillow is hanging.*
• *Place your hands on the bar as before and jump to a Straight Hang (see exercise 317).*
• *This time you will face the free bar with your pelvis over the pillow facing in.*
• *Keep the body stiff and tip the upper body forward, catching the weight on your hands and chest. The legs are horizontal.*
• *Lower the straight legs* slowly *to the vertical and raise just as slowly, three times. Dismount.*

324. HAND WALK

This exercise uses the hands, arms, chest, upper back, and all the shoulder muscles.

• *Mount to a Straight Hang (see exercise 317), one hand on each bar. Simply walk along on your hands between the bars.*
• *Try to keep the body straight, legs together, and toes pointed.*

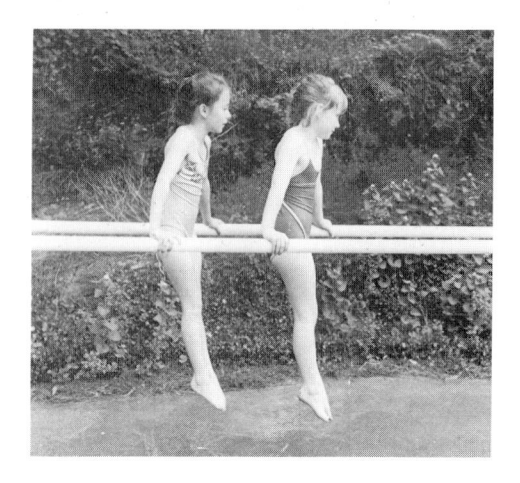

325. SPREAD-LEG TRAVERSE

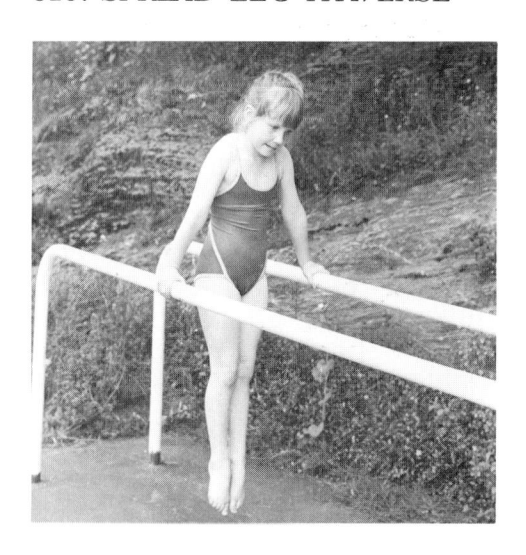

• *Stand between the bars and jump up into a Straight Hang (see exercise 317).*
• *Practice swinging the legs back and forth like a pendulum.*
• *When enough height can be reached, swing the feet above the bar in a forward swing.*
• *Spread the legs wide to land on both bars.*
• *Lean forward to place the hands on the*

Swimming

bars as far in front of you as possible.
- Push the weight forward onto both hands as you lift the legs off the bars, bring them together for a downward swing.
- Carry the swing up and spread the legs and repeat. Progress to the end of the bar.

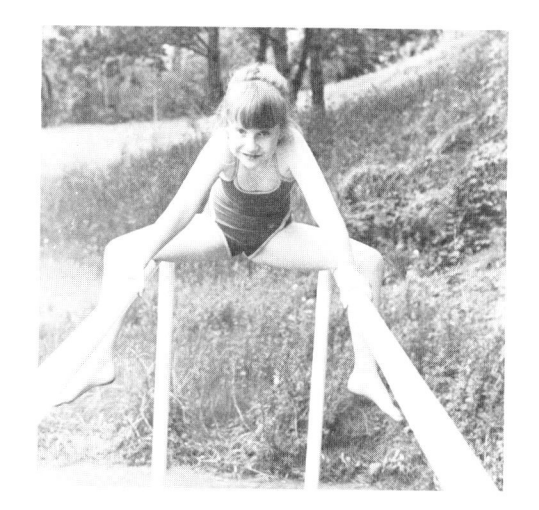

SKIN DIVING

Skin diving comes after the child learns how to swim. It leads into two other exciting sports, scuba and spearfishing. It is a great sport and one that can be shared with parents and even grandparents. When you start children on this sport, be sure the equipment is right. *Don't* buy the handy little packages put together by toy manufacturers as *copies* of what the grown-ups have. Go to a *good* sports store and get the real thing. The mask should fit. *It must not leak,* so make the purchase contingent on its waterproof guarantee. If it doesn't fit, take it back. Snorkels with flexible tubes are better if you intend to do a lot of swimming with your gear, but they also cost more. The rigid snorkel is good enough. The fins should be whole shoes and not "reasonable facsimiles" with buckles. You will not save money that way. It would be better to buy good fins, take care of them (don't leave them lying in the sun), and then pass them on to others in the family or sell them when they are outgrown.

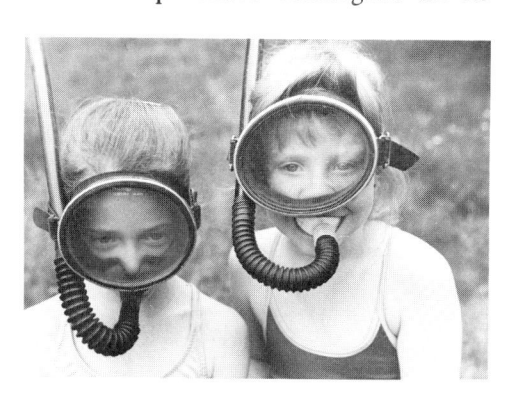

Having bought the equipment, you do not hand it over and say, "Have at it, kids." There *are* children who can get on bikes the first time and sail off down the hill under control. There are first-time riders that stick and first-time skin divers that could make it through the underwater national park in Saint Croix, but you would be wiser to prepare. Let them put on their gear and then work them. Running in place will soon require all the oxygen they can get through the hose. A game of water polo needs eye action as well, and as the whole thing gets sillier and sillier, the giggles will be managed without great gulps of seawater and panic.

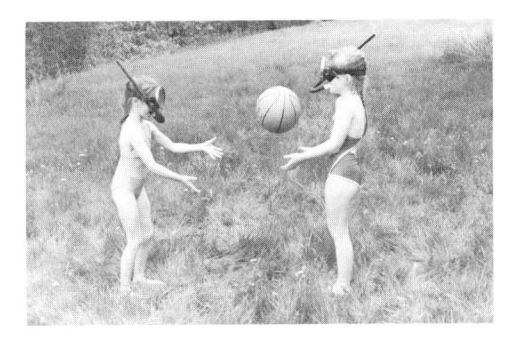

You started preparing for diving when you patterned the child into his or her first somersault, headstand, back bend, handstand, and walkover. Diving is simply tumbling with a different vocabulary.

Don't play dumb uncle and say to a small (often adoring) nephew, "Hey, Dickie, let's see you dive," then step back while he tries to please and plunks in flat as a pancake, stinging, bruised—and embarrassed besides. That's how inferiority complexes are born. You would do better teaching him to slide in headfirst from the last rung on the ladder *after* you had bought him the mask and snorkel set and played two games of croquet wearing yours while he wore your gift. After that you might lose a dozen "favorite" pennies on the bottom, which you can dive for together. When he knows what's down there, he won't worry.

When little folk have had the chance to play in a backyard wading pool (and they are not all that expensive anymore), they won't be afraid of water. They will enjoy being under it, on top of it, or flying into it. *Then* you can feel safe. You have prepared them. Your local YMCA probably has good classes, but good swimmers do best in those classes and instructors like the "best" kids best, most of the time. Grow a "best" of your own—one who can hold his or her own in a class, a dumped canoe, a fall off a lake steamer ... or into a quarry. Of course he wasn't supposed to be near the quarry. Think, did that stop *you?*

The younger a child starts to train and the more time he can spend in the water, the better. In a few years the children will be too old to give *anything* all their attention. If you don't take the time to teach them and play with them now, they will enter that strange waiting land between trusting childhood and trusted adulthood—where you cannot go. Even if you manage to establish a strong bond today, once they take that step, you will often wonder if you were ever really close enough. But if you do your building now, there will come a time when the small son or small daughter remembers. Neither will be small when that happens, and you will be different, too, but you will find that what we call the generation gap is more like a "generation vacation," when *all* of you are on the loose trying to find your various selves. Don't make the mistake of thinking *you* have arrived. You aren't a finished product by any stretch of the imagination and you will change many times. One day, when all of you are free to return from wherever it is we go to grow, happy shared memories will be the signposts that guide you back.

CHAPTER TWENTY-SEVEN
RIDING

There is something completely right about a little girl, a blue sky, a field full of flowers, and a horse. The sight of six-year-old Anna and her gentle friend against a background of August clouds brings back another little girl riding a red mare through a stream a long time ago when neither the mare nor I cared what the rest of the world did—we had each other. Through Anna I can see nine-year-old Petie riding her black mare, Falada, across her grandmother's lawn. It doesn't take any effort at all to call up six-year-old Suzy with long hair mixed with the flying mane of her pinto as the two of them took the back corral fence out in Wyoming.

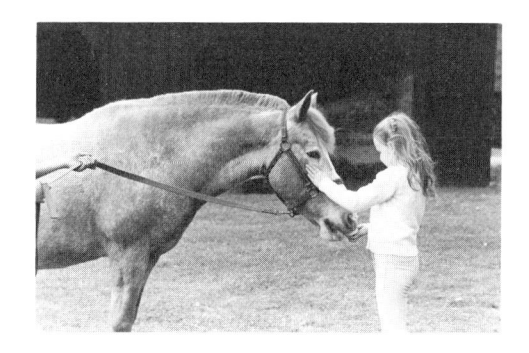

Despite the varying ages, locations, and generations, these children from the past and present have much in common. To start with, all are girls. True, some boys do ride, especially those whose parents once rode or still do, but for the most part horses, tack, stables, trails, and rings—both the dream and the reality—are the province of girls.

If you rode as children, you will no doubt see to it that your children ride, even if only to find out if they really want to ride. However, if you have never had the opportunity yourself, but you do have a horse-struck little girl or boy, it might be helpful to know the right way to get started. The right way is not looking up the name of a stable in the Yellow Pages, making an appointment, and dropping your child off for an hour, saying, "See you later, dear—enjoy the ride." At best you might ruin the child's joy in a wonderful sport. At worst you could be asking for a serious injury, even death. Riding a horse is no more dangerous than riding in a car, statistically much less so, but would you put your child into just anybody's car saying, "Enjoy the ride"?

Horses are very much like people. Some are pleasant, gentle souls, and some are irritable and nasty. If you know the histories of both the gentle horses and the gentle people, you probably find some kind and thoughtful treatment back at the beginning. If you examine the backgrounds of the nasty horses and nasty people, you no doubt uncover some very unpleasant treatment that led up to the nastiness. So when you pick out a stable for your child's great adventure, it would be well to know a great deal about the horses in that stable *and the people who run it*. The person who will teach your child should be someone interested in children *and in horses*. If the mounts are tired, poorly kept old hacks, that tells you that the owner either knows nothing about horses or doesn't care. Neglected horses can be both irritable and ill. If they are rented out to just anyone, they have some horrible habits, one of which is to turn around and bolt for the stable—fast. Get back in the car and drive off.

When you find a stable where the horses look cared for, check the tack. It isn't enough to have lots of saddles and bridles—what is the condition of those saddles and bridles? If leather is not cleaned and tended, it dries out. It would be just your luck to have a girth break, catapulting your treasure with the saddle onto the bridle path headfirst. Make it your business to finger the leather, which should be soft and pliable, and look at the webbing for worn places.

When you look over the owner, find out what his or her idea of instruction is. If it's giving your child a mild-mannered beast and turning him or her into the ring for an hour, leave the place. When this sort of treatment is afforded, it means you have come to a fly-by-night establishment. You *might* get away with turning a child in to a skating rink and forgetting him for an hour (I wouldn't do that either), but horses weigh more than skates, and when they fall on you, you're flat. If there are classes and private instruction, hang around and see what goes on. Here are some things to watch for:

• *The instructor's attention should be on the child being taught, not all over the ring.*

• The horse should be fitted to the abilities of the child. A rank beginner needs a horse that is like a circus horse and goes, stops, and handles almost by remote control. Certainly the little body perched on its back can't do much communicating with the horse—yet.

• Discipline in the ring should be absolute. If others are riding, they should observe the amenities, which means slow, controlled riding *(galloping is something you see on TV)*. When people begin to get too close to the horse ahead, they turn in a tight little circle into the ring and come around on the wall again, but several feet farther back. There is never any shouting or calling or carrying on in a properly run ring. Some horses are skittish, and noise upsets them. Horses are not toys, nor are all of them named Trigger. They represent several hundred pounds of dynamite if something angers or frightens them.

• The instructor who understands animals will also understand the little monkey you have just entrusted to him. The conversation will be quiet and the instruction to the point and applicable to the age of the child as well as to his attitude and physical condition.

• Look for year-round clientele and children wearing hard hats. Hard hats are those domed riding hats that protect heads in a fall, and if you ride, you are going to fall.

CLOTHING

If you are going to take riding seriously, and I don't know any other way, invest in some jodhpur boots right at the start. Rubber boots or sneakers can catch in the stirrups, and heelless shoes can slip through, doing the same thing. If you are going to fall from a horse, you want to be very sure that you and the horse part company with no strings (or stirrups) attached. Out in Wyoming, where my children rode free on the ranges, there was only one law that applied when they were not with us: no saddles. A good solid jolt is one thing; being dragged is quite another. Jodhpur or breeches are comfortable and prevent leg chafing. Hard hats are a must.

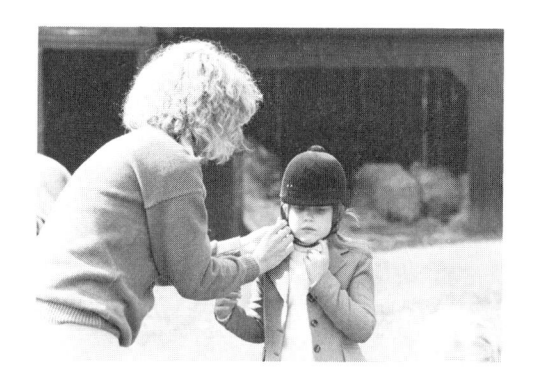

THE LESSON

Private lessons, at least two, should come before class lessons even if your child is a "natural." The instructor will fit the stirrups to the length of the child's legs by having her hang the legs down free and bringing the stirrup to the inside anklebone. A check will then be made to see that they are even.

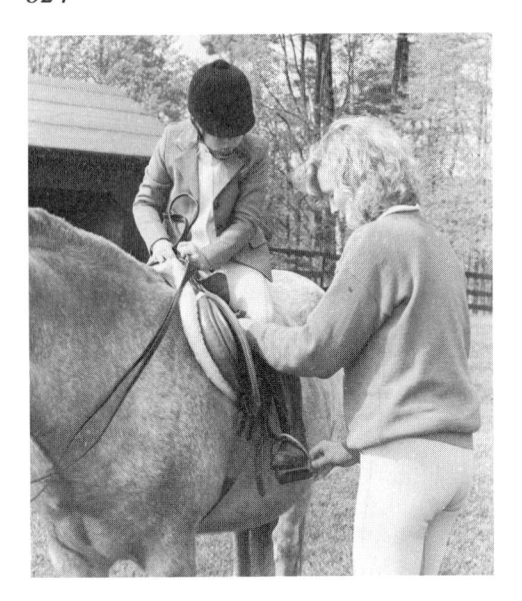

The reins will then be properly arranged and put into the child's hands. You may not hear it, but the child will be told that the reins are for guiding the horse, not to hold up the rider. The hands must stay down and *still*. Flapping arms and wild hands, such as you sometimes see on bridle paths when a group of Sunday riders fares forth, are forbidden. Such activity confuses the horse and ruins its mouth.

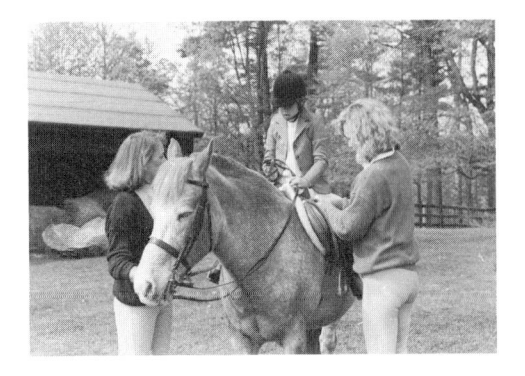

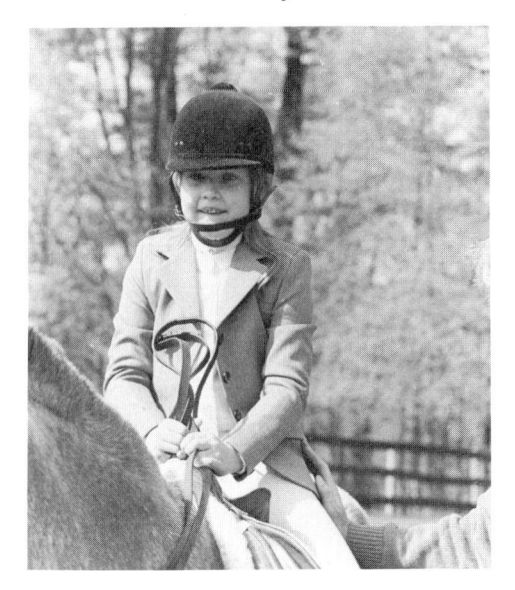

The instructor will take the time to explain that the balls of the feet, not the insteps, rest in the stirrups and that the *heels must be pressed down*. The knees must be "*on*," or pressed against, the horse's sides. If you have given your youngster the exercises in this book, the ability will be there waiting to be taught the skill. The child with the good hands (rope climbing on page 209), erect posture (dance exercises, pages 233–248), strong legs (running, pages 298–306; floor progressions, pages 107–120 and the Russian Series, pages 121–127), and controlled pelvis (exercise 38) has a head start. With a good teacher and a helpful horse, you will reap a rider. *Spend your money at the start* to see that the youngster is taught proper form, posting, cantering, ring riding, change of lead, riding with and without saddle, and the care of horses. As the love of riding and for horses grows, you will find that the "horse-crazy kid" will work hard to earn the money for the hobby. If the job has been well done, the child will not only learn about riding but will develop a fine sense of responsibility as well.

"MY HORSE"

If you have decided to buy a horse for your child, spend at least as much time and effort as you would in buying an expensive car *and get some expert advice before you take possession.* It would be important to know where the horse came from, who trained him, who had him before, *and why he is being sold.* I once bought a beautiful little mare with all sorts of marvelous relatives and background, but somewhere along the way she had had some bad times and developed some very unpleasant habits, which showed up whenever small children wanted to ride her. Later it turned out that *she had been sold because she disliked small children.* Ideally you should buy a horse your child has already met, ridden often, and grown to love.

When your child leads her horse out for the first time for grooming, make sure she walks on the left or the *near side* rather than out in front tugging on the lead. She should hold close to the *head collar,* or *halter,* with the right hand and carry the *shank* of the rope in her left. She will find it easier if she keeps up a conversation. Children quite naturally talk to animals, and this should be encouraged. Horses like it and react to a calm voice. Remember, what you do and the groom or teacher does, the child will learn.

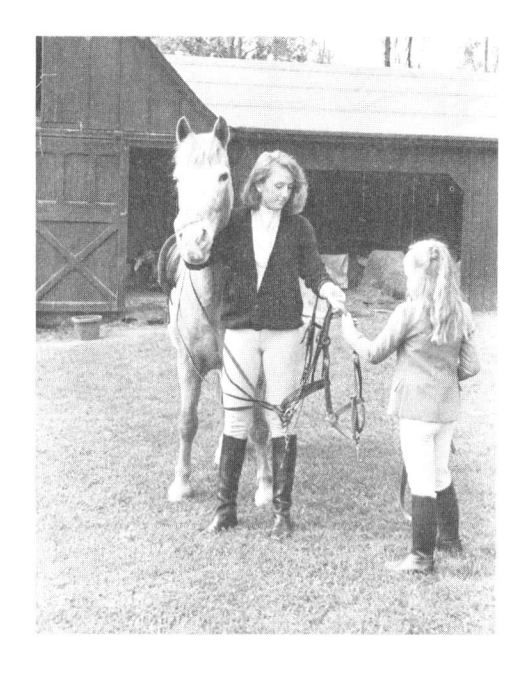

GROOMING

Grooming a horse is more than just getting him clean. It's a sort of love affair. Horse and girl "talk" to each other not only with sounds but with a kind of ESP, which I'm sure was in effect before we had language. Little girls have lots of secrets to share, and horses have a way of looking back the answers. In the heat of summer I used to have quite a time keeping myself in good shampoo. It seemed that Suzy's horse needed it more than I—the horse had told her so. Anna starts with the *dandy brush* and grooms Greylite's neck, talking all the while. She will work her way down over *withers, shoulder, foreleg, knee*, and *pastern* (the part of the leg between the *fetlock* and the *hoof*). As she works her way toward the hindquarters, Anna keeps her eye out for any sudden kick that might come along. Some horses have very ticklish tummies, and just as you can make a dog's hind leg seem to scratch the air as you tickle him, you can get a reaction from a horse—except that the horse's leg has a hoof with a shoe on it. He wouldn't mean to bruise you, but you'd be black and blue all the same. Finally she brushes down over the *quarters*, over the *hind leg, hock,* and *fetlock*. Horses love to be groomed, just as people like their backs scratched, but there is another reason for doing it well: the dirt picked up when they roll in the fields must be brushed off *if the saddle is not to cause a sore back* (see the chapter on Myotherapy).

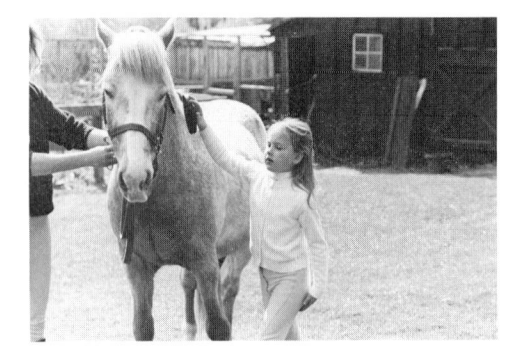

When both sides are brushed and shining, Anna brushes Greylite's face and forelock very carefully, moving her hands slowly and deliberately. Horses are very sensitive around the head, and any sudden move will startle them. If you startle them often enough, they become irritable and jerk their heads back when anyone comes near.

She finishes by brushing the tail. Some pull the tail to the side but still stand in close. If you walk behind a horse, be sure to let him know it's you back there by sliding your hand over him as you go. It isn't *you* he kicks at when he's surprised; it's one of those "horse dragons" he can't see. So make sure he knows who's back there.

FEET

It's those four feet that carry you around, and they must be given every care. Your child will need a *hoof pick* to use on the underside of the hoof. She should carefully scrape out any caked dirt, manure, or tiny stones. Warn her to avoid scratching the *frog*, the soft triangle in the center of the hoof. While she is at it, have her check the shoe with the *pick* to be sure it isn't loose. A blacksmith should check the shoes every six weeks or so. He will take off the shoes, even if new ones are not needed, and pare the hooves just like you pare your fingernails. Then the shoes will be put back on. A worn shoe can cause a bad fall, and unattended hooves cause stumbles that often end in a forward tumble over the horse's neck. Just as you check your car lights, check the horse's shoes. (See the chapter on Myotherapy.)

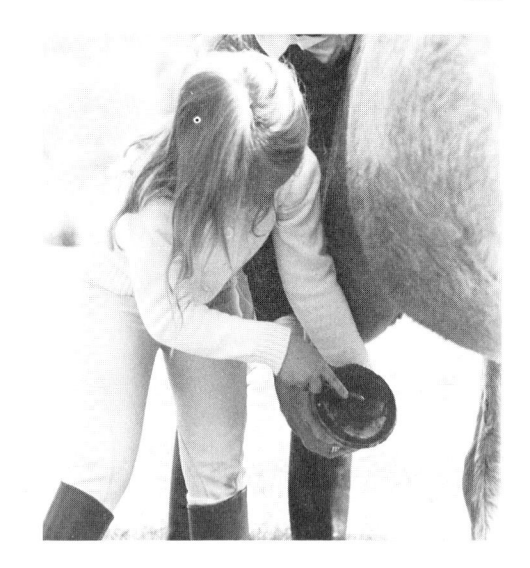

THE SADDLE

Before the saddle is put on, check to see that all the appendages, girths, and stirrups are in their proper places. The stirrups should be pulled up high in the stirrup leathers and the girths lying across the top of the saddle. Horses don't like to be hit with swinging irons and flying straps. Lay the saddle on the horse's back quite far forward *so that it can be slid backward into place, making the hair lie flat as it moves.* As you can imagine, rumpled fur under the weight of a saddle and rider could work up into a pretty sore back. If ever a horse misbehaves for no apparent reason, check—the fault may be yours.

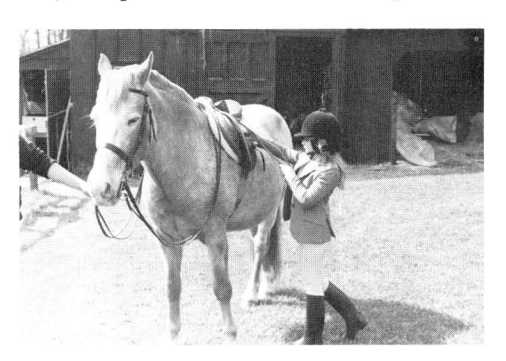

When the saddle is set, push the girths over to fall on the *off side* (which doesn't mean you get off on that side—you always get off on the *near* side). Check to see that they are hanging straight and not in a tangle. Stand on the *near side* close to the foreleg but facing the tail. Reach under with your left hand, grasping the girths by the edge nearest the tail. Draw them through and fasten them up. It is always wise to check again before mounting to see if the girth is tight. Many horses are wise in the ways of girths and may puff up their tummies, pretending that their waists are bigger than they are so that the girth can't be drawn tight. Later they forget they've done it and you can spot

THE BRIDLE

the loose girth, which could spill you on mounting. It is even a wise precaution to check it once more, when you are up, by thrusting your left leg forward out of the way so that you can check for tightness.

THE BRIDLE

In the dictionary one of the definitions for the word *bridle* is "to pull back the head, to resist," and once you have bridled a few horses, you know exactly where that definition came from. Some horses are easy to bridle, just as some people are forever patient and accepting. Then there are others. Slip the *head collar,* or *halter,* over the neck so that the horse remains securely hitched to the fence or post. If your horse is predictable, you can pass the reins over his head, being sure you have a firm grip on them. Hold the bridle by the cheek pieces in front of the horse's mouth. If your horse just doesn't feel of a mind to "open wide," slide the other hand under the chin and press gently on either side of the mouth (there aren't any teeth there) and presto! it will open and you can pop in the bit. Draw the bridle up over the head. Buckle the *throat latch,* and be sure there is room for your whole hand between it and the horse's neck. If it is too tight, it will interfere with breathing and be terribly uncomfortable.

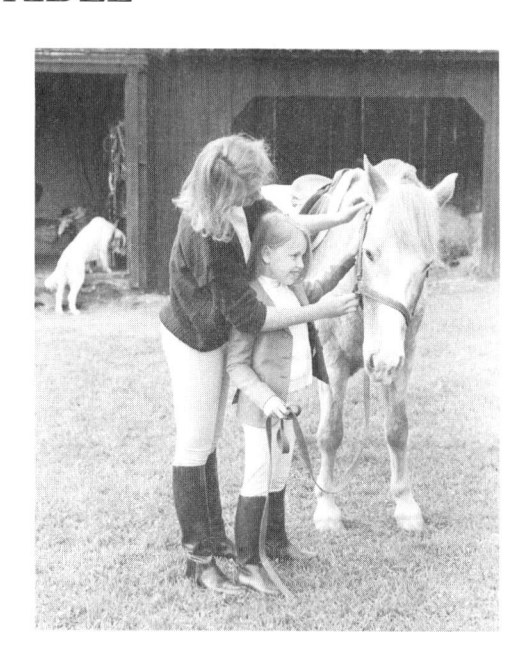

MOUNTING

Very little people are often boosted up to ride in front of the grown-up rider. Then there was the first morning we woke up after arriving at Betty Woolsey's ranch in Wyoming. My husband called me to the window at 6:00 A.M. to see six-year-old Suzy out by the fence. Fully clad in jeans, denim shirt, boots, and hat, she was sitting (like they do in the movies) with one leg hooked over the top board. A cowboy, sitting (like they do in the movies) with one leg hooked over the pommel of his saddle, hat tipped back, was in earnest conversation with Suzy, who was never at a loss when it came to horse talk. Suddenly he unhooked his leg and swung his horse around next to my would-be Grand National candidate. She grabbed his outstretched arm, stepped onto his boot and swung up behind him. Before either of us could say, "Where are you going?" they were gone, cantering down the piny trail, with nothing to show they had even been there but some swirling ground fog.

There have been many times since then that I said to myself, more as comfort than anything else, "She knows how, it will be all right." Most of the time since then she *has* known, and it has been. One cannot say this too often: You can't protect your children from life, *you can only prepare them.* The present adult generation should take this to heart more than any generation I have studied. Your children need more preparation from you because most natural preparations are gone and there is nothing and no one to help you.

If Anna didn't have help for mounting, she would have to drape her reins over her arm while she pulled down her stirrup leathers. Otherwise, she would be standing there with her hat on all ready to go but the horse would have already gone. If you think like a horse (and right now you should), you know that a little girl doesn't weigh much, but it's more fun to run free than to carry a weight on your back. At this early age, Anna's mother and teacher take every precaution, holding the horse's head and giving the little girl a boost as she tries her best *to go through all the correct motions,* just as with tumbling.

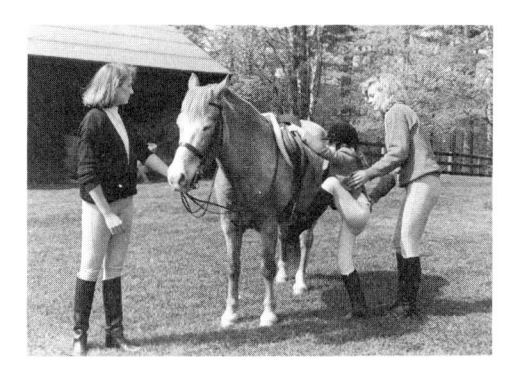

Check the girth one last time, and up we go. Anna is standing too far back for safety if the horse were a stranger to her, and even horses who are ordinarily very good friends can act strangely sometimes if they hurt themselves playing in the field. You will learn what to do about that in the Myotherapy chapter, but in the meantime a better stance would be standing close to the foreleg, but *facing the tail.* Grasp the reins and mane with the left hand and the back of the saddle (*cantle*) and swing up into the saddle.

Check the reins and remind the youngster that the lower leg should hang straight with the weight on the ball of the foot and *heel down.* This "grooving" is the same as putting a child through the somersault over and over again until the body just goes into the action because the muscles feel right doing it. One should never see any daylight between the knees and the saddle either. If there is any space, the legs are not "*on*," and the chance of being unseated if the horse should shy or stumble is good indeed.

The hands are held over the reins

an equal distance on each side from the center buckle. The thumbs are *on* the reins and the little fingers are *outside* the reins. The extra length hangs down on the *off side* of the horse's neck. When the child is just beginning, it helps to pretend she is holding a glass of milk in perfectly quiet hands.

Many people think that to get a horse to go, all that is necessary is a kick in the ribs, a flap of the reins, and a shouted "*Giddap!*" Nothing could be further from the truth. You don't shout impolitely; you *ask* ever so gently with no spoken words at all. Have your youngster hold the reins lightly but with just enough pressure so that the horse's tender mouth feels that something is about to happen. She then *squeezes* gently with her calves. Reins are not used for chinning or holding on—they are merely a way of talking, like a hand on someone's arm.

If the horse is well trained, all your child has to do to stop is sit well down in the saddle, squeeze again with the calves, and at the same time take a firm hold on the reins while keeping the hands down near the horse's neck. The *sitting down* and *squeezing* tell the horse that more is coming. The final pull on the reins says, "Stop." The legs and seat control the rear or *quarters* of the horse. They *collect* or brake. The reins control the front. This is horse talk, and the horse understands it. Can you imagine the confusion in a well-trained horse when a human who doesn't speak the language is on its back? Now you know why a good stableman will not give you his best horses until he knows how much you know—or don't know.

Be sure to keep the legs "*on*" and the reins steady until the message gets through and the horse stops. If you forget this sequence, so will the horse, and performance will be sloppy.

When your child and her horse do just fine on starting and stopping, it's time to try turns. You don't simply pull on the right rein to go to the right as they do in the Westerns on TV. You turn to the right by giving a gentle, steady *feel* on the *right* rein, but more important (and often overlooked), you press against the side of the horse with your *left* leg. If you were to pretend that the horse was an uncooked cruller and you bent the front end to the right and gently pressed the back end to the right (which is what the pressure of the left leg does to the back of the horse), the cruller would look like a half moon going right. If you did that bending, neither the cruller nor the horse would have any choice but to go right. The use of the right rein and left leg (or left rein and right leg in a left turn) is called a *diagonal aid*.

If you are interested in how your child rides and encourage *practice* rather than just riding, there will be both progress and excitement as horse and child begin to understand each other's language.

Easing a horse from side to side is not the same as turning. If you wanted to turn to the right, you would *feel* (gentle pressure) on the right rein and at the same time *squeeze* with the left leg. But if you just want to *ease*—let's say from one side of the bridle path to the other—you would *feel* with the right rein and *squeeze* with the left leg—*but you would also keep a little pressure on the left rein.* In horse language this is, "Move over, please."

When a class is riding in a ring, there will be all sorts of trouble if another use of the legs is not in force. When horses are going in a clockwise direction, a firm pressure on the left rein says, "Stay on the wall." A gentle *feel* on the right rein says, "But keep your head straight." The addition of a *squeeze* from the right leg says, "And keep your body nice and close in."

If you are riding alone in the ring and the horse gets bored and slows down, a quick prod in the ribs with *both* legs will pick things up without confusing direction. If you are riding with others and get too close to the horse ahead, you will want to put some distance between your horse's head and the hind legs of the horse in front. Pull the right rein and squeeze with the left leg, and your horse will turn into the ring. By keeping the pressure steady on both rein and squeeze you will make a small but complete circle and end up back on the wall, but with some distance between you and the other horse.

When your child first starts to trot, she will bounce along most uncomfortably to every step. In time she will learn to post, which is comparable to jumping rope in exercise 86. On one count you jump over the rope, and on the second count you just jump to fill up time while the rope is overhead. When you post to a trot, you sit down into the saddle on the count of one. On the count of two, instead of sitting down again, you rise up in the stirrups. If you can jump rope, you can post. It's a matter of rhythm. This is one reason for learning to jump rope—it improves rhythm and coordination. Watch to see that the child does not support the posting action by pulling on the reins—it won't be good for the horse, and anything that isn't good for the horse is going to react back on the child.

Bareback riding or using either a sheepskin saddle or a felt pad is excellent training. The legs have much more control, and the practice of keeping the lower legs hanging still (not clutching under the belly of the horse) with heels pressed down is something every rider can use. When you bring the horse into a trot, be sure it is slow and controlled, for without stirrups one must *sit to the trot*, which is best done by relaxing and spreading the seat all over the back. The forward direction of the feet helps to spread the seat, and in no time at all child and horse will seem to be all one.

When these several skills are learned, it should be time for games. The *"Basket Game,"* in which you set up a line of baskets down the center of the ring or field is lots of fun. The horse, guided by the child, must weave his way down the line in and out as though through a slalom course. This is excellent practice for *diagonal aids*.

Next place a six-foot stick in ring or field and try to get the horse to cross over the center of it. Left to their own devices, horses will go around either end but not over the center. To correct the easing to one side or the other before getting to the stick takes gentle hands with a very good feel on the approach, and then strong pressure from *both* legs as the center crossover is made. The trick lies in *knowing ahead of time* what the horse wants to do and correcting it before it gets done.

When you walk your horse, its neck will stretch comfortably out in front, but when you trot, the head will come up and the reins must be shortened if you don't want the reins under your chin. Before you trot, you must shorten your reins, but when you teach this to the child, be sure you teach her how to do it so carefully that the horse can't feel it. One of these days your child will want to be in a horse show, and if she is obvious about that shortening, the horse will get the message all right: "My head is coming up—we're off for a trot." However, with all the excitement at the show (horses feel it the same as children do), he won't be able to contain himself and wait for the leg squeeze that says, "All right, let's go." He'll be off before the signal, and she will lose points on "hands."

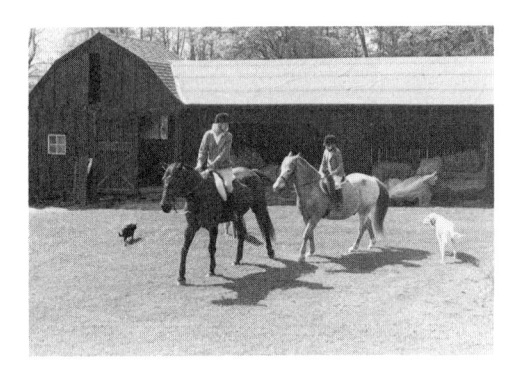

Be sure when you ride out with your youngster that you teach her to watch out for things the same way a motorist watches. The motorist keeps an eye on lights, traffic, children, and animals that might dart out. The rider has a different problem. She must watch out for what is there, of course, but also for what the horse might *think* is there. The horse worries about all those "horse dragons," such as a piece of newspaper blowing across the path, a box, or a post with a hat on it. Once in a while a horse becomes so frightened that he rears, whirls, and bolts for the stable. If the rider is on the alert, she picks up the signs of anxiety: the pricked-up ears, the little snort, the start of a sidewise sashay, and then no one is surprised. A firm hold on the reins, a little reassuring conversation, and a gentle squeeze with the legs averts the calamity. It is always wise to have those legs "on" and a corner of your attention ready for anything. The horse must learn that no matter how he feels about that "thing," he still must go past it. You will help, of course, and you have assured him there is nothing to fear—but pass it he must. He must always know that you are boss, and so must you.

When trotting is second nature, easing and passing scary objects are just part of the ride, and starting and stopping are imperceptible motions, then it is time to *canter*, not before.

Start by walking around the ring. If you are out on the trail, start canters *on the way out*. On the way back it might be just the encouragement a horse needs to take off for home with wings on his heels. Doing it in a ring or closed field makes much better sense if it can be arranged.

Start walking around the ring, let us say in a clockwise direction. *Collect* (shorten the reins) and *squeeze* the legs to put your horse into an easy trot while you post for a few moments. Then, *sit-*

ting down in the saddle and *drawing in on the reins,* come to a slow walk and allow the reins to lengthen for the outstretched neck. As you walk, think this over: *If I were that horse and someone collected me (drew in my head on shortened reins) and turned my head a little to the left or toward the wall, and pushed me forward on my right side—but the bit which he was holding wouldn't let me go forward really—where would I go?* The answer is *up* into a sort of jump, and that is the way you put your horse into a canter and also on the *correct lead.*

The lead is singularly important in circles and on sharp curves. Tell your child to "gallop" around the room. Without any hesitancy she will arrange her one-two gallop beat so that her right foot comes down on *two* if she is running in a clockwise direction. Check it out. It would be far too clumsy to do it the other way, *and she could trip over her own right foot.* Be sure to make this experiment so that both of you understand why the horse must start off correctly. In a clockwise direction it is the *right lead.* If the pressure is on the left rein and his head is turned a little left, he will find it almost impossible to get off with the left foot leading—and there will be no chance of a stumble.

So draw in his head, and with that right leg and your own pelvis (exercises 38 and 42) *lift* him into an *easy, controlled* canter. The *canter* has only two things in common with the "Wild West gallop"— a horse and a rider. You *sit to a canter* by moving your pelvis *with* the movement of the horse. The pelvis moves, but shoulders, and arms and legs are still. Do those two suggested exercises over and over again so that you become virtually swivel-hipped. There should be no separation between your seat and the saddle. If the pelvis moves correctly, the legs don't have to overwork to hold you on; the movement will do a good part of it. One important facet has not been mentioned: carriage. You *must* have a straight back. Do all the exercises for round back even if you are straight as a pole. Do the exercises for shoulder flexibility and also for abdominals— and, odd as it may seem, run.

Like everything else, even the multiplication tables, there are certain steps to be taken *in orderly succession* if skill, self-discipline, and confidence are to be developed. *Don't* let a hurried instructor rush your child through so fast that the fine points are missed. The child will be the loser. She will be able to understand some of what is going on around her in the horse world, but much will be muffled as words are for the partially deaf.

See to it that the first lessons are good lessons well learned, so that for the rest of life riding will be a joy and a way to reach out to nature with all its beauty. Make sure that the job is so well done that when your child has children, they too will have a horse to love.

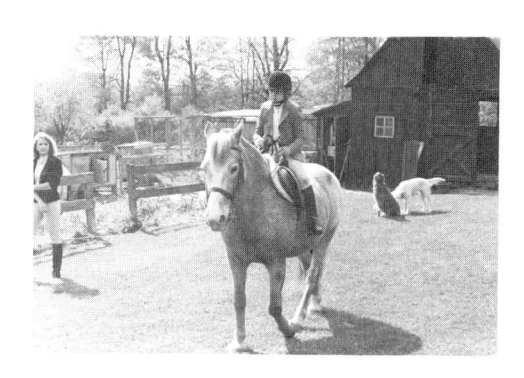

CHAPTER TWENTY-EIGHT
SKIING

Summer slips away, the beaches close, schools open—and children sit down. They sit down in buses, in classes, and in front of TV. They sit down for music lessons, art lessons, and in the library. They sit down in the car and at the table. They sit in the fourth row at the movies. By the time the rains come and the winds whip the last of the leaves from the trees, all the healthy tans are gone and at least three kids in every class are out with sniffles. By the time the turkey is stuffed for Thanksgiving, the storm windows and doors are on, and most of the children are *in* for the winter. Most, but not all. There are the children of skiers, and skiers are different from other people.

The bleaker the November day, the more joy fills the heart of the skier. While other folks are popping corn in the living room, he is down in the cellar checking edges and bindings. The day the man next-door gets his snow tires on, the skier does too—and puts the ski rack on the top. By the time Christmas rolls around and the average family is sitting around amid a sea of glittering wrappings (some of them were on new ski equipment), the skiers are kissing

Grandma good-bye and heading for the slopes. They had fewer presents and fewer wrappings, but they have a nest egg that bears the tag "Merry Christmas to us all and away we go." But the next day when they all fasten their skis on and head out, it won't be the first time for the season, not by at least a month. From Thanksgiving on, and often before, they will have been attending "dry ski school" or holding their own in the backyard. If *you* are a skier, you know about such things, but perhaps you thought dry ski school applied only to racers, not to you and the kids. If you aren't a skier, you may never have heard of it, so now is the time.

Anybody who is in shape can ski, and anybody who isn't in shape should stay away from it until he is. That goes for little kids as well as adults, but for different reasons. A grown-up who puts on skis but hasn't the muscle to manage with is asking for a broken leg and frequently gets it. The little tyke who gets skis for Christmas but couldn't walk to the corner in oversized boots isn't asking for frustration and discouragement; *he's being given it*. You don't ski to get in shape, or to learn how. You get in shape to ski, *and to learn how to ski*.

If you intend to start your family skiing this year or next, try to pick up the equipment in the spring, when there are sales and when parents would like to sell the equipment their children have outgrown rather than push it around the garage for eight months. Watch the ads in the paper and you may be able to outfit everyone for the cost of one or two at the height of the season.

You are not just being a smart buyer when you get your equipment before the season. You are getting it for dry ski school, which begins a month before winter.

EQUIPMENT

You can use secondhand skis, poles, parkas, mittens, caps, and goggles, but you cannot use just any old secondhand pair of boots. *They have to fit.* If you are planning to buy everything new, go to a sports store where the person in charge knows about sizes and makes. Spend your money on the boots and bindings. Less expensive skis will do fine, but if you are skiing on our glazed Eastern slopes, you will need good edges. The old pair that used to belong to Uncle Max just won't do.

Lay the skis flat on the floor and try to rock them from side to side. This will check for warp. If they rock, try another pair. As they rest on the floor, check the camber. Is the bow in the center of each ski the exact match of the other?

The bindings must fit, whether they are for the A racer or the six-year-old beginner. There is nothing so miserable as equipment that doesn't work. In skiing it can be disastrous. The boot must be held flat to the ski, and the foot must be immobile inside the boot. If the child bends the knee into the slope in an effort to *edge* as he climbs, the foot will direct the boot to angle in. The boot in turn should press the ski to the desired angle. It isn't difficult to see what would (or rather would *not*) happen if the boots or bindings were loose.

Poles at this point are not all that important. See that they are the right length for the child and just hope they won't be left somewhere in a snowbank.

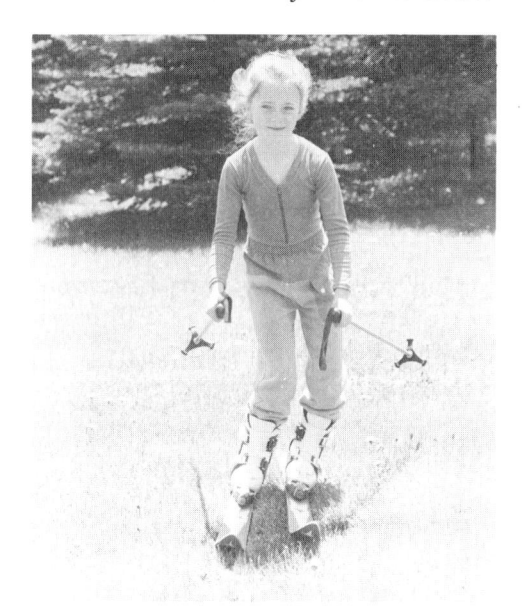

DRY SKI SCHOOL

Most good things come out of a need. The National Ski Patrol was the brainchild of Minot Dole, who got hurt before there were trained people out on the trails to help injured skiers. Dry ski school came about because *I* got hurt on Suicide Six, a racing trail that was tough for racers, which I nevertheless attempted on my first run down ever. The result of being able to ski the distance but not to stop, was a sit-down fall that fractured my pelvis in four places. While I was recuperating, I decided there must be an easier way to learn to ski. That was one need. The second came several years later when some neighbor kids asked me if I'd teach them to ski. Sure. Easy. We could play around on the golf course. In no time they did well. The following year the elementary and high schools asked me to talk on ski safety. Sure again. I also told them that my young friends from the previous year wanted me to talk about forming a ski club and that all of them were welcome. The following day when we met in the lot next to the high school, *there were seventy-five kids, all determined to be skiers!!* Not one had equipment. I called a sporting goods store in White Plains and told the owner that if he would outfit the youngsters as cheaply and as well as possible and give them a 10 percent discount, I'd send him all of our business. He would, and I did. In one week we had skis, poles, bindings, and boots—but no snow. What do you do then? You inaugurate dry ski school. We did the following exercises for an hour a week all through October, November, and December, and when the snow did come, we discovered we had a winner on our hands. *Every* kid could walk across the flat, climb up the hill, turn around, and snowplow down, turning left and right. Most important, they could stop. It took a lot of years before we would discover what a gem we had uncovered. Then we discovered that we had put a thousand children through eleven years of ski seasons without a single fracture and only three knee sprains. (If we'd known about Myotherapy then, those three could have skied the next day.)

One year we set up the ski school in the North Country School in Lake Placid. There were fifty-five children in the school, and fifty-three got the training. Two boys did not. During that snow season there were two fractures, and they happened to the untrained kids.

There were two reasons. The most important one was positive: The other children had gone way ahead of those two boys with their training. They had better form, better speed, and could tackle more difficult trails. The second was more obvious: Those two boys were not up to skiing when the snows arrived. Skiing muscles must be developed, just like muscles for any other specialty. Skiing on the ground is much harder than on snow in one way: You have to do it right or nothing happens. In another way, it's easier: the ground stays put and doesn't slip out from under you.

There isn't anyplace more exciting to be than a downhill ski trail. There isn't a harder, wilder, faster trail beckoning. That will come, to be sure, but *after* the strength, flexibility, and skill are in place.

326. SKI MARCH IN PLACE

When you first start with skis, you will be convinced that they have a mind of their own—and they do. *You* may want to slide straight forward, but *they* prefer the diagonal. If they get the slightest encouragement from a twig or a groove in the snow, they'll turn off to the side and you will fall flat on your face.

• *To teach leg muscles how to direct several feet of ornery material, place the skis side by side and* march. *Keep the tips on the ground and lift your heels to a good rhythm. The poles will help balance, and the "groove" your leg muscles are looking for will be easy to find. Do twenty-five slowly, being sure the skis don't waver.*

327. SKI WALK

• *Place the skis side by side and walk a few steps forward,* sliding them *easily across the grass* straight ahead. *Walk back by lifting the heels but leaving the tips in contact and sliding on the ground. Do several sets of eight.*

328. THE SKIING FALL (DRY)

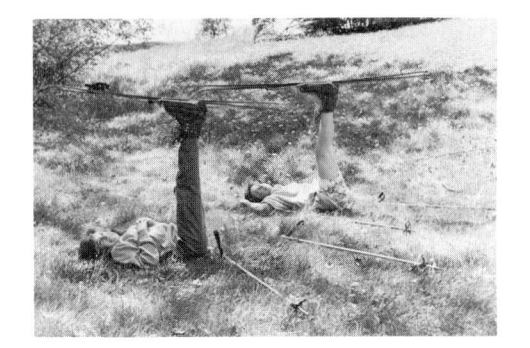

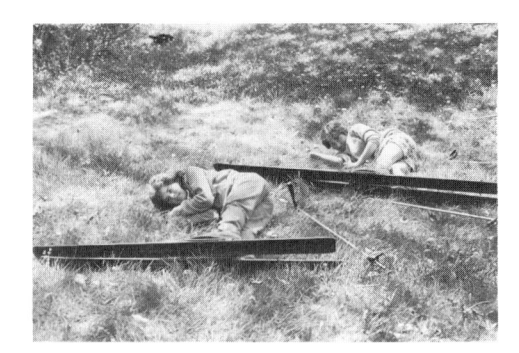

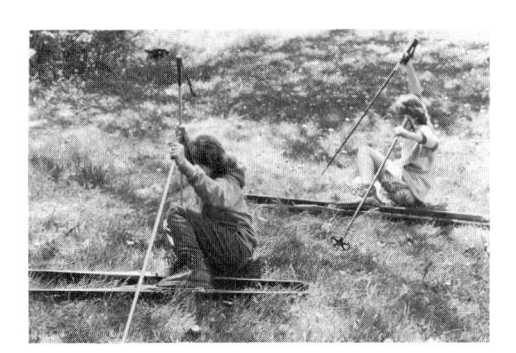

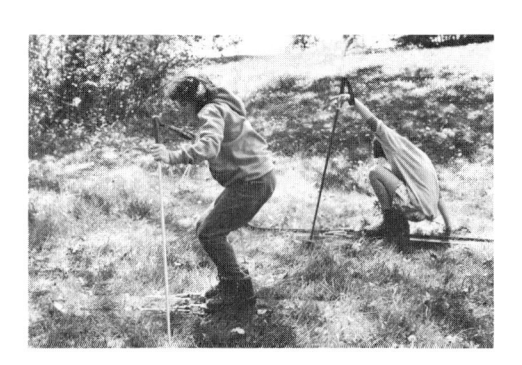

Nobody ever has to learn to fall down. Falling *correctly* and *getting up again*, however, deserve a special section. The beginner who lands in a heap and then proceeds to dig to China as he flips and flops frantically (you would too if you fell in the middle of a slope and could see no fewer than thirty out-of-control skiers zooming straight at your unprotected head) is pretty funny—unless you are the beginner. Learn to get up before you have to and you will have passed the first difficult test. When a skier falls, it's anyone's guess how the legs and arms will come to rest on the slope. Quite often the skier ends up with all four appendages in a tangle and the head downhill. One thing is certain, that skier must get out of the mess—*fast*.

• *Lie on your back on a slight slope. Raise both legs straight into the air and, using your arms, move your body into position parallel with the slope.*
• *Drop both legs together toward the down side. They should land side by side, parallel to the slope.*
• *Draw both legs in close to the buttocks, the under leg a little closer to your body than the top one. Sit up and, using your poles, push yourself to a standing position.*

Try this getting up to both sides and often. That's so that *you* will know what you are talking about. You need not know how to ski but you must know all about *preparing* for skiing. Once you know how to fall and get up and start teaching it, let the youngsters fall into any grotesque forms they wish—it's more challenging to them and should provide more laughter for you.

Impress upon them from the start that *they are never to just lie there.* Very few ski accidents "just happen." Usually someone had to do something wrong. The person who skis out of control is doing something very wrong, but if *you* ski under control and keep a weathered eye out for nuts, you can avoid them. If you are horizontal when you should not only be vertical but out of the way, *you* are doing something wrong. That doubles the chance of an accident.

329. SKI KNEE-BENDS

Knee strength determines how well and how safely you will ski. All summer long and through the lovely autumn, *run.* Seize every opportunity, even if the only chance you have is to run up and down the apartment-house corridors. Also take to the stairs. The more you go up and down that excellent piece of training equipment, the easier you will find it to go *up* and down on the slopes.

• *Using your poles for balance, go into a deep knee-bend.*
• *Come up to a half knee-bend and tuck the poles under each arm. In this position, with weight forward and head low, do eight small bounces.*
• *Stand erect and repeat the set. Do four at the start and work slowly up to twenty. Knee-bends with weights (exercise 194) will help with this one. Knee-bends with heels flat on the floor will stretch the heel cords, another must in skiing.*

330. SNOWPLOW OR WEDGE PATTERN

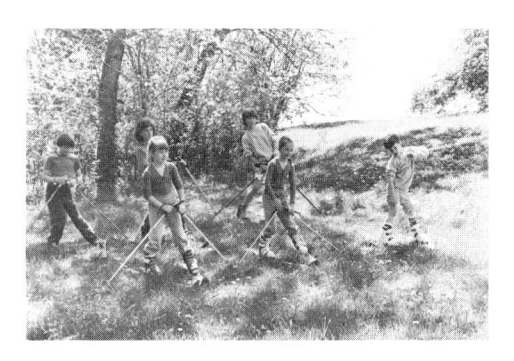

Parallel skiing is all very well, and everybody gets to it eventually, but *first* learn the snowplow; there will be times when it will be your very best friend. Stand with skis *flat*, tips together, and heels apart. Bend both of your knees and *push your seat under.* Holding this position, lean down as if to scratch the outside of your right knee with your right hand. This will pull your weight over the right ski, *where it must go if you are eventually to make a turn to the left.* At that moment play the imagination game. Look off to the left on a diagonal and *see* yourself making that turn slightly to the left. *Keep both knees bent.* The first mistakes the average beginner makes are pushing his seat back, which unweights the tips of the skis and makes steering impossible, and straightening the unweighted leg. If you can *think* those knees bent and seat under while you shift to scratch first one leg and then the other, you're in business and you will ski under control in no time at all. Do twenty shifts *slowly* and work up to fifty. When you can shift the torso weight as if you were scratching the outside of each knee, take up your poles. Try to keep the tips back as you shift.

331. HEEL JUMPS

• *Keeping skis parallel and the tips on the ground,* jump *the heels into the air. Try to keep the skis parallel and lift them the same distance from the ground on each jump.*
• *Start with fairly low jumps and at a medium speed. Do eight and then* march *for sixteen. Repeat the set three times. As the season progresses, increase both height and speed.*

332. HEEL SHIFTS

• *Start as you would for the* straight jump *with poles steady and* thinking *the skis parallel.*
• *Keeping the tips on the ground, jump both heels to the left and then the right. Do eight and then* march *for sixteen. Repeat the set three times. The most important part of this exercise is the rhythm. Keep it steady, and rise out of one bend to shift and drop into the other.*

It doesn't matter whether you are preparing for downhill (also called Alpine) skiing or cross-country (or Nordic) skiing, you need to be able to manipulate two ungainly objects much longer than your feet. You need to be able to climb up hills as well as come down them, ski tows notwithstanding. The more climbing you do, the more strength you will develop, and if you can make it a rule to climb to the top of the easy slope for your first run of the day, you will be warm enough without doing warm-up exercises, at least until you go in for lunch. That warmth won't hold through lunch, so plan on a second quick climb before starting your afternoon runs.

Skiing

333. EDGING

• Stand with skis across a gentle *slope*, feet parallel. Lean away from the slope with your shoulders and into the slope with slightly bent knees. This will press the uphill edges of your skis into the grass. The skis themselves will be on a horizontal line. (If you were to lean your shoulders in, the skis would flatten to the hill and slip out from under you.)

• Place your uphill ski pole up the hill and hold the downhill pole close to the downhill ski.

• Step up with the upper ski while keeping the position with shoulders out and knees in.

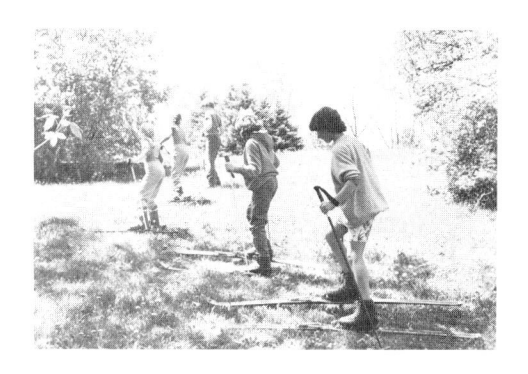

• Bring the downhill ski next to the uphill ski. You will have climbed about six inches. Climb that way to the top of the slope.

334. DOWNHILL MARCH

• At the top of the slope, turn and march straight downhill. Don't try to slide; make it a definite march. If you can, do this on a slope the children will ski on when the snow comes. This is one way to get used to a slope—while it can't slide away. Follow the Downhill March by edging (see exercise 333) up with the other leg in the lead.

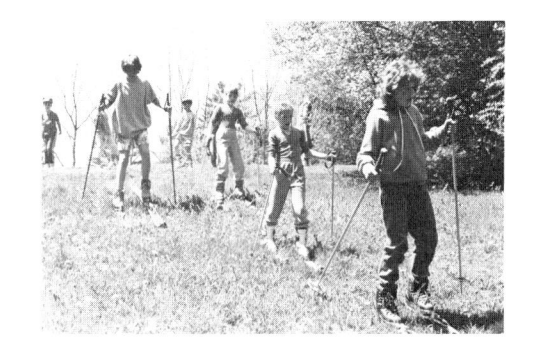

335. EDGING TRAVERSE

A faster way to climb if the slope isn't very steep is the edging traverse, in which you edge up as you did before but each uphill step is also a forward step: Each following step taken by the other foot is also a step forward. In other words, you combine climbing up with going forward on the bias.

• *Edge across and upward until you reach the edge of the slope.*
• *Dig the poles in behind you so that you can't slip back.*
• *Step the fronts of the skis toward the other side of the slope.*
• *When you are facing the other way, proceed to edge-traverse to a point higher on the other side of the slope. Proceed to the top and downhill-march to the bottom again.*

336. HERRINGBONE

Still another way of moving upward is the herringbone, which is especially useful in tight places, such as the approach to the lift. It is also good when the rise isn't steep enough to require one step at a time as you use in edging (see exercise 333), nor wide enough to permit a walk across, as in the edging traverse.

• *Place the ski tips wide apart and the heels close together, the exact opposite of the snowplow.*
• *Bend the knees inward to bring the skis onto their inside edges. They bite into the surface and as long as the angle and knee-bend are held, you won't slip back.*
• *Use your ski poles as an additional insurance against backsliding. You will be able to walk up the slope as though you were on a staircase.*

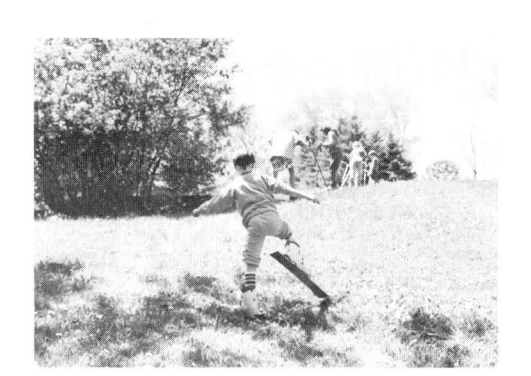

DRY OBSTACLE COURSE

This is where your imagination comes in. One of the chief purposes of dry ski school is to get the legs used to the skis and build the strength and flexibility needed for the sport. You know this and I know this, but the kids don't. They want to put on those things and *ski*. In order to get them to do what you know they must do, you have to make it fun.

Skiing

337. DRY SLALOM

• Lay out dozens of Frisbees on the lawn. Fix them like the gates in slalom racing. Set up your course so that it runs both uphill and downhill.

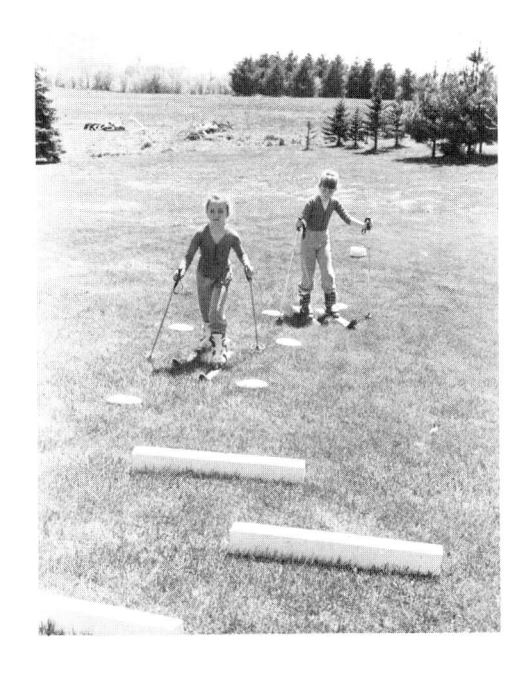

338. DRY OBSTACLES

• Use the railroad ties you made for your "gym." Step over each, leading with the right foot.

• At a given point, reverse direction and lead with the other foot.

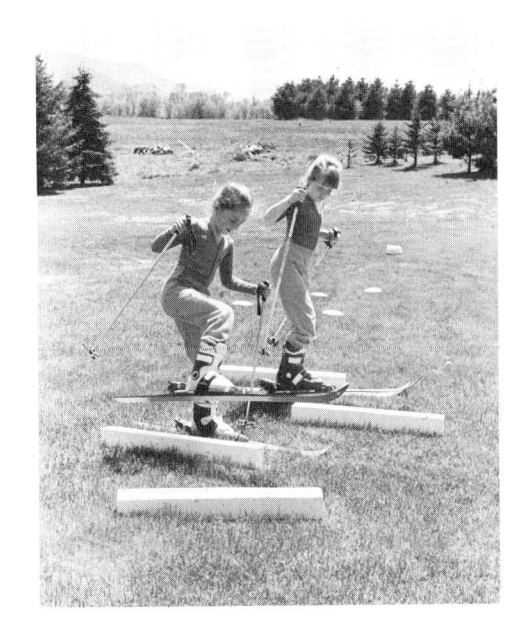

Put anything you can find out on your lawn or the field. Make the children go under, over, and around. If you can make music from your cassette player loud enough, you can get them really worked up and moving. Play "Follow the Leader": Put a marker that means "fall, roll over, and get up," another that means "edge up here" or "herringbone," "edge down here," "traverse up here," "run," "three knee bends," "another fall"—anything you can think of. It all gets pretty hysterical, but the legs get stronger, the skill develops, and soon the skis are just extensions that go along with the rest of the body, not antagonists with mayhem in mind.

ON THE SNOW

And then the snow comes. The first step for everyone in the family should be ski school. For a person who is well equipped with muscles, strength, flexibility, and a certain amount of "grooving" for both brain and body, exposure to a *good* ski teacher guarantees a skier. What is a *good* ski teacher? He or she likes to teach skiing, likes people, and likes to be out in the weather. Not all ski teachers can teach skiing, any more than all English teachers can make a student enjoy English. The *good* ones of either sex and any age *look* at every single pupil and *see* what each is doing that is wrong. Just standing up in front of a class and demonstrating a snowplow, a traverse, or a parallel turn is fine, but that is the least of it. If you get yourself into a class with an incompetent teacher, get yourself out and try someone else in the afternoon. Perhaps the person was just not for you. The racing teacher may not be so hot on the beginners' slope, just as the fellow who is great with the pretty girls may not really have a feverish interest in eight-year-olds and thirty-eight-year-olds.

While the children will profit more from a class, you will get a great deal from a private lesson, and it is money well spent.

The first thing you will need, aside from the ability to walk forward on the flat, is the herringbone you have already learned on your grassy hill. The beginners' class starts out on a gentle slope away from the speedsters, both the kind who can ski and those who can't. One thing you should always keep in mind is that lack of proficiency does not discourage the less nimble-witted from speeding. They always figure they can stop by sitting down—and so they can, which doesn't mean they won't wipe you out in the process. Keep an eye out for comets and bombs; they often appear out of nowhere and in wild-eyed, horrified silence.

Once you have walked out to the assigned place and herringboned up to where the teacher stands waiting, you will be lined up on the side of the slope so that you will be out of harm's way and also in order to keep the slope free of clutter. You should observe this sensible rule even when you are alone or in a small group. If you *edge* your skis as you used to do on the grass, you will be able to stand quite comfortably. The teacher usually demonstrates what he wants you to do and then waits a little farther down to watch how you do it. Each member of the class takes off as his turn comes, and the others edge their way up to the starting point. Try not to edge faster than the person above you; plunking your ski pole on his just as he is about to move can put him off balance. One fall in a line often has the domino effect and ends in a tangle.

Skiing

> Snowplow (Wedge)
> As with many other things physical in the last few years, people have tried to make tried-and-true things seem new by giving them new names. The snowplow (descriptive, but not so chic) is still the same thing but is now called the wedge. The trouble with new names is that they don't tell us much. A snowplow is exactly that; it plows the snow aside. A wedge could be cake, a shoe sole, a piece of steel driven into a split log of wood. Take your choice, but think *snowplow*.

On snow the snowplow position is the same as on grass. Tips in, heels out, skis *flat* until you want to slow or stop, knees bent, *and seat under*. If you have worked well before the season, your seat will stay under as a matter of course, which will keep your weight forward so that you can control the tips of the skis. Remember that where they go, you will go. As you move down the hill, keep the skis flat, then edge them inward slightly as you push both legs outward. The skis will act as a plow, pushing the snow aside ahead of you and slowing your descent. To stop faster, push out harder.

339. SNOWPLOW (WEDGE) TURN

- *To turn to the right, lean down and pretend to scratch the outside of your left knee with your left hand.* Keep your seat under and both knees slightly bent. Look *in the direction you want to go, as you did on the grassy slope, and you will go there.*
- *To turn left, do the same "lean and scratch" with the right hand.*
- *When you have this fairly well under control, play the "waltz game." Make a turn to the right while counting (slow) one, two, three; then left with the same* slow *count.*

As you improve, you will be able to make tighter, smaller curves. Still later they will become smaller and quicker and straight down the fall line. It will take some speed for those, so practice the big slow curves first.

> Here is a teaching tip: There is no better way to learn than to teach. *Have the children lead you.* They will learn to stay with the count so that you can.

340. KICK TURNS

Practice your kick turns on the flat before you try them on the hill.

• *Plant your poles on either side of you a little away from your boots. This will help at the moment of precarious balance, which comes as you kick one ski up and catch its heel in the snow. Let's say that it is the right ski:*
• *Drop the toe of the right ski outward. The heel in the snow will keep it stable.*
• *As the ski comes down, lift the right ski pole out of the way.*
• *The ski should end up parallel with the left, but each ski headed in a different direction. You will look like a ballet dancer in the fifth position (which tells you which exercises will help).*
• *Twist to the right and plant one pole on each side a little ahead in your new direction.*
• *Use the poles for balance as you lean forward and lift the left ski and bring it around. Do it in both directions.*

There are dozens of ways to turn around, and some are fancy indeed. Your preparation in tumbling will make all of them easy to pick up.

341. THE SKIING FALL (SNOW)

We have already said that falls are inevitable, and while the grassy hill didn't offer any resistance to getting up, the snow will. There is nothing quite so embarrassing (or dangerous) as lying out on the hill unable to get up without help. You will be helped, of course, but you won't (shouldn't) feel good about it, because you are a liability. Others can crash into you and your helpers. In addition, you can easily fall into deep powder and just about disappear from view.

• *Find yourself a nice snowy spot on a hill away from traffic.*
• *Fall down and mix your arms and legs up so that you will have something to untangle.*
• *Start by disentangling your poles.*
• *Lie back in the snow and lift your skis (wherever they are) overhead. If one is crossed over the other in the snow, you can't even tell which one is on top until you pull them up into a roof the way you did in the autumn practice.*
• *Maneuver the skis until the heels are pointing downhill.*
• *Drop the heels down to stick in the snow below you.*
• *Now make up your mind which way you want to be facing across the hill when you stand up, left or right.*
• *Allow the skis to fall in that direction to land parallel across the slope.*
• *Draw the skis up close under your body and place the uphill ski pole in close to your seat, the downhill pole in close to your downhill foot.*
• *Push up on the uphill pole. For this you need the training to be had with weights and*

ropes, as well as push-ups and chin-ups. These exercises will prepare you for another kind of skiing—cross-country.

There will come a day when all the practice and preparation are behind you and you and the kids are out on the hills. How well have you trained yourself and your group? Here are a few more aspects of skiing that should be discussed and learned before you hit the trails.

LIFT-LINE MANNERS

Kids who say "please" and "thank you," don't reach past people at the table, do cough into tissues, say "excuse me," and sundry other small things that make life easier all around have been taught those things. Children who stand in line at the lift, wait their turn, and do not try to wiggle past you and seven others, clomp across your new skis, push each other in that icy spot just as you get into it, and whoop and holler and swing pole tips under noses have been taught lift-line manners by somebody. Most children would rather be right than out of line. Most children prefer to be liked than loathed. Most children would do what was expected if they knew what was expected. Where skiing is concerned, what is expected is usually both fair and safe. The little bottom sneaking past to get to the head of the line may be small indeed, but it takes the same size of seat or bar that your somewhat larger derrière will occupy. Don't teach children to be dishonest by permitting that sort of activity. Right now it's just a place in a line he's swiping; ten years from now it may be a place in a car. What's his is his, and what's yours is yours. If the child is also yours, just lean down and tell him quietly that he'd best wait his turn. If he isn't yours, plant your pole firmly between his skis: He'll get the message. Of course this will not endear you to him, but maybe the message will be slightly bigger than "No, wait your turn." Maybe you will get through to him that if he is old enough to ski, he's old enough to obey the rules, even if someone isn't standing right there with a switch. It's a little like not speeding when no policeman is in sight. Kids notice that sort of thing.

TRAILS AND THE SKI PATROL

If your brood has reached the point where a trail is in order, find out which one is suitable for the least expert in the group. The better skiers can enjoy even the easiest trail, but the not-so-expert will be miserable if the trail is even a little too difficult. If the sign says Beginners, be prepared to find beginners on it, and that can mean just about anything. Some will be athwart the trail in the snowplow position, but with skis so sharply edged they couldn't move on a 60-degree slope. Others may be found edging right up the middle as you come around the corner. There is often a cheerful group of know-nothings who have fallen in a heap (always in center trail) and are happily flapping snow and poles in every direction. If you know it's hit them or a tree, take the tree—it doesn't have a steel-tipped ski pole pointed at your eye. Even if nobody is there at all, watch out. Somebody has undoubtedly *been* there, fallen mightily, and gone on, leaving a yawning "bathtub" for you to ski into. The small apertures caused by ski boots when a discouraged neophyte took off her skis and walked down the middle of the trail aren't so harmless either, not if one catches your tip and catapults you into the bushes.

If you are coming down the hill and you hear the call "Track!" move over. Someone is coming and may be faster than he would like. If you find yourself crowding another skier on a trail, say quietly, "Passing on your left" (or right, as the case may be), but don't expect any cooperation. Chances are the sound of your voice will send him into a reverse and he will head for the spot you just said you were using. So after the warning, wait. If all is under control, skim on by.

If you come upon an accident, don't try to move the skier. Climb back up a good distance and plant your ski poles across the trail to warn any descending skiers. Send the first one who comes by for the Ski Patrol, and try to give a description of the injury so that the patrol will know whether to investigate or bring the toboggan. If the injured party is you, don't be a hero. A ride down on a toboggan may be hard on your dignity, but skiing down on a cracked ankle may slow the healing process.

CONDITIONS

Conditions can make a world of difference. The trail you all skied down on Saturday with the greatest of ease may have changed overnight to a slanted ice rink, an interminable stretch of "mashed potatoes," or even that most treacherous of conditions, the breakable crust. *Know the conditions on the trail before you go*, and treat them with respect. Treat with respect the temperature as well. Skiing can be so much fun that quite without anyone's realizing it, noses, chins, cheeks, and foreheads can start to freeze. If anyone in your group has a pale patch of skin, have him cover it with his hand and go into the lodge. *Do not rub the skin with snow.* The warm hand will probably put things to rights before he gets in, but an angry red patch may last for days. In every case, the frozen area will be sore to the touch and be susceptible to freezing for some time after the initial frosting.

If little feet get numb, go in and get those boots off. The thawing process is going to be painful and may be eased by putting the feet in cold water and slowly bringing it to room temperature. Try to avoid this with boots that fit and occasional questions as to how feet and hands feel.

Never let children ski alone. The buddy system in water, in the woods, and on the trails is very important. One child alone can be lost in the woods, hurt, and invisible off the side of a trail, or a helpless target for speeding skiers right smack in the center of a busy slope. A child with a buddy who can call for help or stand above him until noticed by the patrol has a protector. Years ago, when we started the first dry ski school in the country, we called it the Addlepate Ski Club, and you had to be eight to get in. We started teaching first aid and winter rescue to the ten-year-olds, and never have I seen more efficient rescuers. At the sight of an accident they went into action like the best-trained team in any rescue work. One would scramble back up the hill to put up the warning poles. Another would take off for the base station, fast but under control. The third would stay with the injured, protecting him from the wind and pillowing his head. They were trained not to touch anyone who had been hurt unless there was bleeding, and if there was, they knew very well what to do. By the time these youngsters were eleven, all of them had made the Junior Ski Patrol. While they rarely got the chance to exhibit their skill, they were all confident that they knew what to do, and there was always the off-chance that they might be needed. How much better for a child to *know* he is somebody than to wonder if he'll ever *become* somebody.

RACING

Racing is fun, and every time you race, you learn something. It's nice to win, but it's also great to just run the course. If you have taken a group (from two to fifty-two is a group—after that it gets to be a madhouse), set up a practice area off to the side somewhere and put up some slalom poles. Get some six-foot bamboo poles and some squares of red, blue, and yellow sailcloth for flags. Tie the flags to the poles and have the children ski down between them. Set a pair at the top of the run for the starting gate. You will need a pair at the bottom for the finish. Set a pair here and there down the slope so that while the run is downhill all the way, it must be controlled if the skiers are to get through those gates. That's the beginning of racing, the beginning of practice, of "Watch me, then I'll watch you," the start of improving, of learning, trying, striving. Soon there will be bump-hopping, "Follow the Leader," "Best Friends," and all the other kinds of ski fun. You will have given another gift that cannot be left in a will—winter.

There will come a day when the slopes are too crowded and the lift lines too long. That day you will say to your family, "Let's find out what the high mountains are like—let's try the faraway trails." By then you will all be able to ski; but being able to ski isn't enough—you must *want* something more. When you see a book that talks about the wonderful world of winter wilderness, get it. Read it. Talk about it with your family. Plan for it. Who knows, maybe you are just the sort of person who finds the answer to all the discomfort and frustration of modern living in the wilderness. There is some wilderness left. Give it a try.

CHAPTER TWENTY-NINE
FIGURE SKATING

Every skill you give your body opens another door to adventure and excitement. Each skill becomes a stepping-stone for the next, and all reinforce and balance one another. For example, if you have learned to balance on a sawhorse, run a mile in good time, and edge up a grassy slope on skis, you can ski on snow. If you can ski (even a little), ride a bike, and do the dance exercises in Chapter 18, you can figure skate. If you can figure skate and do the various exercises in Chapter 24 on track and field, you can play ice hockey. If you add wind sprints, you can race. It works in reverse too. Any boy or girl who has built good legs with running, has learned to skate well, and then gone to dry ski school will be able to ski. So if you have winter sports on your mind, even if you live far from the high mountains, learn to skate.

As in every other sport, the introduction to figure skating must be carefully planned. Drop a child into eight feet of water with the admonition "Sink or swim" and you *may* produce an instant swimmer. More than likely, however, you will have to rescue a gasping, terrified youngster, who will henceforth have an aversion to a full glass of water. If you take your young hopeful to the top of Suicide Six shouting, "Follow me!" into the teeth of the wind as you push off on flying skis, you will most likely produce a confirmed lodge lounger. Skating does not offer quite the same degree of danger, but if you lace those small feet into Aunt Lou's old tube skates, filling up the extra space with two pairs of wool socks, and then send her ankling out onto a lake in ten below zero, you've done the same thing. You've destroyed a joy.

When you start a child in any sport, give that sport every chance. Begin with pretraining so that the strength, flexibility, and coordination will be available when needed. Next get the right equipment. Finish off whenever possible with a controlled environment. Teach swimming in warm water and skiing on sunny slopes. Skate, when you can, in a rink. Rinks have skates for rent and fitters who know what size a child needs. Also, there are instructors, and the first person to go out on the ice with either you or your child is a *good* instructor.

CLOTHING

Don't invest in any special clothes until you know whether or not you've got a skater in the family (three trips to the rink in one month will tell you). Tights (with feet) under jeans are just fine for both boys and girls, and either a sweater or a parka will look fine and feel comfortable. Rinks are chilly, but only if you are in the observation section. It is prudent to put gloves or mittens on children at least until they get past the falling-down stage. The right clothes do seem to make a difference, however, and if your daughter takes to skating, by all means provide the tiny swirling skating skirt so dear to the heart of little girls.

THE SKATES

Rent skates the first few times, but oversee the fitting as though you were buying. You can frustrate a child by renting poor equipment just as easily as you can by purchasing inferior equipment. Know what good skates should be like, how they should fit and *feel*. Look for those things when you rent, and insist on them when you buy.

Consider first the shoe. It should be of good leather with a steel-reinforced arch support and quite firm around the heel. It is this stiff heel "socket" that will keep the foot flat on the skate so that when the body leans, the skate is forced to lean as well. This will mean the difference between the satisfaction of control and the frustration that goes with never getting things to work for you. The skate blade is about one-eighth of an inch wide and should be screwed, not riveted, to the shoe. It is hollow-ground so that only the two outside edges of the blade touch the ice when the foot is flat. When the body (and foot) lean to either side, only one of those two very sharp sides bites into the ice, and this permits very good control *if you keep the skates sharpened.* The front of the blade is rounded and looks as though it had been trimmed with pinking shears. The little sawtooth points are used for stunts such as turns, runs, and even backward stops.

THE FEEL

Wear only one pair of light wool socks. If the skate fits, more socks will slow circulation. If the skate doesn't fit, no amount of extra sock is going to turn it into a good instrument. Lace the shoe all the way to the top, but there is only one place where it must be really tight: just where the shoe curves upward at the ankle. By lacing tightly at that point you force the heel back into the stiff "socket" and assure control of the skate. At the top the laces should be loose enough to permit the passage of at least one grown-up finger or two child-size fingers. At the other end, the toes should be able to wiggle comfortably. There should be about an inch of tongue showing all the way up the shoe. If the sides touch or overlap, the shoe is too big.

Good skates are expensive, but like the good ski boot, the good tennis racket, or the good saddle, they often make the difference between learning fast and well and quitting in rage or tears. Count your money well spent if from the investment you get a skater, not because it's nice to have a skater in the family but because your child will have a gift from you to carry with him all through life that will be passed on even to your grandchildren.

Care of skates is important. Buy skate guards and see that they are put on the skates after the blades have been wiped dry. If for any reason it is necessary to walk on the skates off the ice, wear the guards. Put a little oil on the blades when they are to be stored for any stretch of time, and be sure the shoes are protected with a good dressing.

THE LESSON

Money spent for private instruction when either you or the child begins a new sport is a wise investment, but there are instructors and then there are instructors. Some feel they have earned their money if they simply hold the staggering beginner in an upright position. Often this is true if the beginner is both clumsy and overweight. There is no need for this to be true in your case.

Long before the skating season you should have been working to prepare for the very first day. When you approach the rink, the basics should be there, ready for use. Instructors are human; they like to succeed. If you and your child are in good shape and ready to learn, you will learn quickly and well. The instructor will be pleased and enthusiastic. An enthusiastic teacher teaches better and gives even more help than is ordinarily required or expected. Altogether it becomes a very satisfactory arrangement. If no instructor is available and the "instruction" is up to you, here are some very basic things both of you should know. As you read them, you may feel they are a little too basic, you "know all that stuff already." That's where teaching comes in. Teachers, too, "know all that already," but they understand that the child does not. If time is taken to explain, show, and help with basics, the rest moves faster and with more satisfaction. The wise teacher says, "My, you stand so straight; it will be no task to get that on the ice too." Without any effort the teacher has encouraged, praised, and reminded the child that *skaters* don't droop. The parents, used to the child's good or bad posture, might not comment. If you are going to teach, then teach.

WALKING AROUND

As in every other sport, the youngster "sees" himself as an expert right from the start. This is a most encouraging habit. If you *see* yourself succeeding, it is easier to do so. If you picture yourself as a flop, you can follow that line too. It is only smart to bolster that happy image, so put on your skates *and guards* and walk over to the refreshment stand and have a cup of hot chocolate. If you need a reason, say *you* would enjoy it. When you get there, see if they have orange juice (not orange drink) instead. The walk over, the standing around, and the walk back will at least give you all the *feel* of a narrow balance beam.

Take off the guards near the rink. Holding on to the rail, lift first one foot and then the other and then slowly walk around in a small circle. *If the ankles bend, it is the fault of the shoe, not the foot; go back for a better fit.*

342. SLEEPWALKER'S POSITION

Arms are very important in skating, just as they are in dance. If they wave frantically, they interfere with balance, so learn from the start to control them.

• *Stand on the floor with skates parallel and stretch both arms out in front a little below shoulder level. Make the shoulders, arms, and hands relax, then lower. Repeat, lifting and lowering.*

Figure Skating

343. SLEEPWALKER'S KNEE BEND

The knees play a tremendous part in skating, and you will be doing all levels of knee-bends. Start practicing while off the ice so that you will know what to do *on* the ice.

• *With feet about six inches apart and the arms stretched forward for balance, go down into a knee-bend and stand again. If you have prepared for this day, you should be able to go all the way down to your heels (see exercise 10) and up without any effort. Do five right there on the floor. If you have any difficulty at all, you need knee-bends; practice at home.*

GETTING ONTO THE ICE

If you are at a rink, getting on is rarely a problem. You simply hold on to the rail and step down *sideways*. If you are outdoors, it is safest to back onto the ice until you know what the surface feels like when you are on narrow steel blades.

344. "FEELING" THE ICE

Once you are standing on the ice, you are perfectly safe; savor it. Nothing can happen unless you move.

• *Place your feet six inches apart and raise your arms forward into the Sleepwalker's Position (exercise 342) and stand straight. Feel your blades on the ice. Feel yourself standing tall.*
• *Relax arms, hands, and shoulders. Have your child feel those things.*

When children are young, they do so without prompting. After all, they have to pay lots of attention to how everything feels in order to learn what their world is all about. Later, when things become automatic, they stop paying attention and they (even as you) lose much sensitivity and awareness and much pleasure.

Your skate blades are slightly rounded like a gentle rocker. Try rocking a bit; get that *feel*. Next go up on the toes and *feel* the bite of the steel teeth into the ice. All else may slip around, but those teeth will stay where you put them.

Posture is all-important. If you lean against the rail or each other, you lose control of the skates. If you round your shoulders, you stagger forward. If you poke your seat out behind, the skates must overturn to the side. Try from the first moment to stand tall and relaxed.

345. THE FALL

You are going to fall. Nobody learns to skate, ski, ride, jump, whatever, without an occasional fall. If you add ice to a sport, you have the perfect fall maker, so it is best to learn how before you need to. The first rule to remember is: *Hands off the ice.* There is only one good piece of fall equipment, and that is your seat. It can neither be broken nor skinned. If you feel a fall coming on, don't put out an arm; *bend your knees and sit down.* Try it now while you don't need it.

• *Stretch your arms forward in the Sleepwalker's Position (exercise 342) for balance and go all the way down into a deep knee bend.*
• *Sit right down on your heels. Then sit off to the right or left, hands and head up. Children do this well—after all, they haven't very far to fall—but you can too.*

You will probably have some unexpected opportunities to practice, so practice a few just to be ahead.

There is some additional information you need to know when it comes to falls on ice. Those falls can be unexpected and *hard.* You or the child may feel sore and bruised for a few days, and if the coccyx, or tailbone caught any of the blow, the soreness may last a while. Then it will seem to go away, and sometimes it does go away. Sometimes, such a fall leaves trigger points, which I discuss in the chapter on Myotherapy. If it does, you can have back pain years later. You can even have headaches and jaw pain due to a fall on the ice. If you have such pain or have had many such falls, read about Myotherapy as a preventive measure for back pain on page 419.

346. THE RECOVER

You don't want to lie around on the ice any more than you do on the ski slope. Those blades flashing around the rink are often attached to feet and legs that belong to people who are neither coordinated nor responsible. They aren't bothering to learn the skill of skating. They just want to skate, and your head is in the way. So get up fast.

• *Roll over until you are on hands and knees with the hands shoulder width apart.*
• *Place one foot between your hands and, remaining in a full knee-bend position, bring the other foot in beside it. Then, tipping up on the sharp teeth of your blades, stand up. The little sawteeth will prevent any slipping and give you a perfect nonskid support. Again you have need of knee-bends, so be sure your knees can bend and recover.*

347. ONE-FOOT BALANCE

Think for a moment about the blades under your feet and remember that each has *two* sharp edges.

• Take the Sleepwalker's Position (exercise 342) and stand first on one foot and then on the other. It may be quite difficult to balance while standing still, just as it is almost impossible to balance on a bike unless there is some *movement*, but for fractions of seconds you can stand there.

348. THE GLIDE

• Take the Sleepwalker's Position (exercise 352) with arms extended and start walking forward. You will have to take very small steps and be sure to lift each foot from the ice as you go.
• Take five or six such steps, which will give you a little momentum, then put your feet parallel but about eight inches apart and glide.
• Repeat that action several times until you know the feeling *of both the* walk *and the* glide. You will be tempted to strike off and skate; don't. Keep up the exercise, and as you glide along, do small quarter and half knee-bends.

349. THE DIP

• *As you walk and glide, go further and further down into deeper and deeper knee-bends until finally you are sitting on your own heels. The only way to get back up, of course, is with the help of the leg muscles you have developed. If you find you need more, do exercise 194, the knee-bends with weight bags.*

350. THE FORWARD SWIZZLE

• Take the "fishtail" position you practiced in exercise 272, heels together and toes open.
• Bend your knees slightly as you did in the plié and extend your arms. Press your skates outward as you bend forward slightly from the hips. You will glide forward, and when your feet are about 2 feet apart, your legs will be straight.
• At that point turn your toes inward and, bending the knees inward, bring your skates back together. Your skate tracks will look oval. Make several linked ovals by pressing the skates out and in.

351. ONE-FOOT GLIDE

Now your foot gets to "ride a bike," and you will see how knowing one skill prepares you for another. You have been gliding on two feet, which did not require much balance. Now try one foot.

- *Extend your arms for balance and take the few steps necessary to gather momentum.*
- *Glide for a short distance on both feet and then lift one an inch or so from the ice and glide on the other.*
- *Repeat, lifting the other foot. Always practice everything to both sides. You never know when you will need the less favored leg. Do several one-foot glides on each foot.*

352. THE T POSITION

When you walk with short steps in preparation for a glide, you can't build up much speed. To really get a good start, you need a base for a "push-off," that is, the T.

- *Take the "fishtail" position (see exercise 272) with heels together and toes apart and then move the heel of the left foot to the instep of the right. The left foot is then facing forward, ready to go. The right is at right angles to the left and presents a firm wall of resistance for the push-off.*
- *Bend the left knee slightly as you push off and glide a few feet, with the right foot just off the ice and the foot turned out. The following leg should be straight.*
- *When you slow down, bring both blades to the ice side by side. Next, twist the right foot outward once more and place your weight on it just long enough to push off with the left foot again. This gives you a scooter action.*
- *Do four push-offs with the left foot leading and then four with the right. Then do three with each foot, then two, and finally alternate feet, doing one with each foot for eight, coming to an almost-stop each time.*

353. SKATING FORWARD

When you alternated and did one push-off to a side from the T position, you were almost skating forward. If you did it with any speed, you *were* skating forward. Try now to alternate without any stop between alternating push-offs.

- *Always bring the skates together and make the pushes strong and the glides long.*
- *Check to see that the glide knee is bent and the following leg straight with foot turned out.*
- *Check your hands for position and check your posture. The knees do the bending; the body is gracefully erect.*

Figure Skating

SKATING BACKWARD

Just as it is easier to do a backward shoulder roll, so it is easier to skate backward.

354. THE SWIZZLE BACK

• *Start with toes together, heels apart, and knees slightly bent.*

• *Hold your arms forward and still as you press the heels of your skates outward with slightly bent knees. When you reach a width of two feet, your legs will be straight and it is time to pull them back in. You will have moved backward and tracked another oval as you did in the Forward Swizzle (exercise 350). Do several linked.*

355. THE WAG OR WIGGLE BACKWARD

• *First refer to exercise 69 in the floor progressions; you will note that the arms and upper body stay still while the action belongs to the hips and legs.*
• *Stand with feet about a foot apart, having checked to see if the way behind you is clear.*
• *Bend your knees slightly and* extend your arms out to the side.

• *Turn both skate heels in the same direction and wag your seat from side to side.*
• *Hold your top half and arms still. Be sure to keep your skates the same distance apart as you go. If they spread too far, you lose control. If they come together, you lose momentum.*

STOPPING

As you begin to gain control, you will also begin to pick up speed, and that necessitates some means of stopping. There are skaters who know of only two ways to stop: sitting down and running into the side of the rink. Both ways are effective, but sitting down in the center of a whirling crowd isn't always practical, and if there is someone between the speeding skater and the rink side, there is apt to be a collision. There *are* better ways.

356. THE SNOWPLOW

In both skating and skiing, knowledge of the snowplow is useful.

• *Point the toes inward and the heels out, exactly like the snowplow that clears the roads.*
• *Bend the knees slightly and press the skates outward.*

If the blades are held flat, the skates will skid outward and no slowing or stopping will be effected. However, if you *edge* ever so slightly by bending the legs inward, the inside edges of the skates will start to bite into the ice, and if there were a light covering of snow, as on an outdoor lake, it would build up under the edges and be swept away. The danger in using the snowplow lies in its efficiency. Edge a little too hard and you will be most efficiently spilled over your own plow. Use it at first only when going very slowly.

357. T STOP

The T stop is easier to control. Take the T position with the right heel pressed against the left instep. *Feel* the position as you stand there with arms out, head up, and body and legs straight. That is the position you will take to stop. As you stand there, unweight the left foot (top of the T) and then replace it on the ice. Do that several times. The left foot is going to act as a brake, and you want that brake to know the feeling of *gradual application*. The right foot, which is to be the glide foot, should also be shown its direction. *Feel* the direction with knee bent. When you have the picture of yourself in the T position firmly in your mind, skate forward to pick up momentum and then glide forward on the right foot. Bring the left foot (the top of the T) in behind the right heel, but do not let it touch the ice. Be sure it is in the braking or T position before you start to lower it. As you lower the blade, keep it absolutely flat and imagine that you are letting down a snowplow blade and are not quite sure when it will scrape the pavement. With both legs straight, lean back slowly and put on the pressure that will bring you to a stop. Repeat with the other foot in the braking or T position. Do several.

358. THE CURVE

When you get to the point where you are ready to start *figures*, you will find that the investment you made for properly fitting skates was money well spent, because curves depend on *lean*, and *lean* depends on shoes. If you were an excellent skater and knew how to do everything correctly as far as body control, balance, and rhythm were concerned, but for some reason you were forced to try your skill in badly fitting skate shoes, your frustration would know no bounds. *You* would lean into the curve, but the blades would not.

You lean into a curve with your whole body from the head down. Take a ruler and stand it up on your desk with the numbers facing you and the bottom edge flat on the desk surface. Imagine yourself to be that straight ruler and the bottom edge the bottom of your skate blade. If you slide the straight ruler from side to side, it will skid easily. Even if you put considerable pressure straight down on the top, it would still skid if pressed right and left. Your skate blade, too, could slide sideward if it were flat on the ice; your forward momentum prevents such a skid. When you want to curve to the right, for instance, if you don't have something to hold you, the skate could skid right out from under you, much as the wheels of a bike slide when the rider leans into a curve on gravel. Tip the ruler to the right and look at the bottom edge. The ruler rides up on one side or corner, and were you to press down, you would be hard put to get the ruler to skid at all. In fact, the harder you pressed, the deeper would be the skid-preventing bite.

There can be no break in the ruler, and there must be no break in you. Bend anywhere at all and your skate bottom will go flat and you will not be able to get into or stay in the curve you are trying for.

Take a few strokes forward, putting yourself into a smooth glide. Bring both feet close together and extend both arms to the side. Now think of yourself as that ruler—*there must be no bend anywhere*—and lean to the right to start a curve to the right. *If* your body is straight, the right edges of your skates will bite into the ice and your lean will carry you around. If you can't get into a curve or if you can't seem to hold yourself in one, you are bending somewhere. Have someone check you over and find it. You may feel as though you are about to fall, and you may even bear the feeling out; falls are to be expected. It may take lean after lean after lean, and you may feel as though you will never get it. Then one day you lean in and you find the "groove"—you'll have it. It is the most wonderful feeling, as though you could go on and on like perpetual motion in a circle. And then you will be on your way to figures on skates, rhythm on skates—and even dance on skates.

These simple exercises are the groundwork, and if they are practiced in order, and carefully, you and your child will be ready for one of the most beautiful and satisfying of all sports, figure skating. It combines grace, skill, and rhythm, and skating, like most of the other sports in this book, can be another link between parents and children in an age when we need every link we can forge.

CHAPTER THIRTY
SUMMER CAMP

Camp is a magical word. To children it stands for campfires, cookouts, swimming, rowboats, canoes, trails, horses, shooting stars, best friends—and freedom. Freedom from parental anxieties, which children don't understand but certainly feel. Freedom from city restrictions (which are just as restricting in suburbia), city patterns, and city clothing. Freedom from school and school buses, heat, dirt, and traffic. Freedom to live for a little while the way people ought to live. That's what the word *camp* means to children. But all too often it falls far short of its promise.

When I was ten, I went to "Camp Manhansack on the shores of beautiful Peconic Bay." Like every other kid taking off for camp the very first time, I could hardly sleep the night before, and I got my parents up two hours ahead of time by arriving at their door fully dressed in my new camp clothes. I could just *see* those canoes and sailboats (they were in the catalog). I could *feel* that water (catalog). I could *smell* the pines and *hear* the wind (all in the catalog). I just couldn't wait.

When I got to "Manhansack on the shores of beautiful Peconic Bay," there wasn't a tent in sight. We were housed in *rooms* in what was called a *longhouse*. That disappointment passed, I faced the first day. We washed up in a communal bathroom, not in a stream as I had dreamed. Then we went down to the dining room and ate a typical American breakfast of juice, dry cereal, and milk. We sang, "Good morning to you, good morning to you, good morning, dear campers, good morning to you."

After breakfast we went back to the longhouse and made our beds, and then, as we would do for two long months, we went down to Camp Sewanaka, also "on the shores of beautiful Peconic Bay," only reserved for the big kids, and had a "sing." Every time nobody knew what to do with us, we had a "sing." Whenever we had a "sing," we knew it was because nobody knew what to do with us.

Most of that first morning was spent in getting settled. After that day, mornings would be divided between "nature" (I learned to recognize a sassafras leaf; it looked like a mitten) and "arts and crafts." Arts and crafts did make one indelible impression, however. Aside from learning how to make a clothes hanger out of plywood that broke the first time I hung anything on it, I learned the facts of life. After the counselor had "set up" our "projects" and disappeared, my best friend undertook to enlighten me. I thought she made the whole thing up. I also thought she was nuts.

At eleven thirty we went down to "beautiful Peconic Bay" (that much was absolutely true) for a "swim." The first morning we spent the whole time separating the swimmers (I was one) from the nonswimmers. After that the "nonswimmers" paddled around close to shore and the "swimmers" paddled around on the other side of the dock a little further out. "Zib" blew a whistle if anyone went out over her head or if we got to fooling around too much. Nobody taught us anything that I remember. In fact, the only counselor with the "swimmers" was "Zib," and she sat on top of a high platform and blew her whistle.

We had lunch and sang, "I scream, you scream, we all scream for ice cream." It didn't do any good, though, because ice cream was served only on Thursdays.

After lunch we had "rest hour," and I lay on my bed reading *Swiss Family Robinson* and wondering when all those camp adventures in which we rassled with nature would begin. "All out for the field" sounded good, but after we had walked up a long, hot, dusty road to a half-cut, hot, dusty field next to a couple of lumpy tennis courts, I lost heart. We were told to choose up teams for baseball, and for this inactive activity we had worn sneakers, knee socks, bloomers, middies, *and ties.* The interminable game went on all afternoon (Sewanaka had the courts that day and every other day except for two), and then we trudged back down the road for our afternoon "swim."

Between swim and supper and for all the many other in-betweens, we were provided with some quoits, a croquet set, and three seesaws. I don't know what Sewanaka did. Supper was typical (same as lunch, only less), and we sang "Down by the Old Mill Stream," with the counselors singing harmony. The assistant head made an announcement after rapping on her glass with a spoon. After she sat down, we sang "For She's a Jolly Good Fellow," and I was so busy wondering how a *she* could be a *fellow* that I forgot the message and had to wait until the next evening to get stationery at the camp store. You wonder how I can remember all that stuff? Kids remember *everything*. That's what's so urgent about teaching them real things when they are young enough to remember. I was wide open and ready—all they had to do was *teach me*. Did they make use of this singularly marvelous time? They did not.

After dinner we hung around the lounge and front door of Sewanaka until "evening activities," which were pretty dull or I would have remembered them better. Then Sewanaka sang "Good Night, Manhansack" to the tune of "Good Night, Ladies," and we headed off up the hill fully convinced that *right then* the adventures were bound to start. I guess Sewanaka thought the same thing when the counselors sang *them* off to bed. The most personal thing that happened that whole long day took place when "Zimmie," our rather pleasant but ineffectual counselor, filled out our health cards. Every night for two months she asked each one of us if we had brushed our teeth and had a bowel movement. About the middle of camp I got so bored with it, I said yes to the teeth and no to the bowels for five straight days, and on the fifth day she looked at me with sudden comprehension and hurried me down to the nurse, who gave me a physic. Well, it was something different anyway.

Once a week we went to "riding," and for this we wore our regular sneakers and camp bloomers. Somewhere I had got the idea that I wanted to ride like a jockey, so I stuck my feet in the leathers *above* the stirrups. Nobody corrected me. The catalog had said "canoeing," and I got into a canoe twice. The first time was when I took my "canoe test" so that I could be "passed for canoes." I had to wear my clothes over my bathing suit, and the kindly counselor who agreed to test me took me out and dumped it over. I got out of my clothes, bundled them together, and helped swim the canoe to shore. The second time I was a "stone-faced Indian" on a float and wore a sign saying I was Chief Peconic. Somebody else paddled, and I, stone-faced, looked into the sunset.

The catalog said we had to have *hiking* shoes, and I sure had mine. They were like moccasins, only high-laced to keep ankles from turning in rough terrain. I got to wear them twice, and neither time on rough terrain. The first time, we walked on the paved road to the Center for an ice cream cone, and the second time we walked down the beach to a cookout at the sandhill. I turned somersaults down the hill, and the counselor snitched.

The catalog had said "overnight camping," and at that time I was reading *Rolf of the Woods*—I knew all about camping. When I spotted my name on the list, I charged up the hill in an absolute lather. It took no time flat to gather my goods: toothbrush, sweater, bathing suit, towel, two blankets, four pins, flashlight, and poncho. I was the first one at the assembly area and had to hang around for *hours* until all the others got there. We were *trucked* to a distant beach, had a quick swim, supper, a campfire with marshmallows—and then off to bed, but not to sleep. With the tireless efficiency of the highly charged, completely rested, overexcited, underexercised young, we gave our counselors one awful night. We tried to slip into "beautiful Peconic Bay" for a skinny-dip and were caught. We got into the food for the next day and were caught. We swapped sleeping quarters and were caught. We listened in on the counselors' conversation and were caught. Knowing what I know now about kids, we must have *wanted* to get caught. We finished off the evening by going to the bathroom down the beach more often than a bunch of soldiers with dysentery, and when the counselors finally got to sleep because some of us dozed off, the others rent the still, predawn air with cries for citronella. After breakfast we were trucked back to camp, disgruntled, disillusioned, and disgustingly wide awake. The counselors were out on their feet.

We got to go out on "beautiful Peconic Bay" in the sailboats, too—once. We had two sessions on the tennis courts (when Sewanaka was off on an overnight), but without instruction. We had one masquerade, several Sunday night "shows" (amateur), a couple of dances (without boys, although Quinepet was less than a mile away), and enough relays and tournaments so that either the blues or the whites could win. The last night we had a banquet, and fortunately a really beautiful, terribly exciting equinox storm broke it up. It tore off a roof, knocked down some trees, and blew three sailboats over to Greenport. At least nature was on our side. She didn't want us to go home without a single great thing to remember.

What kind of camp have you selected for *your* child?

Camps have always had a unique opportunity to help young Americans, even camps that, like Manhansack, were really big kid corrals. They were away from crowded areas, and even the least adequate and posh were usually near some body of water—and in those days the water was clean and swimmable. They had access to enthusiastic and sometimes skilled young counselors who sought jobs with them when schools closed. They still do. Then and now camps had summer on their side, contributing everything from the right temperature by day to the incredible and mystic firmament by night. The children themselves supplied all the hopes and dreams of youth. The trouble was that they often brought all those tender, perishable gifts to Manhansacks.

We now know that children learn most of what they are to learn in the way of attitudes and patterns before they are three years old. We know that even one hour wasted when they are very little people is an hour lost, never to be regained. The younger we expose children to skills, to effort, to creativity, and to discipline, the further they can carry those things. It was Manhansack that could have profited most by anything camps had to offer—it was already late in the day for Sewanaka.

A few years ago I set up a study to see what would happen if children of nine to fourteen were exposed to a real program of physical fitness designed not to entertain and occupy but to develop and challenge. We set up a camp two and a half miles back into the woods. Accommodations were rough: just tents and two latrines. The dining hall was a long walk from bed, and even the activity areas were a quarter-mile apart. Twenty-four young campers were enrolled in a program that was to last three weeks. There was one nine-year-old girl, two boys and a girl age ten, four boys and three girls age eleven, four twelve-year-old boys, two boys and three girls age thirteen, and two boys and a girl age fourteen.

No effort was made to attract physically superior children other than the challenges presented in the publicity releases. In these the aims of the experiment were explained, and it was made quite clear that the program would be both difficult and productive. It was specified that improvement rather than entertainment was to be the major purpose.

While some of the children who registered were physically above average, others were not. The usual quota of tense, anxious children was present. There were a few lazy ones, one was quite hostile, several were overweight, and a few were too thin. All the children had one thing in common: their parents were of better than average intelligence and from professional and executive levels.

Since a large part of the weakness affecting American children today is a result of parental ignorance and anxiety, the fact that the response from this group was favorable was considered very encouraging. Many of them said they felt their children had grown up soft and that it was up to them to see that something was done about it.

Both children and parents were given a complete description of the camp before they were accepted. Its proposed rigors were described in full detail, and they understood that this camp was to be different from all others. The youngsters would live apart in that wooded area, eat a limited diet, and forgo all such customary pleasures as candy, cake, ice cream, and sodas. They were warned that their muscles would ache, that they would often be tired, and that long after the day had ended for the children in surrounding camp areas, they would still be *working*. They were fully aware that they would be expected to finish what they had started, no matter how tired, bored, or miserable they felt. They were told one other thing, and this was kept before them throughout the entire three-week period: If they succeeded in surviving the experiment, they would not merely have spent another period at a camp, they would have *proved* something—something that might help other children, lots of other children. The youngsters understood very well that such a chance does not come often—and seldom indeed to children—and that it does not come cheap in terms of personal effort.

None of the children reacted negatively to the briefing, and all wanted to take part. While this was not entirely unexpected, the attitude of enthusiastic acceptance by the parents came as a complete surprise. The children could not really foresee what such a program would demand of them, but the parents understood very well. That they were willing to permit and even encourage their children to take part in something that would be difficult, trying, and uncomfortable was certainly a departure from what we had come to consider the typical parental attitude of overprotection.

On the first day of camp each child was matched with another as to age, sex, weight, height, and body build. The youngsters in the control group had signed up for a typical camp program and would spend the same three-week period in a camp nearby. Their program would be composed of the usual camp activities: volleyball, baseball, softball, archery, riflery, crafts, swimming, and a little riding. The usual play-off tournaments were to be employed as motivation.

The diet for the control group was to be typical of that in the average camp: emphasis on filling starches and carbohydrates plus daily access to the camp's candy, ice cream, and soda bar.

The physical fitness camp, set back in the woods, was designed to bring the children into close and constant contact with those two important ingredients that have gradually disappeared from the lives of our children: nature and effort. All the area policing and laundry was to be done by the children themselves, and each day they would contribute something of themselves as they worked in reforestation.

A second isolated area, known as the Physical Fitness Center, was set aside, and on it was constructed an obstacle course. It was an exact copy of the one designed by the Institute for Physical Fitness in White Plains, New York. It was brightly painted for eye appeal and graded in difficulty so as not to discourage the weakest or least coordinated, yet difficult enough to challenge the strongest. There were enough stations to keep a group busy and interested for at least an hour at a time.

The course consisted of multileveled balance beams, overhead ladders, slanting walls to be climbed with the aid of ropes, chinning bars, parallel bars, fixed and free ropes, and pits over which had been stretched logs, two-by-sixes, and even taut wires for balancing. Old tires were set in patterns for running exercises. There were graded ramps for jumping, solid fences five and six feet high over which the youngsters climbed for time, and a trampoline.

A record player was provided, and it had enough power to fill the entire glade with full sound. The music was selected for strong rhythmic beat, its ability to excite for difficult stunts, and its ability to provide a throbbing slow rhythm conducive to controlled effort.

TESTS

The program began with a battery of tests, which were to be repeated at the end of the three-week program. The first was the Kraus-Weber test (page

145). The second was the Prudden Supplement Test for Optimum Performance (pages 32–35). Each youngster was provided with a notebook; performance was entered on the first day, and the children were urged to test themselves with one test or another each day *after the fifth*. This precaution was taken to prevent discouragement. Whenever we use maximum effort, the body requires up to four days for recuperation, and testing any time before complete recuperation has taken place will net a poorer score and a lowered level of performance. This is very difficult to explain to a youngster putting out every effort to improve.

Since several campers were overweight and a few underweight, measurements were taken (pages 37–42). And inasmuch as considerable attention was to be given to running, vital capacity was also measured (see page 36). These two tests, like the K-W, were repeated only once again, and that was at the end of the course.

Hearts were tested by a team from Lankenau Hospital to see what three weeks of extreme effort in exercise, running, and swimming would do, or if it would require a longer period to obtain results. (The boys improved; the girls did not.)

THE PROGRAM

The daily program was designed to provide a maximum of controlled activity and a minimum of free time.

7:00 A.M.	Rise, dress, police the area.
7:30 A.M.	Hike two and one-half miles through woods to dining area, where each youngster weighed in.
8:00 A.M.	Breakfast.
8:30 A.M.	Meeting to discuss the previous day's activities and answer any questions that may have arisen. A short progress report from each child.
9:00 A.M.	Calisthenics and tumbling to music.
9:45 A.M.	Juice and one-quarter-mile walk through woods to Physical Fitness Center.
10:00 A.M.	Work out on all apparatus to music.
11:00 A.M.	Hike one-quarter mile to swimming pool.
11:15 A.M.	Swimming and diving instruction. Competition.
12:30 P.M.	Lunch.
1:00 P.M.	Two-and-one-half-mile hike back to camping area.
1:30 P.M.	Rest hour. (Everybody *rested*.)
2:30 P.M.	Conservation work, planting, cleaning brush, etc.
3:45 P.M.	Juice, carrots, and celery.
4:00 P.M.	Modern dance and soccer alternating with weight training.
4:30 P.M.	Swimming instruction and competition.

Summer Camp

5:00 P.M	Free swim time.
6:00 P.M.	Dinner.
7:00 P.M.	Final one-quarter-mile walk back to Physical Fitness Center to work on individual work sheets (homework).
8:00 P.M.	Evening program.

Each camper kept an individual work sheet listing twelve items to be covered daily:

1. Bent-Knee Sit-ups (exercise 1)
2. Spine-Down Stretch (exercise 2)
3. Knee-bends (exercise 12)
4. Six-hundred-yard walk and run (timed)
5. Chin-ups (or Let-Downs if no chin-up was possible)
6. Push-ups
7. Flexibility exercise (exercise 22)
8. Snap and Stretch (exercise 21)
9. Backstroke (exercise 18)
10. Shoulder Shrug Series (exercise 13)
11. Prone arm and leg lift (exercise 27)
12. Spread-leg stretch (exercise 55).

Evening recreation programs were planned to fit in with the day's work whenever possible. One evening the campers were taken to see the U.S. Olympic gymnastic team perform. Another evening they saw a movie depicting the struggles of a group of children in postwar Europe in which much had been expected and asked of the children. The children had lived up to expectations as children do, *if only adults will ask and then have every confidence.* There were discussions on every subject *that interested the children,* and long before there was the furor about relevance, these children asked very relevant questions and even provided some very relevant answers to their own questions.

There were counselors available to watch, assist with daily self-testing, encourage, comment, and praise. These same counselors were as deeply involved in the program as the youngsters. They gave 100 percent of their time when they were on duty, helping the children to help themselves. The running course was well marked, and each child had to run it daily but be timed only when he or she wished. The counselors were available for that chore whenever there was a request.

The swimming coach *taught swimming,* and a second counselor was on duty as lifeguard. The children made no complaints about the amount of work they were required to do in the pool and were delighted that they had any "play" time at all.

Weight lifting was done with weight bags on dowels (see page 189) and only on alternate days. Soccer took the place of the usual baseball game found at most camps, the advantage being that no one ever stands still in soccer.

The diet provided for the campers was carefully regulated. For breakfast: fruit or fruit juices, wheat cereal with wheat germ added, bacon, eggs, and skim milk. Whole wheat toast or bread, margarine, honey, and *skim* milk were served at every meal. Sugar was kept to an absolute minimum. Lunch varied. Vegetable or fruit salad was served daily, as was meat, fish, or cheese. Dessert was always fruit. Dinner consisted of roast or broiled meat or fish and vegetables.

RESULTS

At the end of the three-week period the children were retested. There had been improvement in all areas:

• Fear of height (obstacle course) and physical contact (soccer) had been overcome.
• All K-W failures had been corrected.
• New pride and self-confidence were apparent in all the campers.
• Weight loss was significant, for those who had been overweight.
• Inch loss, denoting improved tone, was significant.
• Endurance had improved.
• Strength, flexibility, and coordination were markedly improved.
• Posture was vastly improved.
• Those who had been underweight had gained.

PUSH-UPS *(see page 32)*

At first testing one boy had been able to do 28 push-ups, and the top performance for girls was 11. Three boys and two girls could do none at all. The combined score for all of them was 160. At the second testing, *all* could do push-ups, and the combined score was 360— *more than doubled.*

WEIGHTED SIT-UPS *(see page 33)*

At first testing the lowest poundage lifted was 4 pounds and the best was 10 pounds. The combined lift for the group was 206 pounds. At the second testing the lowest lift was 9 pounds and the best was 34 pounds. The combined lift was 474 pounds. *More than double.*

CHIN-UPS *(see page 34)*

This test yielded the poorest showing at both the beginning and the end of the period. At first testing the top score for boys was 8, one boy did 6, and two could do 5. *Six boys could do none at all.* The best girl's score was 2, *and eight could do none at all.* The total for the group was 38. At the end of the program four girls still failed to do a single chin-up, but most of the others had doubled their scores. Four boys still failed to do one, but those who were already strong in this area improved noticeably (another reason to begin early). An eleven-year-old who had done 5 at the start increased to 11. The total number for the group increased to 71, *almost double.*

FLEXIBILITY *(see page 35)*

This test yielded unexpectedly excellent results. Inasmuch as inflexibility is tied to tension, it is often very difficult to improve. At the start two boys and one girl failed to pass even the minimum (test 6 in the K-W battery). The girl failed by minus 3½ inches. The best score was made by a thirteen-year-old boy with a plus 5½ inches. Subtracting the minus inches from the plus yielded a score of plus 23¾ inches. At the second testing there were no failures, and one camper who had failed in the first testing had improved by 6½ inches. One had gained 4 inches and a third 3 inches of stretch. The total plus score was 94¼ inches. *The score was quadrupled.*

BROAD JUMP (see page 35)

A fourteen-year-old boy made the longest jump, 6 feet 8 inches. The poorest showing was made by a somewhat overweight eleven-year-old girl who jumped 3 feet 11 inches. At the second testing this little girl took honors for *improvement* with a jump of 5 feet. It was she who went on to become an athlete and a cheerleader at school. The best second jump was made by another fourteen-year-old boy, who had improved his score by 10½ inches to jump 7 feet 2½ inches. The final combined score was 141 feet 7½ inches.

600-YARD RUN

In the first 600-yard run the best time was made by a fourteen-year-old boy with 1:59. The poorest time was turned in by that same eleven-year-old girl with 3:07. The total running time for the group was 58:09. After three weeks the girl who had the lowest score was still lowest, but she had improved her time by 33 seconds. She was second in line for improvement honors. The girl who took first in improvement had improved her time by 44 seconds. The original high scorer was still ahead with 1:51. Two boys had lost ground; one was 5 seconds and the other 12 seconds slower. Another boy maintained the same score. All the others improved. The final total running time for the group was 54:02. An improvement of 4:07.

WEIGHT

All the campers who needed to lose weight lost weight. The total loss for the group was 48 pounds. The heaviest boy lost the most with 8 pounds. A second overweight boy lost 7½ pounds. A third in the same category lost 5½ pounds. The five slim campers gained a total of 5½ pounds. The fourteen-year-old boy who turned in a top performance in everything, including emotional stability, gained 2½ pounds. The youngest camper, a nine-year-old who kept up with the others all the way, gained half a pound.

INCHES

Inches loss was impressive, as was improvement in posture. The fattest boy lost 19 inches, mostly from waist, hips, and abdominals. This in turn had a very good effect on his opinion of himself. A boy who had lost only 2½ pounds lost 12 inches. His fat had been exchanged for muscle. The eleven-year-old girl who had improved so dramatically between the first and second testing lost 2½ pounds and 8½ inches. The total inch loss for the group was 134¾ inches. Three campers gained inches, and two of those three gained weight also—and it was all muscle. The total inch gain was 2¾ inches.

POSTURE

The total gain in height *in three weeks*

was 9 inches. One girl whose posture had been deplorable at the start gained 1½ inches in height as she developed the strength and flexibility necessary for standing straight. This camper's tension had been as apparent at the beginning as her confidence and relaxed attitude were at the end.

Awards were presented to campers for both top performance and improvement. Full reports were sent home to enthusiastic parents.

Certain reactions to the stress engendered by the program are worthy of note. The nine-, ten-, and eleven-year-old boys *and girls* went through the whole program without ever flagging and with considerable enthusiasm. At no time, even when the going got very rough indeed, did they break down, cry, or complain. The girls of thirteen and fourteen had a few weepy days, which seemed to coincide with menstrual periods. However, weepy or not, they did not give up. Major breakdowns and complaints—and these were almost daily—came from the boys of twelve through fourteen. This leads us to believe that optimum effort, concentration, and enthusiasm can be had only *before* boys reach twelve. This may be important when selecting age groups for concentrated programs in the elementary grades. As things are at the present time, the first big push is made in junior high school *or when the children reach the age of twelve.* The golden years, from K through 6, are usually passed over.

When the control group was retested, the results were disastrous. They had even lost ground in the minimum test, and there was no improvement in the optimum test. *We had the impression that the average camp program does not contribute much toward basic physical fitness.*

Naturally, it would not be necessary to have a program as ruthless and extreme as the one just described, although every child from the last to the first declared those three weeks to be "wonderful, and when can we do it again?". But with proper testing it would not be difficult to determine just how much would be needed to augment an already active program, balance a weighted program, and provide a solid physical base for a sedentary program. When I think back on those months at Manhansack, I just wish someone had offered me the chance to sign up for work that was as exciting as play instead of play that was dull as dishwater.

Successful camps today are those that specialize. Some of these are given over almost entirely to one sport or skill, such as tennis, baseball, riding, swimming, gymnastics, or skating. There are camps that specialize in the arts, such as music or dance. There are language camps, tutoring camps, and survival camps. Of late there is a huge boom in camps for the obese. No matter where the interest lies, each of these specializing camps misses a big bet for themselves and for the children if they omit a good physical fitness program as preparation, balance, or carryover.

Four to eight weeks can produce very respectable results with far less effort than that allotted to our pilot camp—and each camper would have some very real and good physical habits to take home, something that could be made to last all year. Young people are the very best carriers of *valuable* information, and a good program begun in camp might even find its way to the whole family. Counselors are often young, too—and today the young want to give their time to something worthwhile.

The camp director who wants to attract the very best young people has only to offer the chance to do something of real value, and the best will come flocking to his door.

CAMP PHYSICAL FITNESS FORMULA

Before any camp can chart the progress of its campers and therefore the efficacy of its program, it must know the condition of the campers on their arrival. It is important to know the fitness level of the entire group and also the level of each child. We always return to foundations. If the individual's foundation is solid, one can always build on it. If, however, there is a weak wall, there will always be severe limitations. Before we can ask for skills, we *must* check the foundations and remedy any weakness discovered at the minimum level.

1. Using the Kraus-Weber test for minimum strength and flexibility, provide each camper with a starting line. Follow up with those exercises that will correct existing weaknesses.

2. Set up self-competition and group competition, using the Prudden Supplement test. Follow immediately with the exercises that provide the strength and flexibility that will allow for improved performances from *everyone*. Competition should be based on improvement, not on the star performances of a few.

3. Give *understandable* reports to both children and parents; these will enlist their continuing support and enthusiasm.

The child who is successful at camp and *knows* just how successful he or she has been, goes home with a better self-image. When a child's self-image has improved, whether the improvement has gone from low to better, good to high, or high to still higher, self confidence and happiness are welcome by-products. If children's confidence and fitness levels improve, academic improvement is sure to follow. With such possible plusses the question of what to do with the long summer months is automatically solved. However, such plusses are not to be found in every place called "Camp." Remember Manhansack. There are far more inadequate camps than there are good ones and even the "best" camp," when it comes to brochures and facilities (remember Manhansack) may house a non-productive program. *Remember, too, that the best years for learning are before the age of twelve.*

Start with the Kraus-Weber Test for Minimum Muscular Fitness (p. 14)

No matter what type of camp or the length of stay, the bottom line and first move after unpacking, should be the Kraus-Weber Test. There are a few generalizations that may help if you know about them beforehand. Children from more or less affluent homes (in America) tend to fail tests 2 and 3. Children who live under more emotional stress than their physical outlets can release, tend to fail test 6. Sports camps can rack up a failure rate as high as 60 percent with test 6 as the only failure. That is due to the stress of competition and poor coaching. When the children can pass the test however, they will be better athletes and less in danger of injury. For athletic injuries, see the section on Myotherapy. For more productive exercise, see the section on Warm-Up Exercises, page 68.

It will be far easier to correct failures of tests 1 through 5 than test 6. However, at camp, as in boarding schools, more progress can be made with flexibility because a great deal of children's stress comes from problems at home which they can neither understand nor handle. Guilt is a well known by-product of such stress. When they are away from home they are called upon to cope with child-sized problems which are perfectly obvious most of the time and with which they can cope successfully.

Function precedes form, which means in essence that if a child cannot do a single sit-up, you cannot expect him or her to belt out a homer or to do a *tour jeté*. The child lacking abdominal strength cannot serve a tennis ball, do a jackknife dive, sit at a piano two hours a day, or even sing a round, full note. The inflexible child *will* be injured sooner or later and the longer the muscles remain in a foreshortened condition, the more severe and lasting the injury. The serious and often career-stopping injuries of college and pro athletes were born before the age of twelve with tension and compounded in high school by coaching built on the maxim, *No pain–no gain.* That maxim, coupled with base ignorance of exercise (called calesthenics) dooms most American athletes at an early age.

ADAPTATION OF THE PHYSICAL TESTING AND PROGRAM TO DIFFERENT TYPES OF CAMPS

TWO-MONTH CAMPS

Two-month camps should test three times: at the beginning, again at midseason, and just before closing. Reports to parents should be made at midseason and again after closing. At that time suggestions should be made regarding the continuance of the program at home.

ONE-MONTH CAMPS

One-month campers should be given two tests plus instructions for carrying on the program at home. If the job has been well done at camp, the child will be sold on continuing. The thought that *you* are interested is often all a child needs to make physical fitness a lifelong goal.

TWO-WEEK CAMPS

Two-week camps should test at the beginning and the end of each session, placing as much emphasis as possible on the progress made by each child. Remember the tremendous value that can be reaped from work with the very young *and from providing that which is relevant to the not so very young.* Physical fitness *is* relevant.

OBESITY CAMPS

If a camp specializing in obesity has one hundred campers, it has one hundred youngsters with at least one problem, overweight. The cause of that overweight is almost never glandular. The children handle their heartaches by filling their stomachs. This in turn creates yet another heartache when they look in the mirror, are laughed off the team, and become the butt of class humor. A stringent diet plus constant activity all summer long *will* reduce weight, at least temporarily. However, since the heartache remains, the symptoms usually return. To make the weight loss permanent, the habit of eating correctly (not necessarily less) must be formed and the feeling of *liking self* instilled. The little eleven-year-old who lost weight and improved her performance and went back to school to make the team and also the cheerleaders' squad kept her lead. Why? She really went back to school a different person. She didn't just lose weight; she became somebody else, *somebody she liked and was proud of.* By keeping track of everything she did, she was so much encouraged to learn that she kept right up with the others. Maybe she wasn't as fast or as good, but every day *she* was better than *she* had been the day before. With her weight and measurement charts she knew to the quarter-pound and quarter-inch what each day's effort netted. There was no guessing; she *knew.* She discovered that it was easier to keep it off than start to take it off all over again—and once *that* lesson is learned, overweight is a thing of the past.

ADAPTATION OF EXERCISE TO EXISTING PROGRAMS

RIDING CAMPS

- *Freedom of motion of the pelvis—exercise 38*
- *Stretched pectorals for straight posture in the saddle—exercises 18 and 21*
- *Powerful upper back for a straight seat and control of the reins—exercise 193*
- *The psoas and thighs—page 27*
- *Flexibility of soleus, or heel cords, so that heels can be pressed down—exercise 12*
- *Arm and shoulder strength—ropes and chin ups*

YOUNG SUPERIOR PERFORMERS

Superior young people are national treasures. We spend billions to locate oil, but unlike the Russians (who *do* do some things right) we spend nothing on locating the "superiors." Someone, and luck, is what we depend on. By the time the someone who would recognize superiority sees it, the best years for really developing it are over.

Another thing: There is no excuse for the fact that 75 percent of the students graduating from music school have developed limiting muscle spasm. There is even less excuse for accepting athletic injuries as part of the game—or compounding them with the "No pain, no gain" premise. Actually no child should suffer muscle spasm (often called "growing pain"), no matter what the cause, including drugs. It doesn't matter *how* the child gets the drugs—from a classmate, a pusher, or a doctor. Drugs, even those taken *for* pain, often cause muscle pain. (See the chapter on Myotherapy.)

TENNIS CAMPS

Tennis is a "spike" activity, requiring quick stops and starts, endurance, and enormous coordination. The trunk must be both strong and flexible, and the body must be relaxed even when under the pressure of competition. The children should develop the following:

- *Trunk strength—exercises A, B, C*
- *Trunk flexibility—exercises 9 and 10*
- *Shoulder freedom and power—exercises 18, 21, 190*
- *Knee strength—exercise 12*
- *Leg strength—see Exercise Index*
- *Endurance—run*

MUSIC, ART, AND DRAMA CAMPS

It is not enough to *want* to be a musician, artist, actor, or actress. Those arts must come through the body as well as through the hands and the voice. The artist in any field will do better work if he can relate himself to space and to rhythm. A *general exercise program* should be employed by every camper who dreams of ever entering these exacting and difficult fields and should develop the following:

- *Release of tension in musicians and artists who must combat the tightness in muscles caused by long hours of concentrated practice—exercises 15 and 16 (to be done every hour during practice to prevent small muscle spasms)*
- *Arm strength and flexibility—exercises 18 and 21*
- *Sense of rhythm use floor progressions—pages 107–127*

BASEBALL CAMPS

Baseball doesn't build a body, but it takes a good body to play baseball. The entire program of exercise, tumbling, and apparatus should be utilized by those wishing to excel in a sport that doesn't need much of anything until it needs everything you have—and you never know when that moment is going to come.

BASKETBALL CAMPS

Basketball players are notoriously inflexible. That is because basketball, like tennis, is another "spike" sport and depends on quick starts and stops. The game itself builds endurance and strength, but it takes away from flexibility. All such sports need exercise 22 often throughout every day.

CHAPTER THIRTY-ONE
HELPING THE HANDICAPPED

I drove up to the school where the "class" for handicapped children was to be held every morning during the summer. The car was so loaded with equipment—ramps, sawhorses, mats, dowels, and a ladder—that it looked like a circus van. There was a small crowd of little children gathered near the school door, and as I got out of the car, a small figure shot away from the group and came racing toward me so fast she looked like a bright blur against the dark green hedge. When she came close enough, I could see Kathy's bright slanting eyes and the little round pixie face one sees on children with Down's syndrome. Seconds later she left the ground shouting, "Bommen Punnin," and I caught her in my arms. I handed her the dowels, and she danced ahead of me crying the news of my arrival as though she had been waiting for it forever. In seconds I was surrounded by all the other little pixie people, all greeting "Bommen Punnin" and trying to help.

In the gym we set up the equipment and put a pleasant record on the player. The volunteers (teenage girls for the most part) were helping to remove shoes and socks, blow noses, and fasten Roger's football helmet. Roger had had terribly high fevers when he was a baby, and now he had difficulty with balance. He'd start out for someplace and suddenly veer off at an angle. If there was a wall in the way, he always managed to hit it with his head. Or he'd set out across the floor and gradually gather momentum until his churning legs just couldn't keep up with his head, and down he'd go. He never cried when he fell, even when he raised a huge goose egg. I guess he had just gotten used to it.

Pat was a Down's child like Kathy, and absolutely startling. Except for a scalplock of blond hair smack in the middle of her crown, which gave her the look of an Oriental chieftain (small size), she hadn't a sprig anywhere else. She was as quiet as my welcoming committee had been effusive. From the very first day when we had put out the equipment, she made it very clear that she would do not a single thing until she was quite sure she could—which meant, in effect, until she had gone over and over in her mind all the moves that went to making up the whole of any one trick or movement. She had the same reticence that some "normal" children display who never say a word for two, even three years. Then, after worrying their parents half to death, they suddenly turn to one of them at the table and say, "Please pass the bread."

Nancy couldn't talk, but she could make herself understood, often all too well. She was three, petite, very pretty, and very willful. It was often hard to imagine that such loud and raucous monosyllabic commands could emanate from something so tiny. The sound was exactly the same for "Pick me up," "Set me down," "Give me that," and "No."

There were other kids there, too, including a pair of boys about five who were not only inseparable but indistinguishable from each other. What one did, the other copied, and the leader seemed to be whichever one was motivated to move first. If one made a statement, the other said, "Yes." They were no trouble, but the volunteers just had to understand that if one went off the ramp, the shadow would be right behind—and prepare for it.

A tall slender girl was no trouble either, which isn't always a good sign. She was very thin and sort of droopy, as though she were just too tired to hold up her head with its masses of dark hair. Unless she was urged to join in, she would just sit. Even when she did get out on the floor, she always seemed to be looking past us at some faraway place we couldn't see. There were several others, mostly kids with Down's syndrome. There were a couple who had cerebral palsy, and all were considered to be "retarded."

This was to be my "class" that summer, and I had promised results. Back in White Plains at the institute we had got results, but I'd had help, plenty of it. We had a "secret society" called the Bellwethers. They had to be unknown so that they could do their work, and only a Bellwether knew who the others were or even that they existed. They were children trained to make other children feel secure and comfortable. When a new child arrived, a Bellwether got the word and dressed next to her in the locker room, went up to the assigned gym with her, and stood next to her during class. If she had difficulty with an exercise, the Bellwether helped. No "new kid" ever had to feel as though he was one against the whole world. I've seen a ten-year-old Bellwether fall laughing in a heap next to a child who had fallen by accident and was both frustrated and embarrassed. They helped each other up and started off with the same exercise, but together. They knew the importance of feeling "good," and they knew who didn't. Once when I'd been away, I found a note on my desk from an eleven-year-old Bellwether named Don: "Dear Bonnie, Jamie smiled today." That doesn't sound very exciting unless you knew, as he did (mind you, there were a thousand people through those doors every week), that Jamie had never smiled, that he was brought alone to class by a chauffeur, helped to dress by that same chauffeur, and then driven away. We didn't know anyone who knew him, but every Bellwether made it his business to *learn* Jamie, and each was as pleased as Don when the first sign of progress was made. Oh, how I wished for my wonderful "secret society"—I certainly needed at least one Bellwether, but all I had to work with was a group of handicapped children.

Well, if we were to get anywhere that morning, I'd best get started, so I put on a slow record, got down on the floor, and began "sealing" (exercise 72) under the sawhorses. Kathy was behind me in an instant, laughing and calling to the others. One by one they, too, began to "seal." The tall, slender girl was reluctant, but not for long. Kathy had her by the hand and was urging her gently and pushing off in front of her, showing her how *easy* it was. The words sounded garbled, but the smile and mime were ever so clear—I had my Bellwether. All that long summer Kathy was like a tireless, incredibly efficient little sheepdog. She rounded up her charges, prodded them forward, held them back, cut out one or another, calmed them, excited them—*and all without a single practice session*. Kathy was a Bellwether by intuition, not training. This was probably for the same reason that Down's children are exuberant and happy when you are happy and are desperately sad when you are sad, even when you don't say a word.

We held little bodies close as the children walked on the balance beam. We, and they, became kittens and crossed on all fours. We were alligators slithering, hippos wallowing, horses prancing, and bunnies hopping. We helped them jump off the ramps, over the ramps, and even from one ramp to the next. They traveled up, down, across, and under the ladder—and they tumbled. For every trick Nancy had another scream, the tall girl waited for Kathy to go first, Roger held tightly to someone, and Pat stood back and watched until she had the whole thing assembled in her head. She established a quota. She would learn one new thing each week, but as the weeks passed, they mounted up.

On the fourth week I brought two attractive young visitors with me, teachers who wanted to see what we were doing. They were sitting on a piano bench just watching quietly when Nancy went over and stood looking up at them. I had told them about her screams and waited for the ear-splitting comment. It didn't come. Nancy turned around and backed toward them, reaching up with both arms. When she was close enough to touch, she said quite clearly, "Lift me up." No screams, no wiggles, no fuss, just "Lift me up." They did, and there she sat, the class demon, looking quite comfortable and no end smug. The only commotion was in the ranks of the staff, who were too stunned to react even when she slid off the bench and trotted over to where I was catching handstands. "My turn," she said, turning bottom up. She had decided it was time to talk.

The successes were not all so dramatic, but they were regular. We started with the warm-ups, and four were able to follow. Kathy and Pat were the mainstays, with the tall girl and Nancy taking part most of the time. After a while we could hold six. From experience I knew that if I made a game out of the exercises, if we played "Follow the Leader" and if the leader were both funny and easy to copy, if everybody had a good time and I stayed ahead of them by constantly changing the exercises, the kids would join in. Sooner or later they all did, and as they learned the exercises and the music, they were like all children with a story they know—don't leave out an "if," "and," or "but." Don't change the sequence, don't change the words. In no time Kathy could lead, and pretty soon so could Pat.

On the last day we had a party, and Roger, happily slurping a cone, headed out onto the lawn, which had a gentle slope. Gentle for us perhaps, but Roger's balance problem turned it into the side of a sharply listing deck, and he started to slip off sideways. For some reason, since we hadn't planned a class, no one had bothered with his helmet, and there he was headed downhill at full tilt and gaining. When the fall came, it was a wonder. Roger clutched the cone tight against his narrow little chest, covering the top with his chin. He looked like a round-backed armadillo as he rolled over and came to a sitting stop. He was delighted: He still had his cone. We were more than delighted: He didn't have a goose egg. The endless "grooving" in somesaults (exercise 97), forward shoulder rolls (exercise 101), and backward shoulder rolls (exercise 100) had paid off.

Roger's adventure had us all on edge, but it hadn't bothered Pat a bit. She was very busy with a project of her own. The ladder was lying across two boxes, and she had started across on hands and feet by herself. Being very slow and careful, she placed each little bare foot on a rung, and then, changing her attention to her hands, she moved them forward two rungs. It wasn't until she reached the end that she was faced with a real problem: There was no one there to lift her off. She looked first to one side and then the other, and one of the volunteers started down to assist. "Wait," I said. "Let's see what she does with it—for sure she won't fall." We waited, four silent people watching a tiny child as she thought through a problem while she was right in the middle of it. No one had come to assist, and like some perfectly normal people I know, she was darned if she was going to ask for help. First she got down flat on her little round tummy and looked over each side, but that didn't get it. Then she got back up on hands and feet and walked her feet through the arch of her arms and sat down with her feet pointing toward the end, but that didn't get it either. Then, with careful deliberation, she turned over on her tummy again, this time with her feet toward the end, and slowly, inch by inch, she wiggled backward until her feet touched the ground. Then, pushing her scalplock back and smoothing her dress, she marched off to join the others. There are those who will tell you that Down's kids can't, don't, or won't think.

That evening we had a performance for the parents, and all the children in the summer program took part. The tall, slender girl waved to her mother from the very center of the balance beam, and she didn't have that faraway look at all. Roger hung from the chinning bar by his knees and had to be coaxed off to do his rolls. They tumbled and did their "warm-ups" in a group, and they moved beautifully. It had taken only a few weeks, but they were so sure of themselves *and so pleased with themselves.*

And all of that happened *before* we discovered Myotherapy and learned that "the dizzies" often come from neck spasms or that turned-in toes come from leg spasms. We didn't know we could often free the little arms and feet of the children with cerebral palsy. When I think what that summer *could* have shown—it's frustrating. Imagine what they'd be like today!

Later we watched the older kids, who had spent most of the time "making things." They had painted boxes and made ashtrays and potholders. Their "activity" had been baseball, the seesaw, and the swings. I felt sick and sad. There they were, big, stiff, and overweight. And just like any other human being who doesn't move, they were tense and awkward and *unattractive.* But there was an important difference. In addition to being unfit, they had the problem of a handicap. It is enough to have the handicap, any handicap, without complicating the difficulty. Almost any child can be made more fit than he or she is, and in the process release all sorts of destructive tensions, which brings us to Elly.

All of this took place *before* the Special Olympics had become part of the national scene. My introduction to those occurred in 1976, when I was asked to talk to a group of parents whose children were being given my program. Four of one class had just returned from the Special Olympics with gold medals, and I was very pleased to hear about their successes—until I thought about it a little further.

Long ago, when the polio vaccine was discovered, there had been some talk about the possibility that the March of Dimes organization might be directed our way to help the half of America's children who were failing the basic fitness test. I was an idealist and thought that surely our kids were valuable and deserved some help. Dr. Kraus, whose test I'd been using, was a realist. "Bonnie, you will be able to raise all kinds of money for damaged children—but never a cent for desperate 'well' ones. They don't *look* the part." Sure enough, the Poliomyelitis Foundation found kids who "looked" the part and the help was turned away.

There in New Hampshire a small group of children with handicaps that "showed" were being given the help that thousands of their fellows were denied because their disintegration was hidden. There wasn't even a way to tell people about it. It's still going on. This summer at Muhlenberg College, where we were training Myotherapists, we met hundreds of the handicapped kids who were there to compete. They were delightful, enthusiastic, well behaved, and had come from everywhere in the state. Each competed and each won something to be proud of. A few blocks away were children who would never be trained, never be helped, never get the chance to compete, never win anything and, incidentally, never feel good about themselves. Who were they? They were the thousands of Allentown, Pennsylvania, children who looked normal and were considered normal. They were the children by the thousands who do not possess even the minimum strength and flexibility needed for living.

Elly was hyperactive. A chemical imbalance before she was born had altered her just enough to make her "different." She was sweet and kind, but she talked all the time and was difficult in class. Finally she was dismissed as disruptive. I met her with her mother in my gym, and as we ran through the tests, she kept up a running commentary. None of it was stupid, but all of it was disturbing. Some of it sounded like the questions I used to ask the dentist to keep him from drilling my teeth. Finally I put on some music, and Elly listened and followed the exercises very well. While her attention was focused on my actions and the music, she didn't talk at all. We tried the equipment. She was just great, and her rhythm was excellent. I told her so, and she just glowed.

We trained Elly's mother in the exercises, tumbling, and apparatus in one of our five-day crash courses, and she went back home to work with her sweet but difficult little daughter. That fall, after three months' work, Elly went back to Duke University, where she was tested for her academic level. The doctors found she had gone up two years in all subjects but arithmetic—in that subject she had advanced three and a half years—*and she hadn't cracked a book.* They also discovered that her eyes had improved sufficiently so that she could be fitted for glasses. The day after she had her glasses, she turned away from her mother's side and walked out on the grounds for a look around. It was the first time she had shown that kind of initiative. That evening back at the hotel when she began her usual exhausting talking, her mother gave her a pad and pencil and said, "Write it down, Elly, and show me." Elly wrote it down and then spent a very happy hour reading back what she had written—*to herself,* while her mother read her own book. Another first.

A miracle? Yes and no. The human body, whatever its hurts, problems, or fears, must find release for them. If release is not at hand, the tensions grow, the hurts begin to swell, and the fears magnify. Then the need to *get it out* becomes acute. If children can get rid of these things through activity, they become pleasant and easy to live with. When they don't, they are painful to themselves and to others. Anything that is normal but denied, whether that be food, water, air, quiet rest, or release, becomes abnormally important. For Elly the need to "get it out" was terribly important, since she had so very much to get out. When her physical outlets were stepped up, when she could move and work to music she loved, she got rid of mounting tensions. Tensions are very much like pain. If you have an operation and are being given medicine to keep the pain *under control*, it will be kept under control, and there will be a minimum of suffering. If you try to avoid the controlling medicine and just "bear the pain," or if the nurse forgets to bring a pill to you at the stipulated time, the pain begins to mount. You become restless and very concentrated on the pain. As it builds on itself and gains momentum, you may even become frightened. When, after what seems like many hours, you give in and ask for the medicine, it may be too late to get immediate relief—and that's the way it is with *any* child when it comes to tensions. As they build and multiply, the need for controlling release through action becomes increasingly important and, after a certain point, less effective. The secret lies in providing release through vigorous activity *at regular intervals* so that there can be no buildup.

Since the work on the apparatus forced Elly either to use her eyes or fall and get a bump, she used and exercised them. When the muscle control improved and the glasses brought her a world that didn't change and blur away, she felt safer and more confident in herself. When that happened, all her curiosity came forward, and she went out to see what there was to see.

It wasn't that Elly suddenly changed from stupid to bright in class. There never was anything the matter with her mind or her ability to learn. She had been learning all the time. But with all the interference (try putting your thoughts together in a combination machine shop, kaleidoscope, three-band rock gathering, snap-the-whip, fun house), she hadn't been able to settle her mind on one thing at a time. You will find a mild form of this kind of disorientation when traffic is heavy and your car radio too loud. You quickly flip the switch for silence and feel more able and secure. When some of the tensions were removed, Elly could give her attention to the job at hand, consider the questions, and sort out the answers. The supply of information had not been augmented. Relaxed, she had time to hunt for the key to the room where the supplies were kept.

John was what is now known as a "holdback baby." The doctor hadn't arrived when the baby was ready to be born, and his mother had been "urged" to "hold back" until he got there. John lost just enough oxygen to damage his brain. I didn't meet him until he was just about twelve. He was very shy and dearly loved his very beautiful mother and one of those aunts that every kid ought to have. It was at one of the five-day workshops, and several mothers of handicapped children had come both to learn how to teach fitness to the handicapped and to provide the children we needed for the training of teachers. Shy John was given a camera and helped to take pictures of some of the teachers working on the equipment—including his mother and Aunt Ida. It was only a short hop and a step until John was assisting first *his* two ladies over the horses, and then *all* the ladies over the horses. John was another Kathy, sensitive, kind, and intuitive. As each teacher thanked him, he began to experience that wondrous balm for the soul—the feeling of being useful and needed. He suddenly realized there was use for his strength and need for his ability to assist.

John's mother took her training back to Long Island, and she took John. When I went there to visit, John had everybody hopping. Enthusiasm is hard to beat and impossible to hold down when coupled with praise. John knew how to say, "That was good," in at least a dozen ways, and each fitted the person and the occasion. Handicapped children need to *feel good* about themselves (as does every other human being), and when they do, they are good-natured, kind, and often very responsible. As John worked with his mother to help exercise the other children, he grew in every way. Now he is six feet two inches tall and writes me two or three letters a year. He works for his father on a truck, loves the work, loves the people, and feels important in what he does. How many who were never injured can say as much for what they do and the people who surround them? John still helps with classes, and he says that of all the things he does, he most enjoys helping other people.

Harold was eleven when he first came to the institute, and he came because he had decided to become an athlete. He had been blind since birth, was a good cook, a good chess player, could play the piano and write poetry, but he had a yen to really move. When he had been down in the lower grades, he had had a chance to use some of the ropes in the gym, and when the other kids had learned somersaults, he'd gone right along—but now that they were supposed to go out for teams, he was sent to study hall. This very often happens to handicapped youngsters. If they have any choice at all, it's between the hall, sitting in the bleachers, or standing out in left field where it's a case of guessing what's going on.

Harold was taken over immediately by one of the best of our Bellwethers, eleven-year-old Danny, who was under a bit of a handicap himself. He had the flattest feet I've ever seen and had gone through the agony of building those feet up from the kind that shuffle and flap to a pair that served him very well. They weren't fast, but they were hardworking and consistent. Danny worked with Harold on the exercises until all he had to do was whisper the name of the exercise and Harold could start at once, not only on the beat but with the right phrasing, so that he was in step with the rest of the class. If Danny ran the track, Harold pumped right along behind him. If Danny went over the obstacle course, he did it twice, once on each piece of apparatus for himself, and then once to get Harold through. In a month Harold needed no help or coaching on anything, including the seventeen-foot climbing wall. If Harold could get his hands on it, whether "it" was a pair of rings or a wrestling partner, he could master it. It isn't that blind kids can't do things; it's just that what is being taught is so often unsuitable. Instead of skills at which they can excel on an equal basis with sighted children, they are asked to swat at huge balls with huge bats, much as we buy a ticket for the sweepstakes—the chances of hitting in either case are slim indeed, but it's for a good cause.

Ideally a physical fitness program should be undertaken as soon as a prospective mother finds out why she feels like she does. (More ideally, of course, she should be in great shape long before she gets married, but few are.) The well-equipped "hotel" that serves a good "table" is the very best place for a baby to spend prebirth building time. If the "hotel" is in *very* good condition, those nine months pass quickly and with very little discomfort. When D-Day comes around, the performance is spelled *Delivery*, not *Disaster*.

Phase two of the baby's physical fitness program should begin as soon as the baby gets home from the hospital, but some babies are lucky. I went up to Vermont when Petie had my number-three grandson, Dick. We had to wait in the hall because the babies (four of them) were in with their mothers for a little get-together plus lunch. Suddenly above the general hospital sounds I heard, "Open your arms. Come on, all the way. Now cross over your chest—that's the boy." It was Petie putting Dick, through his calisthenics, closely followed by three somewhat skeptical Vermont mothers and three very agreeable brand-new Vermont babies. It's hard to say if the others kept it up, but Dick did. His physical development is a delight to behold, but his development of good sense lags far behind his athletic ability. They say he is quite a lot like me. If so, he will probably find that life offers many adventures, which, in his condition, he will be able to embrace. When it's all over, he may bear scars, but he won't have missed very much.

Today in the United States a handicapped baby is born every five minutes. It is often five and even six years before the extent of the injury is known, and by that time the very best years for gaining ground, making up differences, and preparing a wide, firm base for the life ahead are past. *No* handicapped child can use those years to build physically the way a nonhandicapped child can. If you have ever had to be on crutches, you know that even if you are an absolute whiz at getting around on them, the person getting around without them is whizzier. You cannot afford to leave the child's physical training up to him; he doesn't even know he is on crutches when he is little. Then, too, *you* may not know. The best course to follow is one of preparation. Prepare your children for whatever is to come. Give each one the edge of a fine body. Then, if something should happen to set one of them back, they have the magic of that extra margin.

All too often what happens could have been avoided. A child is a little slow, but the overworked mother who already has three hell-raisers is more than a little pleased to have one that stays put and doesn't pull every pot out of the cupboard and chase the cat headfirst down the cellar stairs. Yes, he is a little overweight and, yes, he is a little clumsy, but so is Uncle Jerry, and he's president of Consolidated. When he gets to school, all that will change—but it doesn't. When he gets to school, he becomes tense, anxious, and fearful. The kids tease him and call him "fraidy cat." They grab his cap and keep it away from his awkward hands. He hates to go out for recess, but the teacher insists. She can't make exceptions with forty children to watch. Last week they coaxed him up into a tree, and he couldn't get down, and the teacher had to call the janitor. He won't go out to play after school, just watches TV—and eats. He can't keep up with the class, and he has been left behind twice and is now the biggest (and dumbest) kid in the class.

Now suppose his program had begun when he was seven days old. He *might* still be retarded, although perhaps not to that degree. He might also have a body like little Kathy's—strong, flexible, and coordinated. If he could keep up and perhaps be even a little ahead on the playground, considering the fact that the playground is the place where children earn their places at that age level, think what that would mean. If he was well liked and well exercised, he would feel both secure and relaxed. If he played well, he would enjoy play and keep on moving. This alone would be an asset, since the well-exercised think better. A little retarded, yes, but what *is* retarded? To "retard" means to "slow down," and there are thousands of children who give evidence of retardation. They seem slow, limited, and often difficult. Later it is found that they are not retarded at all. Had they been given a different environment during the early years, they might have perked along quite nicely. They were not born retarded; they were slowed down by environment. By the same token, a truly retarded youngster, given plenty of exercise that "grooves" his muscles into the correct responses, increases his circulation, releases accumulating tensions, and improves his coordination and appearance has a great deal going for him. At the very best, the average man uses less than one-fifth of his brain. If the "physical plant" were such that a child could harness enough energy to tap two-fifths of his not quite average brain, where, then, are the limits?

Melanie was twelve, a big girl with a perpetual smile that vacillated from half to very full. She wrinkled her forehead and squinted her eyes and acted very much like a large, amiable puppy who wanted intensely to do your bidding if only she could figure out what it was. She would nod attentively all the while you were giving instructions, the perfect picture of willing cooperation. Then when you had finished, she would give herself away completely. Whenever she was alone, she would still continue to do exactly what she had been doing before. When she was with a group, she would do whatever they did. Since she couldn't follow them all, it was a matter of luck which ones she copied, and her performance ranged from perfect to impossible. If she was reprimanded, she was patient and repentant, knowing she had offended; however, she never had the slightest idea what it was she had done wrong. Is there anything more frustrating than to offend and not know how you did it?

Melanie had come to the institute with her grandmother, who was big like Melanie but with a governable smile that flashed only briefly to light up her whole face. Melanie's had no light at all. The grandmother said, "I could tell you she was like all the others, and you'd believe me at first, but you'd find out sooner or later, so I'll start off by telling you she's retarded." Melanie smiled more widely and wrinkled her forehead. "She likes other kids and she loves to play, but she always gets the raw end of the deal. They hide on her, leave her behind, send her on ridiculous errands. Last week she was the decoy while they stole a bunch of stuff from the drugstore." Melanie nodded happily and smiled. I asked if she had brought her exercise clothes, and she smiled even more broadly. Her grandmother said, "Your gym suit," and put her hand on the bundle in Melanie's lap. There was an immediate change. The broad grin flashed real for just a second, the wrinkles fled from her forehead, and she nodded furiously and said yes, she had her gym suit. (I had a quick mental picture of myself in second grade when a stern and frightening nun had me up in front of the class doing sums in my head. The minute the numbers doubled up and she asked what 15 and 16 equaled, I went blank. She might just as well have said, "What's pi plus eye?" Those multiple numbers just wiped out my brains. I guess if I had thought that smiling and wrinkling would get me off the hook, that's what I would have done. As it was, I just stood there silent and defiant, working up a stomachache. I never did learn, and even today I'm the slowest adder in the house. Today they would call that problem a block, but in those days it was "inattention" or "lack of concentration" or "stupid.")

"Come on, Melanie, I'll show you where the dressing room is." As I said those words, I took her hand and started for the door. She came right along, and on the way downstairs I picked up Ann, the captain of the Bellwethers, who had been doing special exercises with some younger children. Ann needed no briefing. We had several other retarded children salted in among the classes. The rate was about one to fifteen. I did give her the only clue I had found during our meeting: Melanie couldn't follow spoken instructions. *"Show her."*

It didn't take long to get results, Melanie had a flare for imitation. Why not? It was the thing she did best. She loved music, and if an exercise were done to a theme that appealed, they were forever tied together in her mind. In three weeks she could lead fifteen exercises and lead them well. She had never *led* anything before in her life. All her attention was focused on Ann, who had more good things about her than is said of angels, and Melanie soon picked up the institute rules. With four gyms, an obstacle course, and hundreds of kids on stairs and in halls, there had to be rules. I never saw Melanie break one after Ann had made it clear. Lots of children are followers, and the trouble they get into in such incidents as Melanie's drugstore venture is our fault, not theirs. We don't develop enough leaders like Ann.

It took six months before the constant

reiteration of verbal instructions *given while the exercises were being performed* had its effect. First we noticed that Melanie didn't smile *all the time.* She began to flash on and off like her grandmother. Then she stopped wrinkling her forehead, at least at the institute, where she was sure of herself. She hadn't needed Ann since the fifth lesson, and even when she and the others were blindfolded, she could follow instructions. (Thinking back, I imagine that in time 15 plus 16 would have held no terrors for me if only I had heard it, in a kindly tone, often enough, seen it written often enough, and written it often enough myself—*and if there had been any happiness and acceptance in that classroom.*)

Melanie stayed with us a long time. She would always be retarded (whatever that really means), but she had found something she loved to do and something she did very well. She knew all the exercises and she knew the correctives and she was a gentle, loving soul. She became an "assistant," and she helped with the younger children. She encouraged them and listened to them and made up exercise stories for them. Melanie, the child who was a little "different," had been dropped into a tank full of "normal" youngsters and had taken on their habits, action, and coloring. It also works the other way.

Peter came to visit at the house, and his mother had her hand on his shoulder. When he met me, he looked straight at me and put out his hand. If I hadn't known he was blind, nothing he did would have told me. His body displayed none of the typical "blindisms" affected by many who cannot see: He didn't rock back and forth; he didn't grimace, pluck at his clothing, or rub his eyes. He looked in every way like just an average little boy—but Peter wasn't *average* at all. From the moment he walked through the room with his mother, he could duplicate the path, missing every piece of furniture and stopping at exactly the same spot. Once through a door he could find it unerringly, and he knew whether it was open or shut. He rode his bike with assurance and knew exactly where he had last left it. He could run across a huge open field and end up at the front gate. He could read and write Braille, use a typewriter, and study from records and tapes—and he had never been to school. He had never been because no teacher in his small town felt qualified to teach him, so his mother had done it all with the help of Recordings for the Blind, an organization that will record on long-playing records the textbooks that are needed by students. That was Peter the first time I met him, and he was eight years old—before he went to school.

The school was specifically for blind children and was well equipped with all the latest inventions designed to help the blind get along in a sighted world. The teachers had been specially trained, as were all the volunteers who assisted with activities. Everyone was kind and considerate, and every opportunity was made available. There was one major drawback: *All the children were blind.* For every single child like Peter who has grown up in a healthy, relaxed, *normal* atmosphere, there are *hundreds* who suffer not so much from being blind as from the way the sighted world has handled their problem. There are some who have been so overprotected that they won't move an inch until someone takes them by the hand and leads them. There are others who "circle," turning around and around in one spot. This habit is usually picked up when blind children are confined in a crib or playpen. Most have at least one, and some have all, of the "blindisms" mentioned earlier. The stimulation that the passing scene affords the sighted is denied them, so they provide some of their own through movement. Harold, who had been to a school for sighted children, behaved like a sighted child. Peter, who had never been to school but had played with sighted children, behaved like a sighted child. Just as Melanie took on the actions of the group around her, Peter took on the actions of those who soon surrounded him. When he came home for vacation, he, too, had begun to rock aimlessly back and forth.

When a child (or anyone else, for that matter) is injured, whether that injury occurs at birth, before, or after, the problem is not what has been lost but rather what is left that can be developed. A blind child has merely lost his or her sight. Submarines don't "see," and yet they are sleek and efficient. So long as all the sub's equipment is kept in good order, it can perform in a very satisfying manner. Its design does not permit it to maneuver in shallow marshes or over rocky shoals, since its "hearing" strength, which serves as "sight," is meant for a different environment. The blind child should not try to perform on a baseball field where every disadvantage is his, but rather on the wrestling mat, the parallel bar, in dance and skating. If you have such a child, get my talking book *Physical Fitness for You* from the American Foundation for the Blind, 15 West 16th Street, New York, New York 10011, and get going with the preparation. The earlier you begin and the more skills you provide, the easier all others will be. The greater the sense of security in space and confidence through *real* performance, the more security and confidence will spread to other areas of learning.

Melanie can see just fine, but her craft isn't equipped with a computer. She is like the happy little ferryboat plying back and forth in protected waters. She does what she does with contentment and efficiency, well within sight of land. It is only necessary to see that everything is kept in good order and that she has an opportunity to help others who need her. Computers are not the last word; happiness and service in quiet places often bring greater rewards.

The deaf child sees well, can often add 15 and 16 in her head like a shot, may enjoy using her hands in the arts, can do all those lovely fun things such as work on apparatus, ride, swim, and dive. The only thing that comes hard is speaking, since it is hearing a sound that makes reproducing it easy. Give the body that can enjoy movement a chance to really develop satisfying skills, interesting skills, difficult skills. Don't be satisfied with skimpy little games. *Train the child.* There is nothing in this book a deaf child could not do and well, the sooner the better.

And what of the child who is born without one or more limbs? One year I gave a lecture-demonstration for the Easter Seal Drive in Indianapolis, and the little child whose picture was on all the posters was at the luncheon. She was beautiful, she was charming, and she was lacking one arm. From one sleeve there protruded the metal pincers that are fitted to the stump of the arm, and as she sat on my lap, she explained how she could make them open and close on my finger. When I needed someone for the tests so that the audience could see what it was our children were flunking, she offered (she was four). She didn't fail the test for abdominals, as 24 percent of the two-armed children did. She didn't fail the leg-lift or floor-touch tests, as 12 percent and 44 percent of the two-armed children did. In fact, she didn't fail anything. She couldn't play *real* baseball, though, and it is doubtful that she would ever work out on the uneven parallel bars. However, she was going to start dancing lessons next fall, and she will be able to ski, skate, ride, play tennis, swim, and sail. She didn't even know she had a problem—and so it wasn't one.

If your child is handicapped, give him as good a body as you can manage. The exercises in this book can be adapted for almost any condition, and if a wheelchair is involved, the exercises are on the talking book *Physical Fitness for You* (see Sources). If the child is flat on his back, you can still use weight bags to develop unaffected areas. When it becomes possible, use the horizontal rope across the kitchen floor (see page 207).

Use music with everything, not just because it is more fun, but because *muscles* seem to respond to a beat even when the brain finds it difficult to direct. Any therapy done with music is less boring and even elicits more cooperation. Exercises done in the water to music change from aimless movement to very definite action, depending on the music being played. The walks and runs done in the water (pages 307–319) suddenly have meaning and goals. One hundred running steps done to a beat *means* something; flopping around in the water doesn't.

It may mean a little extra work, but before you begin your exercise program with handicapped kids, get them into uniform. In that respect, as in many others, handicapped children are no different from anybody else—they, too, love costumes. They want to feel that this is a special and exciting time, and there are ways to accomplish that. Clothes, music, a special place, and a special time all contribute. T-shirts, shorts, or just underpants dyed navy blue work fine. Insignia, so dear to little (and big) hearts, can be picked up at any store that sells trimming. If warmth is important, get tights and always make a point of putting on the "cool-off" sweater at the end of the session.

Start with *warm-ups,* just as you would for any class, and do whatever the child can do under the circumstances. For the blind, *all* the exercises are possible. Put him through one at a time, calling it by name. For the deaf *all* are possible. For the retarded *all* are possible. For the child plagued with involuntary movement and spasticity, try to put all parts of the body through the full range of motion each day and check with the Myotherapy section. You would do well to start with *How to Keep Your Child Fit from Birth to Six,* since the same exercises that are designed to develop a good body for a baby, whose motions, too, are largely involuntary, will work for the older child and also for adults.

When you work with equipment, see that it is placed on mats. A fall is not serious, but being prevented from trying is. When teaching tumbling, use your hands to direct the little body through every stunt over and over again until the *muscles* know what to do. Precede the stunt with exercises that will provide the ingredient needed for success. No child can do a headstand without abdominal, back, and arm strength. A handstand calls for the same. A jump from the ramp needs strong legs and feet. Use colored tape on the kitchen floor to improve balance and sensitivity. For children who can see, use a blindfold as little bare feet try to trace the patterns you have stuck to the floor. Allow a few minutes for practice on the square, circle, triangle, or rectangle, and then put on the music and see if they can follow the tape to a beat. When sensitivity and imaginary mapping improve, make your designs more intricate.

The deaf child needs no modification in the program, but since music cannot help any except those who benefit from a hearing aid, the body's pleasure in its own repetitious, almost hypnotic movements is utilized. Set up a good rhythm for an exercise like the waist twists (exercise 9), and do the exercise a little longer than you would for other classes until the rhythm (more than the exercise) has taken hold. Follow that exercise with any others that can be done *to that particular rhythm* and at that particular level—in this case, standing. When you change to a different level (sitting, all fours, prone, and so on), change the rhythm speed and do a series that fits. When you change levels, always change speed.

If the children cannot walk but can sit in chairs or, better still, on the floor, use all the floor exercises that apply. If they have prostheses, use the exercises both with and without them. *Without* will give a feeling of freedom, *with* will develop balance and the muscles needed for the more efficient use of such aids.

Think back to the exercises for tennis and skiing in which you "saw" yourself doing certain things and "pretended" to do them. A similar preparation is used with the handicapped. If you work alone with a severely disabled youngster, put on your outfit and demonstrate for him as perfectly as you can, even if, when it is his turn, you must move his arms and legs for him. In the case of the blind child you have him "feel" what you are doing and then see if he has caught the movement correctly. Later in the day, when time hangs heavy for any handicapped person, have a "think-out," when each exercise is *imagined*, preferably to music.

When you have finished the session, do one exercise perfectly for your pupil, the one he is to do over and over again in his mind for homework. Just be sure it is a good exercise and that it is well done. The mind is a strange thing; it works when nothing seems to be happening. The ski lessons taken this winter may produce minimal results right now. However, if the training was correct and the practice diligent, the learning "cooks" all summer. The second winter your surprise and delight will be boundless. A piano piece properly learned without a single flaw, but played at a very slow speed and then put away for three or four months, can then be played up to tempo without a mistake. Put one away with a single mistake and, like the moth hole in a blanket, it will still be there months later.

Keep accurate records of progress. Check the children with as many tests as you can use: the weight chart, measurements, height, and vital capacity. Check carefully for flexibility, using exercises 43–63 to give you further information.

A handicap is a challenge, something to outwit. Outwit it, and don't complicate it by adding other, even more serious handicaps: a sedentary body, unrelieved tension, and the feeling of inadequacy that accompanies poor performance.

CHAPTER THIRTY-TWO
THE CITADEL

And now we come to the "citadel"—the school, the place where American children spend from six to eight hours a day, five days a week, for more than twelve years of their childhood and youth. Taking the lesser number of hours, six, those hours add up to thirty a week. If we tally up the hours those same children are exposed to their parents' ideals, rules, and personalities, we find a somewhat unequal arrangement. If we narrow it still further and consider the opportunities for influencing children in the average American home today (TV portrayal of the American family notwithstanding), we come off long on the school end and very short on family time. Next question: Who's in charge?

In school there is an immediate and powerful influence—the teacher. When you are a new little pupil, you may think that the teacher is the boss of the entire school, if not the world. Alas, the teacher doesn't feel that way. Like nurses, the average teacher is overworked, underpaid, seldom praised—and held responsible for whatever goes wrong, no matter who is at fault. Like nurses, most teachers develop shoulder, neck, and back pain. Many suffer from headaches, often precipitated by interactions with parents, principals, and other teachers. Like nurses, teachers prepare themselves to do a great job, but rarely get much help from anyone and quite often are subjected to all kinds of hindrances. As with nurses, it's a wonder they stay at their posts as long as they do.

This chapter is addressed mainly to the teachers of American children. They are the people who are supposed to bring some sort of order out of the chaos deriving from our physically deteriorating way of life. There *is* truth in the ancient words *mens sana in corpore sano*. Right there is where the teacher's trial begins.

This chapter is designed to put tools into the hands of that all-important person in every child's life, the teacher. Familiarity with those tools would make parents valuable to teachers. Both groups have the same aim: to help the children. In the world of the physical, both could meet and join forces. The children would profit, of course, but so would the grown-ups.

Here are some facts that both groups should know since they are facts that apply to life as well as school:

• *The physical-fitness level of a child is related to the ability to learn in the classroom.*

• *The physical-fitness level of a child is related to emotional stability.*

• *The physical-fitness level of a child often has a direct bearing on the ability to read.*

• *The physical-fitness level of a child will affect attendance in class and attention to lessons.*

• *The physical-fitness level of a child affects performance on the playground and in turn (especially among boys) the child's standing with his peers.*

• *The physical-fitness level of a child has a great deal to do with his or her ability to release tension quickly, efficiently, and completely. This in turn affects behavior in the classroom.*

All teachers play a part in a child's development, but those who teach first, second, and third grades have the largest and most permanent impact. They come onto the scene just as life begins to crowd even the healthy kids from healthy homes. (Keep in mind that over half the children are not healthy, and the homes of many of them have little in common with health.) The teachers of the first three grades often become surrogate parents for children who are deprived of people who really "parent."

Somewhere around eight or nine, the child begins to find some footing in the world. The leaders stick out at once, often because they are the troublemakers. They could have been identified in kindergarten had anyone thought about leadership. Remember little Kathy, the six-year-old with Down's syndrome who became teacher's assistant? She didn't start right then to be a leader. It was always there. Remember Patricia, the other little Down's child? The one who had to think things out completely before trying anything? She didn't start that at six either. Three is usually the cutoff for that sort of thing. By three, most of us have become what we are to become. It just takes the adults a while to see it.

It is important to identify leaders

early. They can go in any of many directions, and sure enough, there will be a line of followers right behind them. What we are about to show you will use the qualities of leadership and at the same time provide the little leader with a positive direction. Fourth, fifth and sixth grades are dotted with leaders, and it is from those ranks that bellwethers, exercise instructors—and drug pushers come. Nature abhors a vacuum, and if we don't give an energetic (often hurting) leader something of value to work on and with, he or she may well find something very unhealthy indeed to give service to.

Once the child has stepped over the line between young and old childhood, the teacher's influence wanes and becomes virtually nonexistent. This happens at the same time that the parent also loses control: age twelve. High school does not belong to the teacher, just as the "teens" do not belong to the parent. If we wanted to do something real for American children, we would spend more money on elementary schools where children can still be reached, developed, and made healthy. Twelve really is the cut-off age, though trouble may not surface completely until thirteen.

To be sure, there are parents who feel attacked when we talk of the low level of physical fitness of American children. "*My* child isn't like that. *My* child is healthy. *My* child is. . . ." Possibly, but we are not talking about any particular individual child, whose mother may or may not really know him. We are talking about the average American child, and there are *millions* of them. Sometimes teachers can't see that any of this applies to their classes. There probably are teachers with forty marvelous, no-problem, totally balanced children in their rooms, but I have not met any.

Let's take a look at "The New New Math." This particular math deals with children, not with mere numbers. It concerns the well-scrubbed, well-pressed, well-brushed as well as the patched and rumpled, tangle-tressed, green-toothed, gray-kneed "Littles." It has to do with the well-feds who make the team (any and every team) and the overfeds and underfeds, who make no team at all. It has to do with little and big youngsters, happy, sad, and desperate, boys and girls, yesterday's, today's, and most importantly, tomorrow's.

Problem: If you had thirty pupils in your classroom, and all thirty were physically fit—and if physical fitness has a great deal to do with the pupil's ability to handle classwork, which studies prove is true—what percentage of the children would be able to keep up with the day-to-day work of the class?
Answer: All of them, 100 percent.

Problem: If twenty-nine pupils were feeling fit, fine, and ready for whatever you have to offer, but one little person was below par, weak, tired, and not able to concentrate very well, could you continue to teach the others at a good speed and yet have the necessary time to bring the slow one along?
Answer: Certainly.

Problem: What if your class had two or

possibly three slow ones? What effect would they have on your teaching and on the fast, eager, able group? Could you handle three as well as one?

Answer: Not quite. It would take more time, more preparation, and a lot more of you. Still, with extra effort, extra time, and extra preparation, you *could* cope— *but what if there were ten?*

You already know that, indeed, half of the children in your class are below par. Intellectually you know that teaching is hard work. Our studies on occupations and pain show that teaching is one of the toughest; only nurses have as many backaches as teachers do. People who work constantly with computers rival you, but not by much, when it comes to shoulder and neck tightness, the two sure founders of headaches. Nobody, but nobody at all, faces as much runaway energy as does the teacher. Children *are* energy. *One* little one can exhaust a young parent. At her most desperate she should contemplate the lot of a teacher—you.

When you read about the K-W test back on page 12, you discovered what you may have known instinctively—that all was not well with the little people in your care. If you read about the Vanves experiment, you discovered that with help, the teacher could do something about the children, but you didn't read anything about the ways in which the laudable profession of teaching destroys the teacher—it can. Teaching can age you, distort your body, and ruin your disposition. But it certainly doesn't have to, any more than being a world-class pianist has to destroy the artist's hands. There is something to be done about it—and about the children at the same time.

Hold it right there! Don't even think, "Oh God! Not another task on top of all they have given me to do." To begin with, the "task" is pleasant and requires only six minutes a day, and it has successful precedents.

After I had completed the testing of American and European children, I had proof that the Americans were probably the weakest in the world. We knew that at least 32 percent were tense and lacked enough physical outlets to balance their tensions. We had already reported to the president, and there had been quite a lot of publicity. I got a call from the school nurse at Greenacres School, the pride of the Scarsdale school system in Westchester, New York, the richest county in America. She, being a nurse, understood the *teacher's* problems with what we had uncovered. She wanted to know if I had a solution. Certainly we did. It's foolish to present problems to the public if you have not already found an answer. The answer came out of the past, as do so many answers.

Back in the 1920s children went to neighborhood schools. Most of them were red or yellow brick boxes two stories high and boasted a "basement," where the bathrooms were, and a playground, where children released pent-up tensions at eleven, twelve, and three fifteen. America was going through one of its periodic "health scenes," and graham crackers were "in," as were "setting-ups." Fresh air was another attention getter, as were brushed teeth and clean fingernails. Teachers kept combs, nail cleaners, and extra hankies in their desks, and there were setting-up drills.

Setting-up drills were calisthenics, plain and simple, and they came from Europe, mainly Germany, which gives you one reason why they disappeared. America came to dislike and mistrust things German. We never have been awfully good at discriminating between what was keepable and what was disposable. Anyway, "gym" always started with "setting-ups," which in my lexicon have become "warm-ups." They readied the muscles, which were stiffened by long sitting, for whatever sport or game the teacher had in mind. In any case, every child knew how to do setting-up exercises.

In the "olden days" teachers were great at picking out leaders (often the worst kids in class, like Freddie Witz and me) and training them in gym to teach the setting-up drills in the classroom. At every change of classes, the "leaders" all over the school waited in the front of the room. When all the children were in their seats, a nod from the teacher told the class monitor to open the windows. We were to get a change of air. At a second nod from the teacher, the child at the front of the room said, "Class stand." That was the warning. "One . . ." and every right foot in the room was thrust into the aisle. "Two . . ." and every child stood in the aisle next to his or her desk. They had been taught to stand straight in "gym," so they did. "Hands on hips . . ." the warning again. *"Place!"* That got rid of the hands, which always get in the way unless you know what to do with them or have been told. "Mark time . . ." warning. *"March!"* "*One*, two, three, four, five, six, seven, eight, *two*, two, three, four, five, six, seven, eight, *three*, two, three, four," and so on until we had counted four sets of eight marching steps, counting only the steps taken by the right foot. We had been taught how to keep track of sets of eight and we knew how to do marching steps.

"Rise to toes and lower." Then we led them through calf-strengthening toe rises, half knee-bends, waist twists, forward leans (which are now called Flexibility Bounces), chest stretchers (now called Snap and Stretch), deep knee-bends, and fast running in place. It took a couple of minutes. The leaders were good. They could demonstrate, keeping the beat and the count. They had presence, and for the moment nobody cared whether or not they were good students, *nice* children, or even acceptable. There was a reason for what they did, and the teacher's presence was the control. Penalty for misbehaving was to be sent to the hall till the exercises were over. Awful when you are little, and when you are little is when discipline *should* start. The windows, open in April or January, made the "breathing exercises" sensible. They were the last "exercise." "Class sit, *one* . . ." and all the children took hold of their desks, a hand on each side as the near foot was thrust under the desks. *"Two!"* All sat down, starting to assemble the needed materials for class, and the "leaders" went to their seats, their short reign over. The teacher said, "Thank you," which was often the only time those particular children ever heard "thank you."

The gym teacher was responsible for seeing to it that the "leaders" from every class knew the exercises. We met for fifteen minutes once a week at first. Later, each of us was given a slip of paper that designated who was to lead on what days and the order of the exercises. That was it. After a while all we needed were the slips with programs. They were the same for the whole school.

Those exercise vignettes happened three times each morning and once in the afternoons. Afternoons weren't as long as mornings, and we'd soon be out, so once was considered enough. Let's say each session took two minutes. That amounted to eight minutes a day of *action* per child. That's two minutes more in one day than most of today's children get in a week. Don't believe me, teacher? Go watch what happens in a PE class, now that "games" are king. Eight times five equals forty minutes a week of exercises designed to strengthen muscles, improve flexibility, and release tension. I can't remember a single "hyper" kid in my class.

There was the precedent and it worked. Greenacres ought to be a snap *if* it were presented to the right people. The principal was first, because while physical education is given the blame for much of our physical lack, the principal is the hidden help or hindrance. *We* had had Miss Graham, who believed in fresh air, unbinding spirits, and graham crackers. She was a Scottish lady, who ran her school with an iron hand and seeing heart. The Greenacres principal was an ex-college athlete and ex-GI, who had felt that there ought to be a better way to prepare boys for what he had faced at Anzio than the training he had had. He went right along with the exercise—"*if* you can sell it to the teachers."

On a blustery October afternoon, after the school bus had sucked up its full complement of booted, raincoated, and capped little people who wouldn't even get damp in the one block walk from bus to house, I met with their exhausted teachers in the teachers' lounge. I never mentioned the children; they were second in importance, maybe even third. Before help reached them, it had to be extended to these important people and also to the gym teacher—*if* that could be done. "I'd like to talk to you about fatigue and back pain." I hit a nerve at once. There isn't a teacher in the system (any system) who has been there for any length of time who doesn't know about those two things—and headaches. Had I been addressing them today, I'd have said, "Who has a backache right now?" There would have been a show of hands. Then I would have erased every backache, headache, and stiff neck in the room and had their full attention (see the chapter on Myotherapy). In those days we could erase the pain with the right exercise, but it took weeks instead of minutes. Still, I *had* mentioned things that interested them. At 4:00 P.M. most teachers don't want to hear about children, just as one mother said to me recently, "After eight o'clock I don't want to talk to anyone shorter than I am."

I then told them what the tests (see pages 14–17) revealed and what could turn that picture around—two-minute setting-up exercises, done throughout the day. "If you will oversee them, the children will improve in many ways that will make your jobs easier," I told them. "If you will stand in the back of the room and *do* the exercises with the children, you will share in something physical, which makes you special—and you will get rid of your muscle pain and fatigue. Those who wish to lose inches will lose inches as well." They bought it.

Next, the PE teacher. I expected resistance and got none. She was terrific.

But then you have to remember that she was the kind of P.E. teacher who sent little Harold Krentz, the blind boy who grew up to become a lawyer and write *Butterflies are Free,* up the rope, over the wall, through the tumbling line . . . and treated him as though he could see. She would take our exercises and train the "leaders."

So far the teachers didn't have to *do* anything except watch. We had already tested every child in school and provided the corrective sheets so that they could be improved. That's something most physical programs neglect. There was one more person to pull into the program—the parent. These were well-educated parents who didn't like it one bit when they heard that their children weren't perfect. They were like the Swiss educators who, when they learned that the Italian children had a lower failure rate than their children, asked, "What can we do about it?" That's very different from "I don't believe it," or "What in hell difference does it make?" or "It's not my job." Or, as one school supervisor said, "Oh, well, we're no worse than anybody else." We met with the parents and gave them the information you will find in chapter 33 and we were off; that is to say, I was off. I left the job in the hands of the classroom teachers, the little kidleaders of nine, ten, eleven, and twelve—and the physical educator.

One question you may get (we didn't) is "Suppose someone gets hurt?" How can a child get hurt doing simple, properly designed exercises? (not a small arm circle or double leg lift, aerobic dance step, or weight machine in the set-up, and no one is being asked to jog on the road). That knocks out the dangers. The teacher is in the room. That takes care of "negligence." Now put that up against the fact that we have nothing in our schools to fight against heart attacks and yet *98 percent* of today's children exhibit at least one problem that can lead to a heart attack.

You may run into the parent who can't imagine a nine-year-old leading an exercise class. Ask that parent if she has ever met the parent of one of her son's or daughter's friends who talked about that child of hers in glowing terms. "He/she is so *polite,* so *helpful,* so really delightful." Ask her if she wondered who the lady was talking about. It couldn't be *her* messy, noisy, thoughtless, youngster, could it? Of course it could. Kids are often very different away from home, which says nothing against home; it has to do with change and growing— and having been taught what to do and how to behave. If they *had* to behave that way at home to get what they wanted, they would. Nine-year-olds are often far older in sensitivity than grown-ups, and the leaders were born leaders. Salesmen are born, too, as are Olympic athletes and Mozarts. Don't underestimate kids; at nine they already *are*. The future depends on the eyes that see them and the people who will understand what they are—or who will pass them by, intent on other things.

The first change came at Christmas, when the children were retested. They were far better and very proud of the fact. Then the teachers noticed that it was true, they had lost pain and inches, even pounds. In February the nurse reported that absences were way *down* at the very time of year they should have been *up*. Spring brought a report from the office that nobody had been sent to the principal for disciplining in a month. Then came the big surprise: *The academic level had risen.*

Now we have Myotherapy to help. Read up on it in Chapter 34 and see how you, as teachers, can help each other. No child should have to sit through a single class in pain. Tell the nurse about Myotherapy and children's growing pains. Nurses catch on fast. One-third of all the people coming to learn how to be myotherapists are nurses. A goodly number are teachers.

Our next studies were done in the New Hampshire and Vermont school systems and covered everything from one-room schoolhouses to district schools housing children from forty miles away.

In Vermont the mainstays were the Latin and English teachers. (Yes, there *are* schools that still teach Latin!) Our major study was done in a central school in Bethel. The children were first tested. Later they were given the exercise program in the halls in silence. There were six classrooms opening onto the hall, hence the silence. The school was so old they couldn't jump in unison lest it fall down. In six weeks those kids were the equal of the European children.

In New Hampshire there were several levels of schools. Some had nine classrooms and some had as many as seventeen. Some had so-called normal children and some had only the handicapped. Some were introducing "mainstreaming," where both the normal and the handicapped work together. The start came from the teachers of the first grade, who were taking evening classes in the exercises in this book. Enid "Beanie" Whittaker had brought the program to the state. A physical educator, she had left her classes at the University of New Hampshire for a new kind of fitness and had started classes all over the state—for adults. Three of the teachers had asked what they could do to help the children. "Easy," said Beanie. "Get the book for children, *How to Keep Your Child Fit From Birth to Six*, and set up your classes. Success is guaranteed." But there were other teachers, and teachers talk to teachers. A male PE teacher was especially interested. (It only takes one!) He divided his time between two schools and felt frustrated. The classroom program was right up his ally. *He* would train the leaders with Beanie's guidance. By Christmas the failure rate of 38 percent, typical for rural schools, had been brought down to 19 percent by children working with children. By spring the failure rate was 6 percent, best in the United States including private schools.

The usual system involved a series of half-hour training programs for the volunteer leaders. Then the leaders were assigned classrooms. In some schools they'd play a record to all classrooms over the PA system at the same three times during the day. The leaders, who knew how to use the music, led from the front of the classrooms.

In some schools every classroom has either a record player or a tape recorder. The teachers went to the library and borrowed Leroy Anderson's music and taped it for their classes. Sometimes the leaders would bring in their own favorite tapes or records. After the leaders had been trained, they needed less and less supervision, but the key person in all this was really the physical educator.

As more and more schools got involved, we decided to sponsor a Teen Fitness Weekend. We took over a school with a good gym, and well over a hundred kids came to learn. To everyone's surprise there were dozens of teachers in attendance as well. Those were the ones who *did* the exercises and were now strong, slender, and painless.

THE PROGRAM (TEEN FITNESS)

We covered everything we had found to work in our programs with babies, children, adults, the handicapped and the people responsible for them.

1. Warm-up exercises, the ones that can be done in *any* classroom, even the ones where sitting on the floor is impossible.
2. The Kraus-Weber test: how to give the test, record the results and design the needed corrective program.
3. The minimum fitness exercises, which are really the correctives.
4. Discussion and selection of music. If you choose slow music when the exercise needs fast, it will go wrong. It's worse when the opposite is true and the children are trying to do full-range exercises to something that should be used for running around the gym.
5. Discussions of the test and other tests and what it means to children and their

- *Ability to learn in the classroom*
- *Performance on the program*
- *Emotional stability*
- *Ability to release stress*
- *Ability to read (see ladder work)*
- *Attendance at class*

6. Basic equipment, such as is shown here (within the reach of *any* school).
7. How the program applies to teachers.
8. How to interest parents.

Who should come to such a workshop?

- *School nurses*
- *Teacher aides*
- *Principals*
- *Superintendants*
- *Classroom teachers*
- *School secretaries*
- *Music teachers*
- *Physical educational personnel*

- *Art teachers*
- *Guidance Counselors*
- *PTA officers*

All you need for such a workshop is the exercises in this book (as well as those in the book for the next age down, *Birth to Six*). You'll need as much of this equipment as can be managed—the small equipment for sure, but horses, ramps, and railroad tracks will make a huge difference in interest. You will need a *loud* record or tape player and a selection of tapes or records that make people move. *Some* rock is fine, but find other music as well as what is mentioned in this book. The *Teenage Fitness* book is soon to be published as well.

When we first started these workshops, we did not have Myotherapy. Now that we do, we have discovered that the unruined instincts and intuition of young children allow them to do Myotherapy with incredible success. We started teaching six-year-olds in the next class I'll describe. By Christmas, the eighth-graders with growing pains were being made painless by those trained *first-graders!*

It was a small parochial school, where the classes stayed put. If anyone changed classrooms, it was the teachers. We know from our studies that such a school has a high percentage of scoliosis (see page 11). The teacher was not a physical educator, but had attended some of Beanie Whittaker's evening exercise classes and wondered how exercise could be given to her first-graders. No problem. She could use the same exercises as are here, test, and employ her very fertile imagination to make use of what was available in the classroom already.

She started by getting the school carpenter to put the doorway gym (see page 148) into her classroom door. She could use that in all the ways we have shown here during winter recess. Then she organized a leader group made up of every child in her first-grade class. As fast as a child would do an exercise well, she'd put him or her up front to lead it. She ran the children through the warm-ups every time the classes changed from one subject to another.

She used the whole room. She moved the pencil sharpener and had it screwed to the floor. If you wanted to sharpen your pencil, you did it with straight legs. After you finished your stint at the blackboard, you did ten knee-bends right there, holding onto the chalk tray. When the children spelled, they spelled their way down into deep knee-bends— and back up again. When she gave out their papers, they were laid on the floor and had to be picked up while knees were held straight.

She wasn't foolish enough to think that on nice days recess would be enough. Some children run around at recess, but what does that do for a body? Not much. Most lean against the wall, and that does nothing. Outdoor recess was augmented by having to turn a somersault, skin-the-cat, or pinwheel over the doorway-gym bar.

She read the first book on Myotherapy, *Pain Erasure* (see Sources) and had a Mrs. Muscles and Mr. Bones made from cardboard. She taught anatomy. When she decided to teach "seeking massage," she sent home a note saying that the children were going to learn this and would need a bath towel. Nobody complained and everyone came with a towel. The class was a great success. Parents began to write thank-you notes to the teacher.

In parochial schools there is rarely a gym or gym teacher, which makes one feel sorry for those poor neglected children. Don't. The K-W tests showed that while such schools had a 60 percent failure, the public schools with gyms and teachers failed at 58 percent. This particular teacher had *no* failures by Christmas. Never mind the lack of a gym. She turned everything in the room, including her own desk, into obstacles for going over, under, and around, on feet, all fours, and often upside down, just as in the floor progressions (see chapter 10). They gave a demonstration at the first Pain Erasure Seminar, and when an eighth-grader was asked what she thought of what they presented and the way they did it, she sighed and said, "You know, it's hard to believe how much they know and they're only *six years* old. I feel stupid!" We underestimate our children and judge them by ourselves, who were likewise underestimated, as were our parents.

Another parochial school set up a competition. They, too, trained classroom exercise leaders, and once a month each class demonstrated their abilities. One teacher, Sister Patricia, was wheelchair-bound with multiple sclerosis. Today we could have gotten her out of that chair with Myotherapy. In any case, her children loved her and would do anything for her. "Children, we have a visitor (me), and we must show her how we won the banner" (they *always* won the banner). "Andrew, will you hold my book and read for me?" Andrew left his seat, went to the bookcase, and brought her an exercise book I'd put together for classes. He set it on her tray so that while he read it, she could see it. "Michael, will you and Marie lead?" Michael and Marie proceeded to the front of the class and conducted the setting-up drill that Sister Patricia and they had designed. They traded off. When Michael finished one exercise, Marie took up with hers. They never missed a beat. Andrew read from the sheet all four of them had devised for that week. Sister Patricia didn't (couldn't) lift a finger, but her assistants had their hearts in their eyes when she said, "Well, done. Yes, we will win the banner again this month."

That school carried their classroom program one step further. The mothers got together, and we trained them, as well as the teachers. The school allowed them to use the cafeteria on Fridays. The children brought bag lunches and ate at their desks. (Unless you went to parochial school, you can't imagine what a departure that is.) Then the parents gave "mat parties," "equipment parties," and "record player and record parties." Every child got a half hour of tumbling floor progressions and equipment every week on top of a half hour of classroom exercise. Years later, when those children went on to the Catholic high school, it was discovered that almost all the varsity athletes came from that one little parochial school where parents cared and teachers cared and all benefited.

The Citadel

As teaching aids we provided filmstrips, which could do all the leading in the first three grades and kindergarten in case there was no access to child leaders. It is called *Keep Fit . . . Be Happy* and contains two excellent manuals. You will find it in sources. There is absolutely nothing wrong with American children, or adults either, that the *right* exercise done consistently and with pleasure can't fix. The only horse I've ever ridden that kicked and bit had pain. I can't say that for all the teachers who kicked and bit, or at least I couldn't have when they were doing it. Then I gave no time to understanding them, but quite a lot to disliking them. Now that I am grown and know a lot about pain, I'm almost sure that the mean ones used to hurt—somewhere. That does not have to be your lot. If you are painfree and alive and feeling wonderful, *stay that way*. If you hurt, get rid of it. If you are over fifty, know that you are among that enviable crowd, the last fit Americans who built their bodies between birth and six because there was no other way to live. You walked to school and knew nature. You played *kids'* games and were concerned with *kids'* concerns. Lucky you. Read my book about *your* generation (see sources) and learn about yourselves (you are the best we have.) Use that book for work, for pleasure—and for the children. And grandchildren.

CHAPTER THIRTY-THREE
AMMUNITION PTA

When the question of physical fitness comes up at a PTA meeting, don't sit mute. Have an opinion, a loud one. Your children are not getting enough physical training or outlets for stress. Most of them are physical morons, but they weren't born that way; their way of life and schooling has done it. They need your help, but if you intend to speak out in their behalf, you will need some facts to back you up. You will need some proof to offset the erroneous concept that physical education is a "frill." Physical education is anything but. The brain is supported by the body, as was proven in the Vanves Experiment (see page 53), but American educators haven't faced those facts yet. Meanwhile, we've got a nation of sick kids.

The following are examples that prove what you will want to prove when you stand up to speak to the PTA. They surfaced when our study breathed the first whisper "unfit Americans" and then proceeded to prove it. Know this: Nothing has changed. What was bad in the sixties and seventies is worse now.

In 1961 Dr. Richard Pohndorf at the University of Illinois provided statistics showing that

• *About 2 percent of our high school pop-*

ulation has *physical education five times a week*
- *Less than 50 percent of our 12 million boys and girls in 30,000 high schools have physical education even two or three times a week*
- *More than 50 percent have no physical education at all*

James Grimm, director of physical education for the Hamilton, Ohio, public schools, cast a bit of light on just what that might mean when he reported in 1962 on the results of his twenty-year study. It showed conclusively that the performance of those youngsters getting physical education five times a week far exceeded the performance of those getting it only twice a week. It is probably unnecessary to remind you that more than half got none at all and that their performance was not even tested. Which group is *your* youngster in?

What sort of things can we expect from well-exercised children that we might not find in those who are less fortunate? In 1961 Mary R. Carson of Chief Sealth Junior High School in Seattle, Washington, did a study on three groups of girls who had been tested for their physical ability with the following results:

High Group	**Middle Group**	**Low Group**
Seldom absent	The most unpredictable	Health poor
Very competitive	Most difficult to handle effectively	Often absent
Seldom failed to shower	Inconsistent	Panicked easily
Moved faster	Uncooperative	Apt to play poorly for emotional reasons as much as for lack of skill
Efforts to improve were consistent	Satisfied with limited success	Generally cooperative
Group pressure apparent	No effort for perfection	

If you imagine your child with the attributes of the girls in these three groups and apply those attributes to daily living, you will have a better idea of what physical education and afterschool activity *could* accomplish. First of all, if your health is good and you rarely miss school, continuity is better and studying is easier. If you *feel good*, concentration is better and so is absorption.

The competitive person is highly motivated, enthusiastic, and attentive. Studying is more exciting and interesting for such a person; for the inconsistent, uncooperative, difficult child, it's a drag.

When a child has a low level of physical conditioning and health, he or she cannot make effective use of such physical outlets as are available, and there is little opportunity for the release of tension. Emotional problems multiply, and as in the case of the children who play poorly for emotional reasons as well as lack of skill, poor performance often limits participation, and the vicious cycle is established.

True, you will say, it would be great to be in the high group with all those built-in advantages, but a nonathlete is a nonathlete, and at the junior high level isn't it a little late? Gertrude Shaffer, supervisor of girls' physical education in the Johnstown, Pennsylvania public school system, tested two schools with the Kraus-Weber test (pages 13–17) and found that in the fall one school that had had some conditioning exercises fifteen months prior to testing had failure rates of 47.22 percent and 45.91 percent for eleven- and twelve-year-old girls respectively. A second school, which had had no conditioning exercises but did have a strong "games" program, failed at the rate of 80 percent for eleven-year-olds and 56.97 percent for twelve-year-olds. By providing the girls with *two exercise classes each week for only part of one semester,* Mrs. Shaffer was able to bring the failure rate of the girls at the first school down to 14.28 percent for the eleven-year-olds and 22.77 percent for the twelves. The second school, with the same time allotted to exercise, dropped to 16.66 percent and 10.46 percent for elevens and twelves. *Any child can improve with exercise, and exercise can be taught almost anytime and anywhere.*

A high level of physical fitness affects classroom work, too. A study done by Reagh Wetmore at Phillips Exeter Academy proved that it is quite possible to improve a brain while developing brawn. At Phillips Academy the boys had two physical-education classes a week in the morning, and every afternoon they participated in a full athletic program. Several faculty members felt that so much physical activity was unnecessary and might even be detrimental to academic work. In order to prove that the morning classes had value, or at least did not take anything away, Mr. Wetmore was permitted to conduct an experiment. Half the freshman class participated in the morning classes and half did not; the average IQs of the two groups were comparable. The results must have given Mr. Wetmore no end of pleasure:

• *The general academic average for the participating group improved; the average for the control group declined.*
• *The number of honor grades for the participants increased; the number for the control group decreased.*
• *The number of failing grades decreased for the participants; this number increased for the controls.*

Immediately after the foregoing report was released, the *Physical Education News Letter,* which is put out by Dr. H. Harrison Clarke at the University of Oregon, printed a report from Germany made by psychologists Lienert and Paterkiewiz entitled "Exercise and Mental Fatigue." In the study, 309 twelve-year-olds were tested. The procedure always began with either a gymnastics lesson or a biology class. Each such lesson was followed by a ten-minute break, and then the children took a thirty-minute written exam designed to test concentration. The children's power of concentration was about 12 percent higher after the gymnastics class than after the biology class. This margin was even higher, 23 percent after the gymnastics class, when the same test was made with a math exam. Could release from the stresses of sitting and concentrating, plus increased circulation and a fresh supply of oxygen from time to time, have anything to do with thinking?

What happens to a child in nursery school is largely dependent on what went before, at home. The experience is then reinforced by what happens during the elementary school years, which in turn are influenced by the early years at home and in nursery school. High schools make demands of elementary schools and junior highs without realizing that those demands can be met only by those whose backgrounds were adequate from the beginning. Colleges make similar impossible demands on high schools, and the feelings of hopelessness, pressure, and failure crowd in on thousands of young people, who never had a chance from the start. Remember, more than half of them flunk the very barest of minimums when it comes to physical fitness, and physical-fitness levels do dictate limits—both ways.

Dr. J. Stuart Wickens at Groton School in Groton, Massachusetts, proved that the brainier boys were also the brawnier. For "brainy" he used the names of boys who eventually made Phi Beta Kappa. To rate as "brawny," the boy had to have won a school athletic letter.

- *Of 124 Groton graduates elected to Phi Beta Kappa in college from 1890 to 1959, 52 graduates, or 42 percent, had received a total of 71 letters in football, baseball, and crew.*
- *Six of the above had captained letter sport teams.*
- *Of 125 boys graduating from Groton with honors between 1947 and 1960, 59, or 47 percent, won a total of 72 letters in football, baseball, and crew.*
- *One hundred of these "honor boys" represented the school in interscholastic competition in the so-called minor sports. Representing Groton in outside athletic contests from this group were 9 out of 11 with summa cum laude (82 percent), 35 out of 40 with magna cum laude (87 percent), 47 out of 56 with cum laude (84 percent).*

It is not necessarily the "advantaged" youngster who develops the body that supports the brain. I have seen fine exercise classes being conducted in the poorest of schools, in basements, in corridors, and in classrooms. It is not necessarily the private schools that get all the financial gravy when it comes to physical education. I have seen better equipment and more interest and concern in the Powell, Wyoming, public schools than in the finest of private schools. It isn't always the public school with the greatest reputation in the country that has the best program. I've seen a parochial school, scarcely three miles away from one such public school, with an infinitely better physical-education program—conducted in classrooms by nuns whose closest contact with phys. ed. was a good exercise book, and on Fridays in the cafeteria by volunteer mothers. What usually determines the quality of the program and the number of students to be included is the energy, understanding, and devotion of a few dedicated people who want better fitness levels for their children. All the great things have been done by a few—and often against overwhelming odds. Don't wait until you have proof positive, through some failure in *your* child, to investigate what is being done about physical fitness in *your* school. Do it now. Back up your PE teacher; talk to your school board; ask for more time, more space, and if necessary more teachers. If these reported studies are right, more physical education could mean less time spent in academic work but with a higher level of accomplishment. You might be able to achieve a higher academic level with fewer teachers of academic subjects if the children attending class had the bodies to support concentration, absorption, and thought. In these days of overcrowding, double sessions, exhausted teachers, and burgeoning taxes, anything that might speed the process of learning, lessen the time needed for both teaching and sitting immobilized within four walls, and at the same time improve the level of health would be worth a try. The time is past for letting George do it—George is up to his neck trying to keep the whole thing from collapsing over his head. Physical fitness isn't the answer to everything, but it's a darned good start, and it's the last chance at a good start that children between six and twelve may ever get. It won't just happen—you are the key.

CHAPTER THIRTY-FOUR
MYOTHERAPY: A WAY TO GET RID OF PAIN

All through this book you have been reading about Myotherapy. It has been referred to in connection with pain, with athletic performance, with concentration, and with studies and classroom work. So what is it?

Myotherapy is a vital piece in the puzzle called Pain. For millions of years, certainly as long as man has been able to connect cause (a stubbed toe) with effect (Ouch!) he has sought methods for relieving pain. Millions have died as a direct result of the medications they have taken *for* their pain. Often the medication is as deadly as the disease . . . only faster. Today, Americans spend over twenty percent of their money for OTC (over the counter) medicines.

Anyone who has held a suffering baby or rocked a weeping child knows there is no special age for pain. In the end it isn't the accumulation of years that causes the distortions called aging. . . . it is pain.

Myotherapy is a way to erase, and even to prevent, pain without any invasion of the body or limitation of its functions (through braces or bed rest). It works 95 percent of the time.

Myo means "muscle" and *therapy*

means "fix it." *Most* pain is muscle related; good examples are the baby's colic and teething, children's growing pains (often called arthritis for the older set), anybody's headache, shoulder pain, backache, jaw pain, wrist pain, elbow pain, menstrual cramps, spastic colon, "trick knee," arthritis pain, and even the pain connected with diseases like multiple sclerosis and cerebral palsy.

Muscles are involved in other problems as well—weakness and poor balance—and they have everything to do with coordination and endurance. Muscles determine the level of athletic ability, the quality of the dancer's, singer's, or musician's performance, and much more. Muscles can determine the quality of life.

In the mid 1940s I was a topflight athlete, performer, and teacher—and I had back pain. There are many kinds of misery a performer can turn off and ignore, but back pain isn't one of them. So I did what almost everyone does: I went to the doctor for heat treatments and pain pills (mild ones—at first). I tried everything. I tried cold and I tried heat. Then I tried alternating them. I went to bed, per force on a mattress on the living room floor because I couldn't get up the stairs. I had the GP's X rays and then the orthopedist's X rays and then the neurologist's X rays. None of the doctors seemed to trust the others' X rays. I was told how to lift things, how to sit, how to stand, and how to lie down. I was told to think "sick-disk." I wore a steel-and-leather brace, a lift in my shoe—and took stronger pills.

Like other people of that time, I had no idea that my chronic back pain was due to stress and was telling me that my life needed an overhaul. In those days "stress," other than for bridges, wasn't understood. Dr. Hans Selye, the Canadian "discoverer" of stress, hadn't even begun to publish his findings, which later led to today's interest and understanding.

My stress continued, and so did my pain, so I took even stronger pills and kept going. One day while rock climbing in the Shawangunks near New Paltz, New York, which was then an unknown heaven for climbers, my partner on the rope, Hans Kraus said, "I think I may be able to get rid of your back spasms." That was the first time I knew I had "back spasms." Everyone else had talked about "unstable fourth and fifth lumbar vertebrae," and "discogenic disease," "disintegrating this" and "degenerating that." That climber was not only the best climber I knew, he was also a "sports" doctor while that title still meant dealing with sports and was limited to those who really did specialize. (Eventually he was to take the title *physiatrist*, the medical arm of physical therapy.) I agreed to let him try.

The technique he was going to try was called Trigger Point Injection and was pioneered in this country by Dr. Janet Travell, whom I was to meet many years later. I knew full well what injections were, but I certainly wasn't prepared for the spinal "probe" he got ready to use.

"What's a *trigger point?*" I quavered as my bottom was being swabbed with something that smelled like iodine. He explained that *it was an irritable spot in a muscle that got there when that muscle was* damaged and that could throw the muscle into spasm, which causes pain. "I think you've got several," he told me. I had several all right. I went to him a couple of times a week for what seemed like forever, but I got better. I got better and I'd stay better for months at a time. Then, out of the blue, the pain would be back and I'd be back on the table and that dagger would be hovering over my back again. It took many years for me to discover that there was a connection between my muscle spasms and my stress level. It took even longer for me to accept the fact that there was a connection between my stress level and the people in my life.

Over many years I've worked with doctors designing the therapeutic-exercise programs that would precede or follow operations and sometimes prevent them. One morning in 1976, I was searching a lady's neck for the trigger points that were causing her torticollis, (neck spasms). I had been working for some time with a doctor who was interested in trigger points. I had had a lot of experience with them in thirty-odd years, so I would hunt them down, mark them, and then he would inject them. I'm not sure even now what happened with that lady's neck. I may have found the chief bandit, I may have pressed at just the right angle—whatever it was, she screeched, and I jumped back. Her head snapped up straight, and she said, "Oh thank you. That feels just fine now." After that one "hit," her neck was straight and there was no pain whatsoever. I had discovered (by accident, which is how many discoveries are made) a way to reach and defuse a trigger point without injecting *anything*. I had found a way almost anyone could do the same thing, including the six-year-old granddaughter of my patient if she learned where Gram's trigger points nested.

When you think of just plain people doing work on muscles without years of anatomy study, you have to consider that work as you do swimming: Kids do a dog-paddle, clumsily and hit or miss, but still afloat. Then there are the Olympic swimmers, who have lots of background and training (like the certified Myotherapists we turn out after fourteen hundred hours of training.) In between are all the other levels. Whatever the level, *most* people could use this muscle work somehow, just as *most* folks can swim.

In 1979 I wrote the first book on Myotherapy. It was called *Pain Erasure: The Bonnie Prudden Way*. When it came out in 1980, no one had ever heard of Myotherapy. The doctor I was working with, Dr. Desmond Tivy, gave it the name and wrote both the Foreword & Afterword. That book recently went into its twelfth printing. Hundreds of thousands of people know about Myotherapy through that book alone, and that was just the first. In 1979 I opened the Bonnie Prudden School for Myotherapy and Physical Fitness. We started with fifteen students—one more than Harvard started with. The difference lay in money. Harvard had many backers, the Bonnie Prudden School had only me, and I had only my mind and the ability to work hard.

In 1985 we brought out the second book on Myotherapy. And we had learned a great deal since its discovery five years before. The first graduates from the school were now out in the world, and several had their own clinics. The name of the second book was *Myotherapy, Bonnie Prudden's Complete Guide to Pain-Free Living*. The "quick fix," a way to get rid of pain quickly, was one of the new things we put in that book, along with information about what kinds of damage particular occupations and sports do and how to make one's own fitness center that really works.

Those two books told people something they hadn't known: that chronic pain has a reason and a message. They also gave the message that pain could be erased without drugs and invasion and that ordinary people could take charge of the pain and their lives. In 1986 *Bonnie Prudden's After-Fifty Fitness Guide* reached the bookstores. Older people are discovering that (a) they are the last fit Americans because they were active as children; and (b) pain is what ages people; they can manage, and erase, their own pain and therefore the rate at which they age. Also in 1986 a complete revision of *How to Keep Your Child Fit from Birth to Six* was published. In it there is a chapter on Myotherapy, even as there is here. The message in all of these books is that *you don't have to hurt* most of the time and you can *prevent* pain for yourself and your family.

So now we come to you. You already know that a trigger point is an irritable spot in a muscle and that it gets into the muscle when that muscle is damaged. When it is "on" (like an electric-light switch), it has the power to throw not only its unwilling host into spasm, but muscles far away from its residence as well. Spasm causes pain, and pain causes more spasm, until you develop a spasm-pain-spasm cycle that must be interrupted if the pain is to ease. Heat, cold, drugs, and sometimes surgery are all methods used in breaking that cycle. Myotherapy, too, breaks the cycle, but leaves no after- or side effect other than an occasional bruise.

There are five major events that put trigger points into muscles, and you have seen them all, but usually with uneducated eyes. That is about to change right now.

• *The first event is birth. Being born isn't all that easy on the baby, and until recently nobody seemed to understand that fact.*
• *Next come accidents. Every accident can lay down trigger points, and most of them do.*
• *The third is sports: Every sport has its own map of trigger points. The soccer player can have them anywhere and, like the skater, has mobs of them in the thighs. The road runner's trigger points start in the feet and lower legs, but in no time at all they attack knees, lower back, and ultimately the floor of the pelvis. Tennis, of course, like basketball, is a "spike" sport, demanding quick starts and stops. That means trigger points in the thigh muscles that control the knees. Then there is the overworked elbow, much like Little League shoulder.*
• *Next in order is probably the most important (since one cannot give up a job as easily as we can a sport): occupations. One's occupation at the age of thirty can determine the pain one will suffer at the age of sixty. It is easy to understand that digging up the street with a pneumatic drill might give a*

person a backache. It is harder to see how being a dentist with a tiny drill is even more certain to do the same thing, but it happens.

• *The last place to pick up trigger points is disease—any disease. Trigger points remain in the neck after swollen glands; asthma puts them in the muscles of the chest and upper back. High fevers not only leave trigger points in many muscles but light up existing ones. Trigger points ride in with multiple sclerosis, lupus, and arthritis.*

For some time now some doctors have known that trigger points cause pain. What has been overlooked are the other criminal acts that can be laid at their door.

• Trigger points interfere with strength. We apply that old myth "The legs go first" to older athletes. The legs didn't "go", they were loaded with trigger points due to extremes of effort over a period of years. Cleared of their accumulation of trigger points, those legs usually "go" quite well. Often we see children who can run neither long nor well, although there doesn't seem to be any reason. A thorough search of the little legs with seeking massage (page 426) would reveal numerous trigger points that throw off the child's coordination.

• Muscles in spasm can put a clamp on circulation, and that can endanger feet. Muscle spasm slows healing after an injury and puts the feet of diabetics in double jeopardy. Any injured extremity—for example, a burned hand—will heal more slowly and less efficiently if trigger points are present in muscles between them and the source of the hand's nutrition.

• At the first sign of the flu, trigger points light up like the Fourth of July; the sufferer's muscles ache from stem to stern.

• Growing pains are neither inevitable nor unavoidable. An occasional seeking massage can clear legs, back, and arms even before the "pains" show up.

• Musicians start to collect trigger points as soon as they begin to practice assiduously. The constant repetitions of micromovements demanded by the art as the rest of the body maintains a static posture leaves microwounds in muscles, which then produce microscars. These seem to attract trigger points with even more ease than large injuries do. The more skillful the little musician becomes, the more certain trigger points are to appear. This is true even of young choir boys; for them the throat is the instrument, a delicate, easily injured instrument.

The main thing to remember about trigger points is that everyone collects them. They can be at their howling worst when they cause pain, but they can also do a very thoroughgoing job silently when they limit normal function and cause both substitution and poor posture, such as kyphosis (round back), scoliosis (spinal curvature), and lordosis (swayback.)

Trigger points usually lie dormant until some form of extreme emotional or physical stress turns them on. They then "turn on" the muscle by throwing it into painful spasm. What, then, do we do about it?

First let me show you a trigger point on yourself. Lay one arm flat on the table in front of you. Make sure the palm is down. Look at the crack caused by the bend in your elbow. Locate the spot on the top surface of your forearm about ½ inch down the arm toward the wrist. With a knuckle of the other hand, press into that spot hard. Pretend you want to press straight through the arm to the table. There will be a painful spot in that area. When you have located it, hold the pressure on for five seconds and then release very slowly. You have now erased that trigger point or defused it or put it out of action for the time being much as doctors do with acupuncture. Now comes the other half of what must be done to alleviate pain. Stretch that arm straight out *in front of you* (see exercise 16). Rotate your hand counterclockwise until the thumb points to the ceiling. At that moment you are *stretching* a kink out of the muscle. Relax the stretch by rotating your hand clockwise until the thumb points out toward the side. Do three. Now, drop your arm to your side and feel the difference in your two arms. You will find that the treated one feels warmer or lighter or both. Why? There is almost always a trigger point at that spot because all of us use our arms a great deal and often overwork them, as when we drive long distances. The trigger point keeps a slight spasm going in the muscle of the forearm. When you defused it, the muscle relaxed. It also relaxed its hold on the arteries and veins traveling the length of the arm, so you felt a sudden increase in circulation. Had you been in pain, it would have taken more than one defused trigger point to get rid of it, but the result would have been the same: a warm feeling, one of lightness—and painlessness.

The major pain complaints of the six-to-twelve crowd are growing pains, strains and sprains, stomachaches and headaches—so let's begin with those. Growing pains are really muscle pains, and they are basically the same kind of pain suffered by Grandpa who used to play football for dear old Watershed U. They call his pain arthritis, however, and he probably accepts that. He shouldn't. Let's say that your youngster has calf-muscle pains. They are the same as Auntie Ruth's calf cramps at night, and the child (or you) can get rid of both those cramps, and Grandpa's "arthritis pain" by doing the following.

LEG PAIN

Before you begin, explain to the child what a trigger point is. Make a deal with the child. Tell him or her that you are pretty sure you can get rid of the ache if he or she will *direct* you. You will find the point and the child will tell you when the pressure is too much. With adults we work on a pain scale of one to ten. Ten is the last level before *too* painful. Three or four wouldn't be much discomfort. Six or seven would mean "I've got a live one." Eight and up means, "Don't press

Myotherapy: A Way to Get Rid of Pain

any harder." With children I use finger signals. One finger raised means "It hurts, be careful." Two fingers mean, "Don't press any harder." Those signals should be as respected as The Ten Commandments, or the child will not trust you. If he learns at the outset that you are as good as your word and won't press any harder, then the two of you become a very productive team. Once the child really *knows* you won't press too hard, he will stand more. The fact that every move you make is slow and controlled is another plus. That means that the child has a chance to stop you before it really hurts. The first time is the worst time, and there is no hurry. A little done every week, as with seeking massage (page 426) will not only get rid of existing pain, it will also prevent future pain *and athletic injuries.*

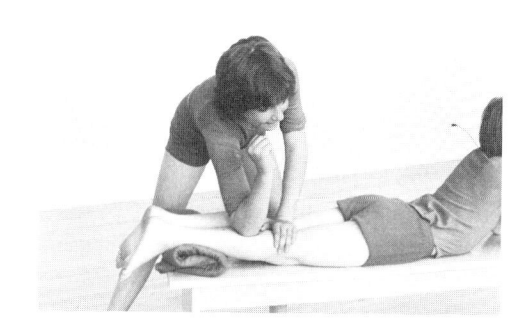

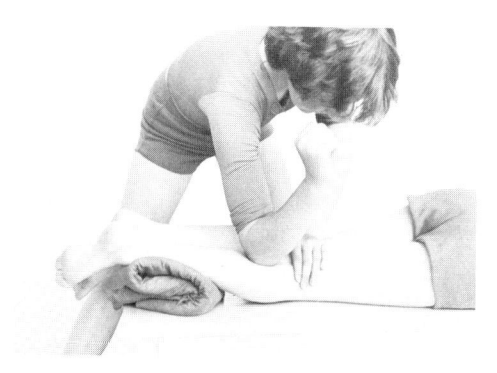

• *Have the child lie prone on a flat surface with a rolled towel under the ankles to prevent strain in the ankle.*

• *Take a felt-tipped pen and draw a line down the middle of the lower leg from the popliteal (the space behind the knee) to the achilles tendon (the heel cord that attaches to the heel).*

• *Place your elbow in the exact middle of the lower leg, right on the line and halfway between knee and heel. You are on the* gastrocnemius *muscle. Press in* slowly ... *watch for signals. You will be alerted quickly, which means you have found the trigger point; hold the pressure for seven seconds. There is nothing magical about seven, five might do as well on a little leg. Remember, when the "Hurt" sign goes on, don't press any harder.*

• *Move down the line at 1-inch intervals right to the heel. Hold at each spot where a trigger point is found.*

• *When you reach the heel, go back to where you started and do the same "search and knock out" action at 1-inch intervals up to the popliteal.*

• *Draw a second line down the leg about an inch and a half to the* inside *of the first line. This one will go over another calf muscle called the soleus. You will be pressing along its edge, which is one of the most sensitive spots in the body, so go easy.*

• Have the child roll slightly *to the side so that the line is on the top surface of the leg.*
• *Begin your search at the top of the lower leg where the top edge of knee socks would be. Go down the line to the heel at 1-inch intervals. Remember, this line is very sensitive.*

• *Draw a third line down the back of the lower leg, 1½ inches to the outside of the center line.*
• *Have the child roll back to the prone position. Reaching over the leg, go down this line the same way you did the other two. (We rarely find much on this line, but it helps to be sure.)*

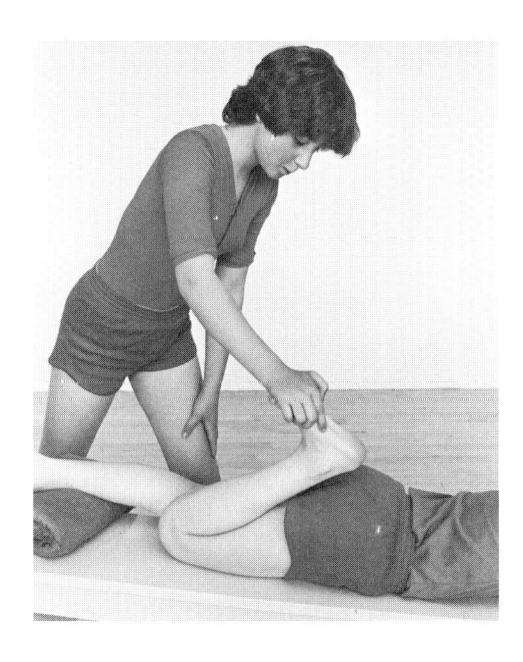

359. CALF MUSCLE STRETCH

When you have found the trigger points in a given area and defused them, you have completed one-third of what is needed. The next step is the *stretch* to get the kink totally out of the muscle and start its reeducation into healthier habits.

• *Holding the ball of the foot, press the heel back toward the buttock as the child bends her knee. Press down on the ball of the foot so that the calf is stretched.*
• *Relax the leg by bringing it to the vertical.*
• *Bend the knee again as you press down on the ball, but this time rotate the foot outward to stretch the soleus.*
• *Relax the leg and bend again with the foot rotated inward. That makes up a set. Do three.*

Do the same work on the other leg, even though only one leg may hurt. You have now completed two-thirds of what is needed. The third step is continual stretch and strengthening exercise for the calf: heels-flat knee-bends (exercise 12). See that the child does this exercise often. One session of Myotherapy should get rid of the growing pains—but suppose it doesn't? Why didn't it and what do you do about it?

When Myotherapy fails, it is because we have not found the trigger point causing the pain—that is, of course, if the problem is muscular. Make sure of *that* by asking a doctor.

The next step would be to draw a continuation of your first three lines right up the back of the leg from knee to buttock and then do the same 1-inch-at-a-time hunt for trigger points up each line. That should get it, but suppose it doesn't? The next step would be the seat, which houses the trigger points causing most backaches.

BACK PAIN

Back pain is often attributed to deformations of the spine, even in children. It is in fact almost always due to muscle spasm. Once your doctor has ruled out fracture, tumor, and similar horrors, think muscle spasm. Since the seat muscles are at the tops of the legs, we think of that connection next. If we were looking for the trigger points for back pain and didn't find them in the seat, we would think legs, and then groin, which is the front of the back and therefore connected.

• *Have the child lie prone on a table or bench and go over the pain signals so that they are fresh in both your minds.*
• *Pretend the child is wearing blue jeans and visualize back pockets. You will find three or four trigger points where the back pockets would be.*
• *Reach across the body to place your elbow over that back-pocket site. Press down first and then pull in, with your elbow. If you find nothing,* hold the pressure *and move your elbow around very slowly.*
• *If you find a point, hold for ten seconds and move on. If you find nothing, just move on. Pick the elbow up and move it somewhere else in the back-pocket site and repeat. You should find at least one trigger point. If* the child is an athlete or has had a fall on the seat, as in ice-skating, you may find many. Do both sides to complete the first third of the work.

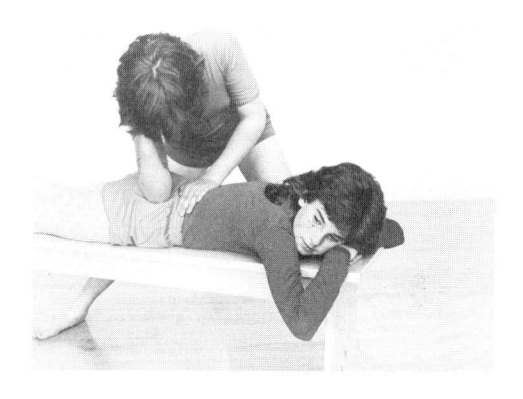

360. SIDE-LYING STRETCH

This is the single most important exercise for back pain, and it doesn't matter whether the person with the pain is a baby (babies also get back pain and often reveal it by disliking drafts on their backs), a child, a grandparent, or a teacher.

• *Turn onto one side and draw the top leg up to the chest as in exercise 42B.*
• *Extend the leg full length about eight inches above the resting leg.*
• *Lower the leg and relax for three seconds. Repeat four times with each leg.*

SIDE LEG PAIN, SCIATICA

Pain has different names according to the age of the sufferer. If the child has back and leg pain, it will be called growing pains. If an adult has the same thing, it will be called *sciatica*. If, when you have done the seat work, there is still back pain, or if the person has been diagnosed as having sciatica, the next trigger point will be number 11 on all the charts in books I've written on pain erasure.

• *The child (or anyone else) lies prone. The person doing the work reaches across the body again, but this time at waist level. Number 11 is about 3 inches out from the spine on the belt line. It lies between the ribs and the crest of the pelvic bone. Press down and then pull in. Hold the required 7 seconds. Do both sides.*
• *Next pull the child a little way onto her side and pretend she is wearing warm-up pants with a nice wide stripe down the outside.*
• *Start to put elbow pressure on that imaginary stripe up at the waist and work at 1-inch intervals all the way down the leg. The worst spot will be about 3 inches up from the knee. This is especially true of athletes and teachers with knee problems from standing. Do both legs even if only one aches.*
• *Do the Side-Lying Stretch (exercise 42B).*

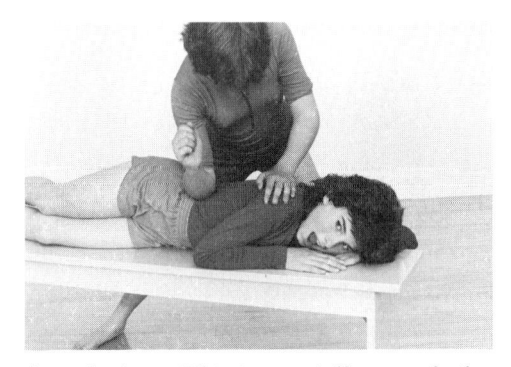

BACK OF SHOULDER

The third place to look for the cause of back pain is the scapula, or shoulder blade.

• *With the child prone again and the far arm resting at her side, reach across her body to find the number-13 trigger point. This is*

Myotherapy: A Way to Get Rid of Pain

another awful-awful, like the soleus. Find where the seam would be that joins the sleeve to the shirt. That is the guideline. Then find the spot on the seam that is midway between the shoulder top and the armpit. Now slide your elbow to rest right there.

• *Press down and then pull in. Be careful; this is a really sensitive spot. Hold for the required seven seconds.*

• *Hunt around in that area for a second and third sensitive trigger point; then do the other side.*

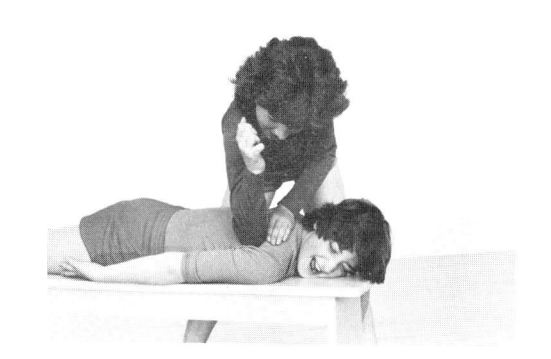

361. MYO-STRETCH FOR SHOULDER

• *Sit up and stretch the arm straight forward as you did after you found the trigger point in the arm. Rotate in and out three times with each arm.*

To keep trouble out of the shoulders, do the shoulder shrugs as well as the shoulder rotations often throughout the day. If a round back accompanies the pain, do the Snap-and-Stretch (exercise 21) and the Backstroke (exercise 18) *often*.

Those are the three places we look for back pain immediately, and what you have just done is what we call a "quick fix." If the pain is still there *somewhere*, we head for the groin.

THE GROIN

The groin is the front of the back. It is one of the anchors for the abdominal muscles, which play a starring part in little kids' stomachaches that are not due to green apples but rather to stress. Many years ago, I was approaching a divorce but didn't know it. One married for keeps in those days and thought about divorce only when all other avenues had been tried. We didn't know then that the damage to children is done *before* the divorce and is only recognized afterward. Every evening, promptly at seven, my little daughter Suzy threw up.

First she would say, I have a stomach ache; then her freckles would stand out, and two minutes later it would happen. Seven o'clock was when her father came home from the office and that's when the tensions went on like lights. Nobody ever quarreled, nobody ever spoke sharply, it was just *there*. For months it went on. Later in the winter, when we were visiting the grandparents in Florida, and we would all be ready to go out to dinner, we would have to wait until seven so that Suzy could get "that" over with. One certainly couldn't blame her father; he was in New York.

When I got home, I took her to a pediatrician. After examining her he said, "How are you and your husband getting on?" I said, "Oh, we manage." He was quiet for a minute and then he said, "No, you are *not* managing, and here is the sign of it." That's when I knew I'd have to face it and admit defeat. There was, after all, something I simply could *not* manage, even though I thought I was doing it *for* the children.

Lots of little people are caught up in adult stress and they get the stomachache habit. Years and years later, long after they have forgotten about those "childish" reactions, they come down with "spastic colon," "menstrual cramps," and sometimes jaw pain, or TMJD (for temporomandibular joint dysfunction). They are often all tied together. If you have a bellyacher, or were one, think groin.

• *Have the little person lie supine for this hunt.*
• *Reach across the abdomen and place your thumbs on the* inside *of the hipbone on the other side. The abdominals tie in there, and trigger points are often found at attachments. Hold for seven seconds.*
• *Standing as you were, use your fingers to find any sensitive areas on the near hipbones.*

The next two anchors run north and south from the symphysis pubis, the bone in front at the base of the pelvis, to the ribs.

• *Press with your fingers or thumb right into the front of the pubic bone at its midpoint. Hold for five seconds.*
• *Move your fingers out one inch to the left on that bone and press again.*
• *Move 1 inch to the right and repeat.*

The next two are rather hard to find, but with patience, you will. They are right over the psoas muscle, which plays an enormous part in back pain (which in turn plays a part in stomach and abdominal pain).

• *Pretend that your subject is wearing bikini pants that have the slanted French cut. About midway between the bottom of the leg seam and the top, right on the edge of the*

Myotherapy: A Way to Get Rid of Pain

pants, you will find a very sensitive point. Go easy but hold for five.

• The ribs are fairly easy. Just imagine that you are a tailor and you have to pin the abdominal sheath to something solid like the ribs with pins just under the edge. Everywhere you would pin, you have the potential for a trigger point. Move your fingers under the ribs from sternum (breast bone) to the bottom of the ribs' curve on one side at 1-inch intervals. Do the same to the other side. Now get out your felt-tipped pen.

• Draw a line from the bottom of the breastbone all the way down over the abdomen to the symphysis pubis, that bone in front.

• Now draw a second line straight down, starting at one nipple. Do the same on the other side. Again you are faced with three lines and 1-inch intervals.

• Make a rigid mitten of your hand. If you have long nails, you have to make a choice: Either cut them or get someone with stubby nails to do the job while you direct.

• Start just under the breastbone and press the fingertips straight down into the abdomen slowly. Everything inside is very adjustable and will move over for you. Just go slowly. If you find a sensitive spot, stay there for seven seconds. Mostly you will find nothing. Your major problem will be giggles with ticklish children. If you do find trigger points, hold.

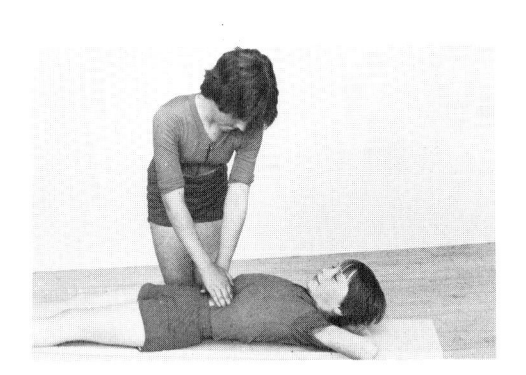

362. ABDOMINAL AND GROIN STRETCH

The back-bend exercises (pages 105 and 138) will work to stretch both the abdominal muscles and the groin, and these two areas are essential when it comes to stretching. People often think that round back can be corrected by telling a child to stand up straight. It can't. There are muscles that have foreshortened, and they are *pulling* the shoulders forward. *They are the chest muscles, the abdominals, and the thighs.*

• Ask the child to slide over to the edge of the table and hang his leg over the edge. Gravity will pull the leg down to stretch the abdominals and groin to a degree.

• He should try to relax as you stabilize the pelvis by pressing down on the hipbone opposite the hanging leg. Then, pressing down on the hanging thigh in short, easy bounces, the groin, abdominals, and thigh can be stretched. Do both legs.

Follow the above exercises with exercise 60 and exercise 111.

Lots of children suffer from "stitches" when they run any distance, jump rope, or do anything calling for sustained action. Use the groin-and-abdominal hunt for trigger points and the stretch shown above. The worst trigger points will be up under the ribs, where the stitch pain originates.

SHOULDERS

Shoulders are a mine field for Americans. Most of our daily routines revolve around the shoulders. We drive long distances, which puts strain on both arms and shoulders, tightens the chest, neck, and low back. We work at desks and computers, on telephones, and with gadgets. Children do not do anything to stretch the arm and shoulder muscles, and nothing to strengthen them, either. Since we live with stress, the shoulders are constantly being tightened without relief.

• *You have already worked in the area of trigger-point number 13 on the scapula in connection with the back. Now we are concerned with the shoulders. Start with # 13 and take out any trigger points you can find. Follow with exercises 15 and 16.*

ARMS

Hanging from the shoulders are the arms. It is their muscles, and those of the chest and upper back, that cause most of the pain called bursitis.

• *The subject lies supine with arms at the sides and palms flat. Start by pressing with knuckle or elbow into the forearm just below the elbow crack. Imagine that the three lines you drew on the leg have been moved to the arm. Start at the top of the forearm and press in every ½ inch down the center of the arm to the wrist.*

• *Using knuckle or elbow, press down the other two lines, elbow to fingers. It is very unlikely that very much will be found, ex-*

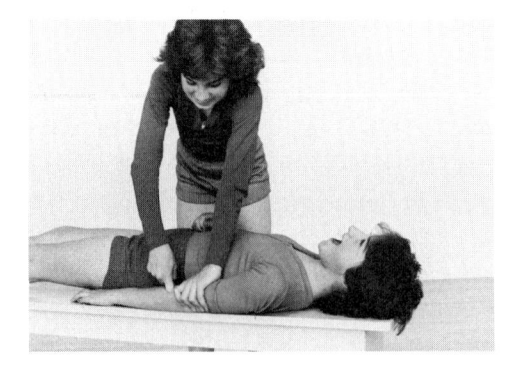

Myotherapy: A Way to Get Rid of Pain

cept in the arms of little musicians, baseball players, or gymnasts.

• Turn the subject to the prone position with arms at sides and palms up and repeat the three-line search for trigger points, elbow to wrist.

• Follow with exercises 15 and 16.

THE CHEST

The chest muscles, or pectorals, are also a part of the shoulder girdle, and many have large crops of trigger points picked up from bouts of coughing, falls onto one or both arms, and sometimes from being yanked about by adults or other children.

• *Pretend that the child is wearing a tank top. Using the fingers of both hands at one time, press in all along the armholes of the imaginary top.*

• *Have the subject rest the hands behind the head, which exposes the axilla or armpit. There are many trigger points there. Pretend that you have laid a washcloth over the whole area. The washcloth is imprinted with a crossword puzzle. Press into every square. Some will be real zingers. Hold for the required seven seconds.*

• *While the arms are still bent and behind the head, do the entire chest by starting at the sternum (breastbone) just below the cla-vicle (collarbone). Draw imaginary lines across the chest about an inch apart. Press from the sternum to the outside edges at the chest on both sides. Cross on those lines, always at 1-inch intervals.*

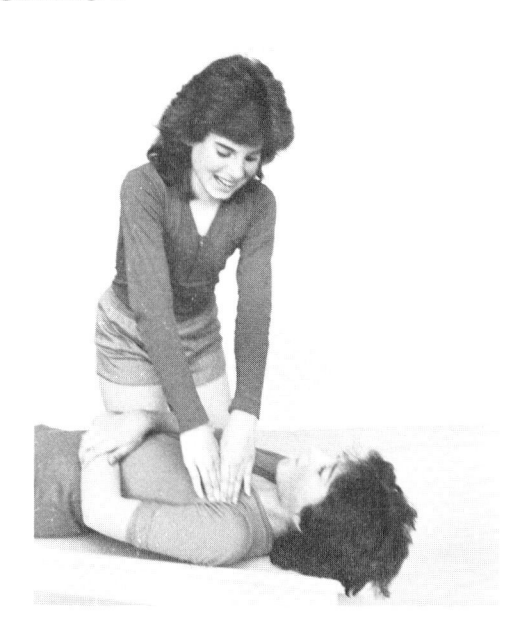

HEADACHES

Children have headaches, toothaches, small aches, and general achiness. It has been our habit to give them a child-size aspirin or something else the size of a pill. Try not to. It's easy to use a pill, but it's better for them if you give them your time, yourself, and Myotherapy.

Try the next trigger point hunt on yourself first and then on the child. It will be helpful for you to know the feel.

- *Put your fingers on your spine at the back of the neck just at the hairline.*
- *Slide the fingers halfway to the ear on the hairline and you will find a hollow spot up under the eave of the skull.*
- *Press up under that roof,* hard. *In all probability you will find a fiery little trigger point. Hold it for five seconds.*
- *Slide your fingers halfway down the neck on that same vertical line.*
- *Press into the neck. If you get headaches at all, you will probably find one there, too.*
- *Slide the fingers down to where the neck joins the shoulder. There will probably be one there, too.*
- *Now comes the one that usually causes the headache. Stay on the same line, but slide your hand a couple of inches down over the edge of the back. That spot, right there, is usually awful, but you can't reach it on yourself.*
- *Sit in a chair and bow your head. That muscle (the splenius) is now on the stretch. Let someone else put his or her elbow in that spot and push: It will feel like a shock. Hold for seven seconds and then do the other side. In all probability, if you had a headache before, you won't have one now.*
- *To stretch, use exercises 13 and 15 and 16, to retrain the spasmed muscles.*

You now have some idea of what myotherapy is and does. In order to use it to best advantage with your family, you need one of the two books that describe the procedure fully (see Sources).

SEEKING MASSAGE

We use seeking massage with athletes and performing artists either before or right after a performance. Let's say that we are interested in an eleven-year-old tennis player who will play in a tournament tomorrow. As would be expected, he is tense and doesn't want to spend much time on Myotherapy.

- *Cover both legs with a light coating of massage oil and then pretend you have drawn the three basic lines on the back of each leg.*
- *Place the athlete facedown on the table. Making a hard fist, run your knuckles slowly down first one leg and then the other, buttock to heel.*
- *If the little athlete complains of a tender spot, stop and press for seven seconds and then continue.*
- *Do both legs, both arms, and the back. Take out every point that shows up. If there are any that are especially sore, mark them.*
- *Just before the match, check for the matrix trigger points you discovered the night before. Be sure you press them out and then stretch the muscle before the real warm-up.*

Seeking massage will show up anything that is tight and in danger of tearing when the stress of performance or competition comes into the picture.

The following is a list of problems children are heir to—conditions that can be avoided, prevented, erased, or at least minimized with Myotherapy.

ANKLES, PRONATED

Children whose shoe heels wear on the inside edges, like misaligned tires, often have ankle pronation. As with knock-knees, the trigger points will be on the stripe of the warm-up suit where we found the trigger points in sciatica. They may also be in the seat, where we looked for them in back pain. Do the ballet exercises (pages 232–248) and all of the foot exercises (pages 82–85). Watch to see that the knees cover the toes in all knee-bends and pliés.

ARTHRITIS

Children do get arthritis, and it can be very painful. In a medical dictionary you will be told that arthritis is joint inflammation. What pulls on joints? Muscles in spasm pull on joints. If your young ones come down with arthritis, work on the muscles that connect with the joints and see that they are free of spasm causing trigger points. Use music with the exercises. If the child is unable to do much for himself at first, get *How to Keep Your Child Fit From Birth to Six* (see Sources) and do the passive exercises with the child *after* you have taken out the trigger points. Keep after it so that you don't give up any gains.

ASTHMA

An asthma attack is awful to listen to, worse to watch, and usually it's in the middle of the night. When all is well, clear every trigger point out of the chest, arms, and upper back. Don't leave even one hiding between the ribs. Pay special attention to the sternum and both sides of it. Myotherapy has been known to abort an attack that has already started, but rather than count on that, clear the child's muscles on a regular basis. An asthmatic child can enjoy many of the exercises and activities in this book. Exercise is one of the key releases for stress, and asthma thrives on stress. Use seeking massage on a regular basis.

BACK, FLAT

In a flat back there is less than a normal curve in the lower back. When the little person has his or her back to you, it *looks* flat and the clothes seem to be pasted on a straight piece of cardboard. Do lots of the Angry Cat, Old Horse (exercise 34) with special attention to "the horse." Do all the back bends, walk-overs, and pelvic tilts (pages 78–139).

BACK, ROUND

By the time children are six, those who are going to have round backs have usually begun to develop them. They come from tightened chest, abdominal, and groin muscles. Spend some time with myotherapy, locating the trigger points that cause the problem, and with the Snap and Stretch (exercise 21), the Backstroke (exercise 18) and the Abdominal and Groin Stretch (exercise 362).

BACK, SCOLIOSIS

This means a lateral curve of the spine, and it rarely shows up until the child is about eleven. There is a test for it on page 17. If you find one, don't be upset. What pulls bones out of line? Muscles in spasm do that. Your children are young enough to get rid of those muscle spasms and straighten the back. Check with the book *Myotherapy* (see Sources). In addition to getting rid of the spasms, get the child into *bilateral* activities, in which both sides of the body are used equally—gymnastics, dance, swimming, and riding. For the time being, don't push tennis.

BACK, SWAY

For this you will need the pelvic exercises 19 and 38, the Angry Cat, Old Horse (exercise 34), and the corrective for the psoas, the Spine-Down Stretch (exercise 2).

BALANCE

If your youngster has trouble with balance, don't think she walks like her uncles on her father's side. Those are her very own trigger points causing imbalance in the muscles. Do Myotherapy on the legs, feet, back, and abdominals. Help with the warm-up exercises (see chapter 6) several times a day. Do the floor progressions (see chapter 10) with her and build strength with long walks uphill and downhill. There is *always* something to be done about balance, and now is the best time to do it.

BRACES

Braces on the teeth are irritating and often cause jaw and neck pain and headaches. The work done on children can sometimes contribute to TMJD (temporomandibular joint dysfunction), which attacks later. Use Myotherapy, as described in the pain books (see Sources), *before* the child goes for the first fitting. Be sure to do inside the mouth as well as the face and neck. When your child comes home and complains of aches, do it again. It *will* ease the pressure.

CANCER

Myotherapy cannot cure cancer, but it can relieve muscle spasm. When a child is very ill, there are many causes for spasm—the disease itself, the drugs and procedures used to combat the disease, plus old injuries brought to light by the disease. Myotherapy can lessen pain, improve balance, prevent weakness, and keep joints functioning to full ROM (range of motion.)

CEREBRAL PALSY

The earlier you get after the trigger points (immediately, please), the better the results will be. Use one of the pain-erasure books (see Sources) to clear the little person and then note the changes. First, the body will be more relaxed, have better balance, be better coordinated. Posture can be altered almost at once. Myotherapy not only works against what the disease has already done, but it is a preventative against further incursions by the disease. In adults it relieves pain just as it does in adult scoliosis.

CHARLEY HORSE

This is another name for growing pains and muscle stiffness after exertion. Later, when the person is older, it will be called arthritis. It responds at once to myotherapy, and you can prevent it with seeking massage (page 426).

COLDS

No, you can't cure the common cold, but you can make folks feel less miserable. Use myotherapy for headaches and check with one of the books on pain (see Sources) to discover what to do about stuffy sinuses. Do the whole body for the aches and pains that seem to be part of nasty colds. A seeking massage (page 426) would help, followed with some stretching exercise to relieve the stress that takes the form of misery.

CROUP

This is a word that can mean many things. It includes any condition of upper-respiratory obstruction, especially acute inflammation of the pharynx, larynx, and trachea. Sufferers usually have a brassy, strident cough and difficulty with breathing. Myotherapy can do wonders. Do the same areas as for headaches and teeth braces, both the neck and chest and the axilla.

DYSLEXIA

You would be amazed if you knew how many people who have done wonderful things with their lives have dyslexia. Some people do the best they can with it, but some use it as a crutch. Working with the equipment, tumbling, and floor progressions will help with problems of eye-hand coordination. Try to do everything that demands "Look . . . see . . . report back to the brain."

DIABETES

Exercise seems to be one of the best aids for the diabetic, and there is plenty of it here. Myotherapy can help, too, especially with keeping nutrition going to the feet and also to the head. Use it at the sites where injections are given. Trigger points gather where there were wounds, and injections are wounds.

FLAT FEET

This condition means that there is a depression of the arch in the sole of the foot. A child can be born with it or can develop it later. Like the foot with the long second toe, the flat foot is something less than perfect, but it can be given the power to do a great job for its owner. Exercise 78 will help enormously. Every foot exercise in the book, and that means all the floor progressions, is essential. You want to make and keep the anterior tibialis muscles on the outside front of the lower legs strong and limber. The more running, skipping, jumping, and hiking the better.

FRACTURES

Most of the fractures children sustain are called "green-stick fractures." They don't splinter the way old bones do and they heal well and quickly. One of the reasons is a lack of trigger points that limit nutrition to the bone. The doctor will set the bone and apply a cast so that the bone will remain undisturbed until it has knitted, usually in about six weeks. What is rarely addressed, however, is the tissue around the fracture, which was also injured and is now in the grip of spasms acting at the behest of old and new trigger points. Those trigger points will contribute to pain, swelling, and slow healing due to poor nutrition to the fracture site. This is particularly true if the break is in the lower leg, the tibia. Do trigger-point hunts above and below the cast to any exposed flesh. This will help with both pain and swelling.

When the cast comes off, the bone will be healed, but the tissue around the site will be in just about the same state it was when it went into the cast. The extremity will be sore, weak, and atrophied. Do the entire area, remembering that toes begin in the hips and fingers begin in the shoulders. If the hand is injured, start your work in the shoulder. If the toes have been mashed, start in the hips and groin. Find every trigger point and eradicate it; then go for full range of motion with exercise.

FORWARD HEAD

The forward head is a posture problem that's caused by another posture problem. When the chest muscles shorten and pull the shoulders and back into what we call round back, round shoulders, or, at its worst, kyphosis, the forward head will be one of the side effects. The neck is part of the spine, and when the back rounds, the head has to go along with it. Thus it tips downward. Unfortunately, it's impossible to see what's up ahead while staring down at the ground—so the victim lifts his or her face. The only way to do that while the back and neck are rounding down is to thrust the face forward. This puts a tremendous strain on the muscles at the back of the head, neck, and shoulders. Unfortunately, what affects the *back* of the shoulder girdle has an echo effect that can be felt as far away as the heels. That works in reverse, as you will see with the long second toe (page 435). *Everything* that affects one part of us affects all of us. *Every* posture anomaly should be corrected, just as the owner of a rare Rolls-Royce would check a veering to the right. What could it mean? he would ask. A tired, bent, or broken axle? The owner doesn't know, but he will jolly well find out—*today*. That Rolls is worth *money*. So is bad posture. It will lead to the expenditure of a great deal of money one day, not to mention the cost to the self-image, which is just as important, if not *more* important, since it dictates what one does in life.

All the exercises that work to stretch the chest and strengthen the upper back should be used constantly until the child (or you) stands straight *naturally*. See the exercise index.

HERNIA

If a child develops a hernia, he will probably require an operation, which in itself is nothing very special; the stay in the hospital is minimal. What is not minimal in a hernia operation, as in any of the more serious operations, is the scar tissue that will form when the wound heals. Scar tissue attracts trigger points, as you know, and trigger points can cause muscle spasm. Look for them at the scar area and neighboring areas, such as the seat, groin, and legs. When the child is dismissed, begin an easy exercise class and do seeking massage (page 426) to keep the area clear. When all is well and the scar is completely healed, stretch exercises for the whole area will be necessary.

HIPS

Hips make up part of the pelvic area, which is the center of balance and power. The little one who bats only with the power in his arms sends the ball dribbling. The skier who tries to turn without the pelvic shift keeps going straight. The child on a horse who cannot use her pelvis to lift the horse into a canter, keeps trotting. In the book *How to Keep Your Child Fit From Birth to Six* (see Sources) there are two little girls, Anne and Sue. When they were babies, the doctor discovered a kind of roughness when he put their baby legs through an ROM (range of motion) test. The examination led to X rays, which revealed that the children had hip dysplasia. Each wore a harness and one a body cast for the first year of life. Both are now straight and strong with excellent and beautiful legs. The only side effect from the cast is the increased strength of Anne's shoulder girdle, which she built dragging her immobile body around the house.

If there is something wrong with your child's hips, you will see it in his or her walk. You will hear about it when they talk about school sports (if any). Do not attribute any anomaly to something that's in the family. It's there all right, and there may be a familial tendency, but each child is separate and deserves the best body you can give. Check for trigger points in the groin and in those "back pockets" on the seat. Check the little legs with seeking massage. Treat that little body the way my neighbor Mary treats her million-dollar horses—with great care. Mary doesn't have any children to worry about, and she worries about her horses far more than she does about herself. I recently had to send a Myotherapist over to fix one of her beautiful Irish hunters in order to put help within reach of Mary, whose shoulder was aching. Your children are your million-dollar hunters, and if one of them is standing with a head tipped even *slightly* to one side, *pay attention*. There are several differences between expensive, extraordinarily beautiful horses and our own children: Familiarity. We are around them all the time and we don't notice subtle changes, but every posture anomaly and many injuries begin with subtle changes. The seeking massage is your greatest ally. Like a kind of night-vision camera, it can see what you can't. Use it.

Incidentally, fat, wobbly hips are anathema. Whole books could be written about seats and what they reveal. You want tight, strong little rear-ends on yourself and the children. Climb stairs and mountains.

IMMEDIATE MOBILIZATION

This is the "new" way of looking at injuries and operations. When I was a child and the little boy down the street had a hernia operation, he stayed in the hospital for two weeks. When my young friend Lori, the chief instructor of Myotherapy, had her hernia, she spent the night. Period. The little boy took weeks *to get over the hospital and the immobilization that went with it.* Lori was back at work by the following Monday and lost neither strength nor vitality. Bed rest is something to avoid whenever possible.

If you are interested in sports and read the paper, you will often read that this or that athlete *sprained* or *strained* this or that part of himself or herself and is expected to be sidelined for so and so many weeks. The treatment for these valuable people is at least sixty years behind the times and is given an acronym so you will remember it: RICE. The *R* is for Rest which is the *last* thing you should be thinking of in either a strain or a sprain. Then comes *I* for Ice. That's the old standby where any injury is concerned, and one can say this for it: It's not as bad as heat. The third letter, *C*, stands for Compression and means taping. Trainers spend years learning to apply tape to injured joints, which causes more swelling and thus prolongs the healing process. The letter *E* stands for Elevation, which is what the person does after the first three methods have made the injury so painful there is nothing else to do.

The people who are the main proponents of Immediate Mobilization, are athletes of the more rugged kind—wilderness skiers and backpackers. When someone like this gets hurt, there is no X-ray machine around the corner. He learns early on to distinguish a break from a sprain. What is a sprain anyway? It is a temporary dislocation, which is easy to get in a football game, but jumping from rock to rock while climbing four days from civilization in the Wind River Range is just as good for one. The injured joint returns to its normal site, but the tissue around it has been torn to a greater or lesser degree, and swelling starts immediately, as does the resultant pressure (which has more results than you can believe at first).

Coaches, trainers, physical educators, and therapists all know these things. What few of them know is that every trigger point, from the sprained ankle north to the hips and groin, has lit up and thrown resident muscles into greater or lesser spasm. In effect that means that a whole bunch of fists have closed over every passageway in the leg. Blood flow has been slowed down, and so has the passage of healing nutrition. What's more, the highways and byways by which waste products and fluids make their way north to be disposed of in the main body close down too. Result

Myotherapy: A Way to Get Rid of Pain 433

of that: the swelling. Any backpacker, as well as a lot of other people, know that if you sprain an ankle and have to keep walking, you can. It hurts, but ambulation is possible. If the bones were really fractured (I don't mean hairline fractures, the real thing), you'd have to be carried and you'd know it. Now, what happens to the sprained walker when it is possible to sit down? The swelling increases because the muscles of the legs are not being used to squeeze the fluids past the encroaching spasm. When, a little while later, the sprained leg is placed on the floor and told to get going, there is so much pain that it can't. Resting got it to that point. Then comes the ice, which may or may not help a little; it certainly keeps the athlete busy. The taping merely compounds the tension. What could you do?

1. Forget the hurting ankle. If you are in the wilderness, you don't have a choice. If the accident happened in the mall, on a court, or on local ski slope, there will be a doctor with an X ray machine nearby. What you want to know is, is it busted? If it's just a sprain, you don't want tape, aspirin will increase the bleeding and the pressure, and sitting with your leg up is a waste of time. Get rid of the trigger points.

2. Your ankle begins in your groin and hip, so start there to detrigger the muscles. Work down on *all* sides of the leg using seeking massage (page 426). Take out every trigger point you can find as you move down *to*, but not *on*, the ankle. Check the foot as well, particularly the instep. Don't press hard, just enough to surprise the system.

The first thing you will notice *if you are looking* is that the swelling will go down—way down. That immediately eases the pain. You can't see it, but the leg's circulatory system has been released, and healing has already started.

3. Now comes the *mobilization* part. *Point your toe down.* Then, keeping the leg straight, pull your toes up toward your knee. Third—rotate the foot (not the knee) inward and then outward. Surprise, surprise. You will be able to do those things without much (if any) pain. Do that *gently* five or six times. It will squeeze more fluid and vagrant blood from the injured site.

4. Now we need to squeeze the muscles a little harder, and for that we use resistance. Your companion, who has been de-triggering your leg, will now have to provide that resistance. He should stand facing your foot sole, take your heel in one hand, and put his fist against the ball of your foot. You point downwards again, but against his resistance. The resistance should be strong enough to make you work, but not so much that it hurts.

5. When you are at full point, he places his resisting hand across your instep. You pull the front of your foot toward your knee. The resistance is applied again.

6. Now you must rotate your foot inward against the resistance of his hand. Then rotate outward. Do those four movements three or four times against resistance.

7. Stand up and put the weight evenly

on both feet as you hold on to a table or a *friend*. Bend both knees *slightly*. Straighten. Do a dozen of those movements. If something protests, find the muscle doing the talking and hunt for an active trigger point and defuse it.

8. Keeping your weight evenly distributed between your two hands (which are resting on a table or some other support), rise to your toes. Don't try to be a ballerina; a little lift is adequate. Feel for the sharp protest again and defuse its cause. Do a dozen or so lifts.

9. Hold on to a friend if one is available and take four unlimping steps *backward*. You will be able to do it. When you walk forward, you may limp. Your brain has said you must. Walk backward and forward for roughly thirty seconds. Then sit down with a good book for half and hour. Repeat the whole thing. It will be no time till you are painless, unswelled, probably very colorful, but able to function.

The same goes for the wrist, elbow, knee, toe, finger, and so on. What you don't want to do is immobilize, but suppose you have to; say the tibia is really broken and the cast is in place. Find as many trigger points above and below the cast as you can and keep the rest of the body as active as possible. When the cast comes off, don't grab your crutches and a taxi home. Do exactly the same *immediate mobilization* as you would have done for a sprain, because what you are faced with are the same sort of problems that attend sprains. You will be limpless and functioning well in a couple of days. Use the seeking massage.

I have presented this to you as though you were the patient. With your child you will want to be more careful. Ask your doctor what sports *he* does. A skier, mountaineer, white-water canoeist would be your best bet if you want understanding. A no-exerciser, golfer from a cart, is the worst. Age doesn't seem to matter; some of the most open-minded are older, as are some of the healthiest. I have been the guinea pig for a great deal of Myotherapy and I have found that it works as nature does—naturally. My mail from people who read the pain-erasure books talks of miracles. Nature *is* miraculous, and so are we and our children. The mistake we have made is to move away from nature's way, but we are moving back. Listen to your body. *So* many answers are there for you. Immediate mobilization is one of them.

JAW PAIN

Listen to little kids chew and watch them. Some of their jaws click and some of them chew with the sideways motion of a cow. If the children are girls, they will most likely suffer with menstrual cramps. Sometimes the jaw clickers squint, have neck pain and headaches. For you adults this jaw pain is called temporomandibular joint dysfunction—big name for jaw pain. Look for trigger points in the seat and groin. Start your work there. When you reach the collarbone, start again with seeking massage in the hands and work up the arms to the armpits. Do them carefully, then the chest and neck. The head as for headaches comes last. If you need more help, use one of the pain-erasure books (see Sources). You will find that most jaw

KNOCK-KNEES AND BOWLEGS

Sit on a table and dangle your legs. Now stretch the right leg straight out in front of you as you pretend to be a puppet operated by a master puppeteer. There will be two strings running down your legs, one on the inside and one on the outside. If the puppeteer (you for now) pulls the string in your groin, your feet will turn in. If you pull the one on the outside up at the top of your leg, the foot will turn out. Right now, without going any further, you should be able to see the causes for both pigeon toes and turned-out feet: tight strings on one or the other side of the leg. Think. What could a tightened string represent? Could it be a tightened muscle? Indeed it could. To get rid of the pigeon-toe habit, clear the trigger points in the seat and all down the inside of the leg from groin to foot. To get the turned-out feet on the right track (forward), go after the trigger points in the seat and all down the legs on their outsides.

Now, puppeteer, lock the knees of your little puppet and substitute strong piano wire from anklebones to groin on the inside and anklebones to hipbones on the outside. Use one of those gadgets sailors use to tighten the ropes to the mast top and slowly tighten the wires on the outsides of both legs. What will happen? Any kid could tell you that you will have two bows you could use for archery, and the top of each arch would be a knee. Now you have knock-knees. To straighten them out, get rid of the trigger points doing what those wires are doing. They are on the outside of the legs, hip to foot.

To straighten bowlegs, you only have to see the wires tightening on the *inside* of the leg, bowing those knee-locked legs, and you'll know where to work. You already know that getting rid of the trigger points is only one-third of myotherapy. Stretching the newly freed muscles and re-educationg them is the second. Lastly, an exercise program. Floor progressions build strong legs, as do walks in the country and swims in mountain streams and walloping surf. What makes good legs for a child? A chance to use them.

LONG SECOND TOE

This is a structural anomaly that millions of people live with. It is also called the Classic Greek Foot and Morton's Toe. The nice thing about it is that it can be taken care of simply. The bad thing about it is that it can cause anything from agonizing pain, bunions, hammertoe, and practically useless feet to jaw pain and headaches at the other end.

In a so-called normal foot the heel strikes the ground when you take a step forward. A split second later the body's weight is transferred to the ball of the foot just behind the big toe on the inside of the foot as well as on the outside of the foot near the little toe. That arrangement provides a nice solid tripod. The long-second-toe foot is different. The heel strikes as in the normal foot, but as the weight is transferred to the front of the foot, it goes on a single straight line, to be caught in the middle of the metatarsal arch under the joint of the second toe. There is a knife-edge support instead of the solid tripod. The foot, instead of plunking down with all sides on the ground, so to speak, wobbles precariously. The muscles of the foot are forced to work overtime and in ways for which they were not designed. So are the muscles of the leg, especially the anterior tibialis on the outside front of the lower leg. The results are soon apparent. The foot doesn't run or walk well, and the ankles are unstable, which endangers the knees and ultimately the hips. The toes, trying hard to maintain the balance against millions of wrong movements, are subjected to muscle spasms. They bend up, as in hammertoe, or are pulled out of line, as in bunions. They develop neuromas. If it weren't so easy to help, it would be a tragedy because walking is one of man's best fitness aids and usually the major way to reach nature.

The name Classic Greek Foot was applied by Dr. Janet Travell, who pioneered Trigger Point Injection Therapy and who noticed that *all* the Greek statues in museums had the condition. Why no hammertoe and no bunions? For one thing no sculptor would have wanted to use them as models, but there is a better reason: The ancient Greeks wore sandals. Going barefoot or wearing sandals allows the foot to behave normally because the toes spread out and take the weight all across the base rather than in the middle. You can see the results of that shoe-caused limitation on older women: It's a huge callus. Men usually get theirs on the outside edge of the big toe. Men's shoes, being wider and flat-heeled, do less damage.

One thing you can do is to find out if you actually have this condition. Lots of feet with even toes have a long second toe. It isn't the length of the toe that counts so much, but where the joint is in the foot as compared with the big toe. Bend all your toes down with one hand and with the other use a felt-tipped pen. Draw a circle around the big knuckle of the big toe at the end of the foot. Now draw a circle around the knuckle of the long second toe. If that one is further forward in the foot, even a little, you've got it, the LST.

We use what we call "the $1.80 cure." Of course nothing is "cured." The bone structure came with the body and needs a little help. Get a pair of Dr. Scholl's inner soles. At the same time pick up a sheet of adhesive foam for an extra pad. Cut two circles the size of a quarter from your foam and stick them one on top of the other on the bottom of one of those inner soles right where the ball of the foot behind the big toe will rest. Be careful: None of the pad should encroach on the middle of the metatarsal arch. What this pad does is to lift the weight *off* that spot where the callus shows up. That will give you a tripod enjoyed by those with normal feet.

Check your children for this anomaly and keep them shoeless or in sandals as much as possible. That goes for you, too. High heels are good-looking and fun to wear, but when you are *not* wearing them, think sandals.

MENSTRUAL CRAMPS

These usually come from trigger points in the abdominal and seat muscles. See page 279.

PERFORMING ARTS

Check with the exercise index.

PIGEON TOES

See Knock-knees and refer to the exercise index.

POSTURE IN GENERAL

Refer to the exercise index under Posture.

RETARDATION

There are many grades of retardation, and sometimes there is accompanying pain, weakness, poor balance, and co-ordination. Often these things manifest themselves through withdrawal. Back on page 378 you read about Kathy, my "aide." She had a father who was an engineer and refused to think of the material that went into his daughter as waste. He was right. He took what she brought him and made a lot out of it. So can you. You know how to lessen the problems of handicapped children. Try to remember that the earlier you start, the better will be your results.

SHINSPLINTS

These are muscle spasms in the *front* of the lower leg. Use the same system as that shown on page 417, but on the front rather than the back of the leg. Shinsplints often come from exercise without sufficient warm-up. Don't be guilty of that.

SINUS PAIN

Sinus pain is sometimes called sinus headache and often accompanies a cold. Get one of the pain-erasure Myotherapy books (see Sources) and use the headache technique. Don't say to yourself, "He's only four, he won't understand." He will understand just fine and will use the finger-control for pain as you work. Don't be surprised if he starts telling you *exactly* where to press. Children have not yet been corrupted by old ideas and limitations.

SPASTICITY

This can range all the way from what looks like a "little clumsy," to "My child can't do those things; she or he is spastic." A new baby who is born with cerebral palsy may look as though it had spent its first days strapped to a board. The legs cannot be spread at all. Later, when those children try to walk, they progress on their toes, which are turned in.

Find every trigger point you can with seeking massage (page 426) and then re-educate the muscles. You will be amazed at the changes.

TORTICOLLIS

This is a very stiff neck and is often caused at birth. It may not be heard from for years and years, or it may show up in a tipped head at once. Watch your little people's necks and keep them clear of trigger points. People do not "grow out of" problems; they just shelve them for later.

There are volumes and volumes written on the physical problems we humans can develop. My grandfather wanted to be a doctor so badly that he apprenticed himself to a German shoemaker so that he could learn the language because in his day, Germany was where medicine was at. He had to give up his studies because there were so many diseases and he began to think he had them all. One short trip through a children's hospital can almost throw you into despair. *But,* keep in mind that almost all injuries and diseases have one thing in common: pain. You already know something about preventing and easing pain. You could learn a lot more and be of great value to the other people in your life. Pain takes all the color and warmth out of the day. There is no need for a lot if not most of it. Believe that, and do something about the pain little people suffer from mashed fingers (trigger points start in the shoulder) to mouth pain from braces (trigger points in the mouth, face, and neck) to aching knees (the thighs and calves), and so forth. *You* are their key; not the druggist.

CHAPTER THIRTY-FIVE
HOW TO HELP A FRIEND

I was giving a Pain Erasure Seminar in Pennsylvania many years ago and a lady in the front row sat all day with a cardboard box on her lap. There were air holes in the box, and every so often I heard somebody who was in the box give a small, impatient snuffle. Somebody didn't like it in there. As we broke at the end of the seminar, I asked the lady who was in the box. Notice, I didn't say *what*, I said *who*. She opened the box carefully to expose a slightly dirty white mop of a dog. It was the kind that has to go somewhere before you know which is the bow and which the stern. It seemed to be about a foot long, and by the way it moved when she set it on the floor, I knew that every inch of that foot hurt.

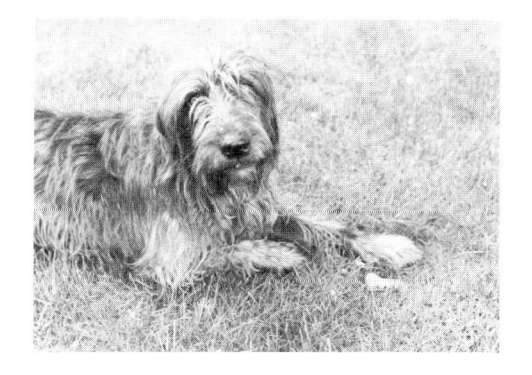

"Mopsie has arthritis," the lady reported, "and you said on TV that where pain is concerned, dogs are no different than people. Can you help her, she's all I have?" I didn't know for sure, but I was certainly going to try.

Mopsie hadn't moved very far from her mistress. She just stood there, all humped up, the way people do when they hurt a lot. When her mistress spoke, she took two tentative steps with her front feet and then gave a halfhearted hop with the two back ones at the same time. That was it. She'd made the effort. I picked Mopsie up, but not before explaining to her that I was going to make her feel better. Don't laugh. People who don't discuss things with animals, babies, and small children don't get very far. I even told her I was going to look for trigger points in her back muscles and her legs.

I started with the muscles in her back just outside the spine. I pressed gently and waited for her comment. She just looked at me. I went all the way up the back, pressing at half-inch intervals about as hard as I would have pressed on a baby's face. By about the fifth press the little dog laid her head down with a kind of resigned air, which said quite clearly, "Okay, go ahead."

When I finished the back, I did both back legs the same way I do the legs of little kids who have growing pains. I finished with the groin, the inside tops of each little thigh. Only once did she squeak, and then she pretended she hadn't by looking away. Then I stretched the legs, first one and then the other. As the second leg was stretched *she* took over and stretched all of her. She grew several inches right there before our eyes—as people do.

Nobody was prepared for what happened next when we put Mopsie down on the floor. At first she just stood there and then suddenly she was off! She became a wild streak of white fluff tearing around the gym as though dog demons were after her and closing. She circled twice before her mistress could get her to stop. When she was finally snuggled into the welcoming lap and the discarded box had become a thing of the past, she busied herself wagging furiously at one end and kissing the lady's tears away at the other. I still get Christmas cards from Mopsie, who is still pain-free due to a little Myotherapy and a lot of exercise.

Then came Delilah. Delilah is an English mastiff. You can see the breed on Babylonian bas-reliefs dating back to the year 700 B.C. There they are hunting lions and wild horses. Although they are great watchdogs, they are even better friends and allies. Marco Polo reported that Kublai Khan had five thousand mastiffs around just for hunting purposes. Henry VIII used them as war dogs. Those were Delilah's ancestors— and she behaves as though she knows it. She races over the fields, and her great stride carries her magnificent self as though she were leading the pack after the king of beasts. The best we can turn up for her is a rabbit, but the instinct is there, as is her affection for her friend, man—or, as in my case, woman. Delilah was not always so exciting to watch. There was a time when to watch her try to move would bring tears to a person's eyes. When I met her a couple of years ago, she was going to be "sacrificed" to see why her muscles were spastic, why she had to drag herself around, and why, when the weather was inclement and she was kept indoors close to the fire, she got so much worse. She had had all the examinations, tests, and X rays, and nothing had been found. I asked my friend Eva Olsen Fisher, who raises mastiffs in Virginia, if Delilah had ever had an accident or been strained in any way. Well, she loved people and spent a lot of time waltzing around on her hind legs as a puppy in the kennel. Let someone appear, and Delilah was the greeting committee. "She was a big puppy," said Mrs. Fisher, "and maybe her legs were strained then." I went on that assumption when she was brought to where we were standing in the windswept driveway. I hunted at one end of Delilah while Eva kept the other end busy. She was a bigger dog now, and I wasn't sure about the end with the teeth. A mop is one thing, a mastiff something else.

In five minutes she was better—not well, but she could walk better. That night when I got to Washington, I called and asked if I could send one of my students who loved to work on dogs down to "fix" Delilah. We got permission. In fact, Eva sent the dog north for me. What a gift! At first we had to carry her up the three stairs to the door. If she got down on a polished floor, there was no way she could get up. If she did walk, she dragged the tops of her front paws and had to be watched lest she skin herself. Helen Haskell, the student, worked on her every day, and in a few weeks Delilah was a mastiff again. When Helen graduated, she decided to treat animals as well as humans and is now putting as many show horses and dogs back into the ring as people back into jobs. She was followed by two students who became the first licensed equine myotherapists; they work with racehorses. Myotherapists are helping veterinarians all over the country, but you need not be either a myotherapist or a vet to help your horse, dog, cat, or even bird. *They* know what you are doing. No Myotherapist has ever been bitten, kicked, stepped on, or even spoken crossly to.

Delilah tells us when she needs Myotherapy. If a prospective Myotherapist is sitting in a chair, Delilah will walk in front of him and rest her huge chest on his lap. The Myotherapist is *expected* to reach over, as we do with humans, and take the trigger points out of her back legs, outside and in. Delilah then stretches the worked leg as long as she can and walks away. But she's not dumb. In seconds she has approached from the other side and is now resting her chest in the person's lap again, but with the other side exposed. I have never known her to settle for one side. When the second side is done, she will stretch and move away to rest on the floor at the Myotherapist's feet. It seems to be a way of saying thank you.

The next problem, after clearing her muscles, was exercise. She needed a lot, and after a while she was ready for speed. How to take care of that? Beggar took care of that. Dogs are pack animals and they not only want company, they have to have it for health and happiness. Beggar moved in. She was seven inches long and needed a friend. She didn't just move into the house, she moved into the space between Delilah's paws, and Delilah began to bloom. Beggar is the kind of dog that says, "What shall we do now? I know, let's . . . ," and away they go. All I have to do is take them to the fields and Beggar takes over. Delilah can't chase lions, but Beggar is a reasonable facsimile. She is also company, and sometimes when dogs seem sad and droopy, it's because they are lonely, which is a form of stress. Stress soon causes old injuries to flare up, and a shoulder injured in a jump from a porch at age six months can be called *discogenic disease* in an older dog. Prevent old trigger points from taking over your friend.

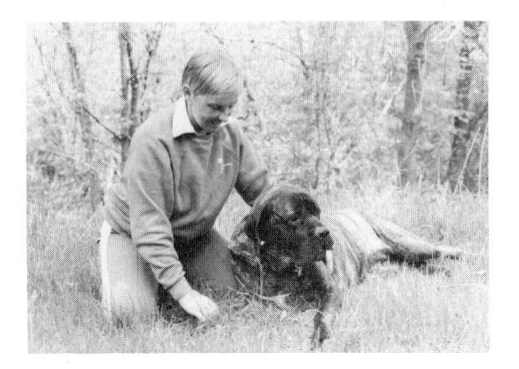

Big dogs are often injured as puppies, before they develop the strength to handle their size. Do the exact same work on them as is described in all my books and don't be concerned if the dog has a diagnosis four words long.

A few weeks ago one of our Myotherapists was asked to help a goat named Ariel. You dog and horse people may not feel too much for goats, but this goat's mistress cared very much about *her*. The vet said she had cuprine arthritic meningitis and that while Myotherapy probably couldn't make her well (goats usually die of that particular disease), he thought it might ease her last days. It took two people to get her on her feet. The Myotherapy was done just as I described for Mopsie and Delilah, and little Ariel was laid on clean straw, hopefully eased. Her gravesite had been chosen before her mistress went off on a business trip. The next day, when the Myotherapist paid a return visit to ease Ariel's last hours, Ariel could not be caught. She had risen from her death bed and was leaping over hay bales and water troughs. Her vigor was restored, and she was not about to lie down and die—not that day or the next. The grave waited, empty. Ariel is well, her mistress is happy, and Myotherapy has another convert.

Then there was "That Damn Bird."

"That Damn Bird" didn't have a name. It was one of those rare species that has to be quarantined for a number of weeks before being turned loose in these United States. Somewhere along the way it had hurt its wing. Not a good thing to happen to a valuable bird in a government facility. That's why it was known as "that damn bird." Every day it would get up on a perch and make unseemly noises that announced an attempt to fly. It would flap both wings unevenly, dive off, and fall on its face. "That damn bird . . . it's going to break its neck, and then who'll pay for that?" This had been going on for several weeks when Myotherapist Moira Dorsey arrived as a summer replacement at the facility. Mostly she cleaned up after the birds, changed water dishes, and fed her exotic charges. In addition she told everyone about Myotherapy and what it could do for animals. "What can it do for That Damn Bird?" was asked one sunny morning. Moira didn't know, but she said she'd give it a try. She and That Damn Bird went out into the courtyard, and she sat it on her lap. She did Myotherapy as if he was a baseball player with a pitcher's wing. It took about twenty lovely minutes while the bird looked at her as the dogs and horses do (we haven't tried it on a cat yet that I know of). Most of them get dreamy-eyed and sleepy. Then Moira stretched the injured wing very gently, not wanting to hurt or frighten him. Out it went like Delilah's leg—and in again. Once, twice, and then she stretched both at the same time. Whether it gave That Damn Bird an idea or what, no one had time to find out, because right then in the sunny courtyard it stretched both wings and took off into the wild blue yonder, free and fabulous, several thousand dollars worth on the wing—*both* wings.

Last there are the horses. Horses are so big you'd think that myotherapy, to be effective, would have to be applied with a baseball bat. Helen Haskell, who learned on Big Delilah, knew differently. If a fly lights on a horse, the horse's skin flickers. Her first patient was a beautiful show horse headed for extinction. There wasn't any reason not to try myotherapy. It couldn't hurt and maybe would make the poor twisted animal feel a little better. Six months later the horse was back in the ring taking blue ribbons.

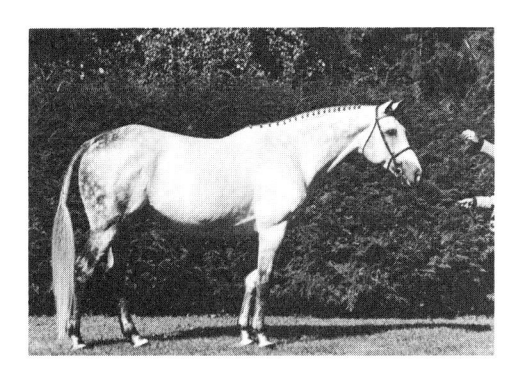

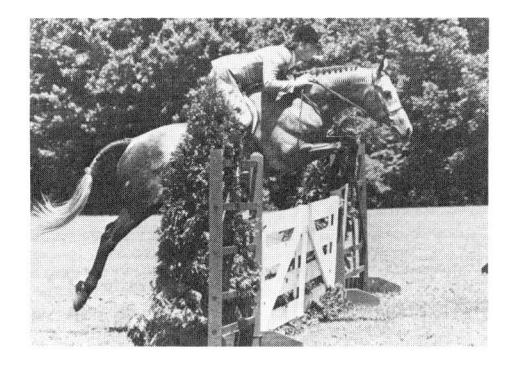

At Mary Stokes' nationally known stable, every horse has had Myotherapy at one time or another, and some at crucial moments just before competition. Horses are really funny under the hands of a Myotherapist. They never bite, push, squash, or shove. They know exactly what's going on and will even move to make reaching "the spot" easier. Their eyes get dreamy and sleepy, and their necks stretch longer and longer. From time to time they blow great gusty sighs of contentment and gratitude as they make faces like Mr. Ed. How do you do a horse? The same way you do a person. Look at the pain erasure and Myotherapy books with their charts of human anatomy (see Sources). Notice where the trigger points are for people and think horse. If you put the chart on the floor and get down on all fours to look at the chart, you will see where the points would be on your temporarily four-footed self. Moira found That Damn Bird's key point in the axilla, right where you would find it on a tennis player or baseball pitcher. Press about the same way as you would for a child and use seeking massage (page 426) any time the horse behaves skittishly or seems to be in a bad temper. The key is in the muscles—as it is with all of us.

The key to all of us is painlessness and exercise. The keys to both are in this book, and you are the Keeper of the Keys. What a wonderful thing to be! Keep in mind that from six to twelve are the last best years in which to build a body, get close to a child, and walk in that garden between the dawn and the daylight—when everything is magic.

SOURCES

BOOKS

There are two books which you as the parent of a child, no matter what age, from birth to fifty, must have and they are about pain, its erasure and control. Almost more important, its prevention.

Pain Erasure the Bonnie Prudden Way. New York: M. Evans & Co., Inc., 1980 (hardcover). New York: Ballantine Books, 1982, (paperback).

Myotherapy: Bonnie Prudden's Complete Guide to Pain Free Living. New York: The Dial Press, 1984 (hardcover). New York: Ballantine Books, 1986 (paperback).

Those two books can prevent a great deal of pain and misery and help you improve both your child's self image and your own. No child should be denied two active parents if that can be avoided . . . or two active grandparents.

The Children's Trilogy:

How to Keep Your Child Fit From Birth to Six. New York: Harper & Row, Publishers, 1964. Revised edition, New York: The Dial Press, 1983. Second revised edition: Ballantine Books, 1987

Teenage Fitness. New York: Harper & Row, Publishers, 1965. Revised edition, New York: The Dial Press, 1983. Second revised edition: Ballantine Books, 1988.

Your Baby Can Swim, New York, Reader's Digest Press, 1974. Revised edition, *Teach Your Baby to Swim* New York: The Dial Press, 1983. Stockbridge Massachusetts: Bonnie Prudden Press.

At least twenty years ago I started the first Baby-Swim-and-Gym classes in Y's all over the country. One-baby-one-Mommy. Soon fathers began to take an interest. Then, as with anything "new" the Nervous Nellies got into the act and tried to stop baby swims. They failed. The book tells you how to teach your baby or grandbaby to swim and presents the facts about baby-swim, which are all positive.

In addition, if you have a handicapped baby or know of one, baby-swim and gym is made to order for that child *and its parents.*

As your children grow and as you grow with them you and they will need to find ways in which to use the wonderful bodies you have developed and you will want to do that as a family.
How to Keep Your Family Fit and Healthy. New York: Reader's Digest Press, 1975. Stockbridge, Massachusetts: Bonnie Prudden Press.

As your children approach the teens you will need to know a different way to present sex from that offered by the schools. No one can do that better than you, but there are some guidelines that prevent the children from saying, "Aw, we had that two years ago in school." The next is a gentle book about feelings, sensuality and loving. The dual exercises can be used by all of you. While they do improve bodies for sex (you don't have to tell anybody) they also improve golf and tennis scores, make horseback riding easier and banish fatigue.
Exer-Sex. New York: Bantam Books, 1978. Stockbridge, Massachusetts: Bonnie Prudden Press.

Today's grandparents are the last naturally fit Americans. They walked to and from school and everywhere else. They played out of doors, they knew and played all the kid's games that have been forgotten. Grandparents have much to impart. Give them a chance to help with your children's fitness as they reclaim their own.
Bonnie Prudden's Guide to Fitness After Fifty. New York: Villard Press, 1986 (hardcover). New York: Ballantine Books, 1987 (paperback).

TAPES

Tapes are available for pre- and post-natal programs, babies, general exercise, skiers, executives, and teenagers. *None of these tapes will injure* and all of them build excellent bodies to excellent music.

AUDIO CASSETTE
How to Relieve Pain.
This is a forty minute audio cassette tape explaining Myotherapy and taking you step by step through fixing a backache or a headache.

FILMS

Prudden, Bonnie, *Your Baby Can Swim*, Stockbridge, Mass.: Institute for Physical Fitness, 1972.
15mm, color, sound, 12 minutes
Complete instructions for teaching babies to swim. A companion to the book *Teach Your Baby to Swim.*
Also available for VCR.

Alive and Feeling Great, New York: Harvest Films, 1974.
16mm, color, sound, 14 minutes
This film was made with the cooperation of the Pittsfield Girl's Club in Massachusetts and provides a complete exercise program for girls five years of age and up. The right music, the same equipment as is in this book . . . and routines you can use. It was funded by a grant from the Reader's Digest.

Sources

VIDEO CASSETTE

Your Baby Can Swim—This lovely cassette shows babies swimming in and under the water ... with emphasis on *under*. Their wide-open eyes, smiling faces and actively churning little bodies make viewers comfortable about babies swimming. *Water is the baby's medium.* No baby can walk, but every one of these can swim—and should, for safety's sake, as well as for enjoyment.

You can use the cassette for public relations and as an orientation tool before you start a swim class. This is also a training cassette and helps prepare teachers of babies to handle both babies *and* parents. Use it with the book *Teach Your Baby to Swim* for a successful program for class or family.

VHS color, sound, 12 minutes

FILMSTRIPS

Prudden, Bonnie. *Keep Fit ... Be Happy.* Stockbridge, Mass.: Institute for Physical Fitness, 1971.

Five color filmstrips for use on manual or automatic projectors.

Five 12-inch long-playing records providing exercises, directed by Bonnie Prudden to Orff Music. The Teacher's Manual outlines a complete physical fitness program which can be conducted in any classroom. Delightful cartoon children teach exercise to the class leaving the teacher free to check performance and make corrections where necessary.

DOORWAY GYM©

For information about a ready-made Doorway Gym, contact Bonnie Prudden, Inc., Stockbridge, Mass. 01262

WARNING

This is the second book containing Myotherapy for children. That means that soon imitation "myotherapists" specializing in children will appear. Why? Because it works. Why again? Because many babies and children are in pain. Be sure you select a *Certified Bonnie Prudden Myotherapist*cm for your child. They have been trained by Bonnie Prudden and her staff for 1400 hours in both Myotherapycm and exercise. They have taken and passed board exams and the name Bonnie Prudden is your guarantee that they know what they are doing. Ask to see their papers showing that they are updated and in good standing. If you have doubts about anyone or if you want a Myotherapist, contact the office of Bonnie Prudden, Inc., Stockbridge, Massachusetts.

EXERCISE INDEX

#1A,B,C,	Abdominal Correctives	26–27
#362	Abdominal and Groin Stretch	423–24
#321	Abdominal Hold Parallels	317
#322	Abdominal Stretch	317
#96	Alternating Forward Thrusts	127
#262	Alternate Shoulder Shrugs	234
#34	Angry Cat, Old Horse	91
#80	Apart-Together Jump	116
#256	Apart-Together Rebound Jump	226
#161	Arm-and-Leg Hold, Sawhorse	172
#279	Arm Circles, Ballet	243
#121	Assisted Keel Walk	153
#6	Back and Hamstring Stretch	30
#172	Back Bend on Horse	177
#111	Back Bend	138
#60	Back Bend, Prone	105
#289	Back Extension With Lift (ballet)	247
#224	Back Flip, Interrupted	212
#293	Backhand Patterning (tennis)	253–54
#120	Backing Across Plank	152
#125	Back Keel Walk	155
#282	Back Point and Retract (ballet)	245
#264	Back Stretch and Bend (ballet)	235
#18	Back Stroke (warm up)	77
#117	Back-to-Back Lift	143
#115	Back-to-Back, "M"	141
#123	Back Track Walk	154
#173	Back Walkover (horse)	177–78
#100	Backward Shoulder Roll	130–31
	Back Yard Track Meet	286–97
#247	Balance Beam	222
	Ballet	231–41
	Barre	241–48
#285	Bent-Knee Back Extension	245
#284	Bent-Knee Forward Extension	245

#	Exercise	Page
#283	Bent-Knee Side Extension	245
#1A	Bent-Knee Sit-Ups	26
#1B	Bent-Knee Sit-Ups	26
#1C	Bent-Knee Sit-Ups	27
#271	Bent-Knee Toe Rise (ballet)	238
#193	Bent-Over Row (wgts.)	193
#310	Bike (swim)	312
#185	Bird Landing on Lake (ramp)	185
#231	Bird's Nest (rope)	214
#251	Block Balance	223
#290	Bow (ballet)	248
#127	Bridge Walk	156
#129	Bridge Walk, Crossed Feet	156
#128	Bridge Walk, Crossed Hands	156
#219	Caboose (rope)	208
#359	Calf Stretch	359–60
#113	Cartwheel	139–40
#147	Cat on a Fence	165
#139	Cat on a Ladder	161
#90	Change-Level Side Extensions	122–23
#169	Chest Lift Over Horse, Prone	176
#210	Chin-Ups	202–3
#211	Chin-Ups, One Hand	204
#210	Chin-Ups, Reverse Hold	202
#220	Climb to Sit/Stand (rope)	209
#223	Controlled Back Flip	211
	Correctives	26–30
#74	Crab Walk	114
#306	Cross-Country Running	304–5
#241	Crosses Clockwise (garage)	220
#239	Crosses Foreward/Backward (garage)	220
#242	Crosses-Fours (garage)	220
#236	Crossover	218
#240	Crosses Side to Side (garage)	220
#54	Crotch Stretch	103
#192	Curl (wgts.)	195
#46	Curl...Extend...Curl	100
#358	Curve (skate)	360–61
#5	Diagonal pull-back lift	28
#349	Dip (skate)	357
#303	Discus (track)	294
#296	Dodgeball (tennis)	257
#249	Dog on the Ties	222
#70	Dog Run	112
#238	Double Jumpers	219
#73	Double-Leg Jumps	113
#84	Doubles Runs, Backward	118
#83	Doubles Runs	117–18
#85	Doubles, Crossover	118–19
#334	Downhill March (ski)	341
#141	Downhill on the Ladder	163
#338	Dry Obstacles	343–44
#337	Dry Slalom	343
#154	Duck Walk on Fence	168
#27	Edging (standing)	84–85
#333	Edging (skiing)	341
#335	Edging (traverse-ski)	341–42
#26	Elevator (standing)	84
#291	Eye Exercise	251
#345	Falls (skating)	356
#328	Falls (skiing)/(Dry)	338
#341	Falls (skiing)/(Snow)	346–47
#344	"Feeling" the Ice	355
#150	Fence Mount	166–67
#142	Fence Walk	164
#146	Fence Side-Walk	165
#145	Fence Walk on toes	165
	Figure Skating	351–62
#217	Fish on a Line	208
#272	Fishtail Turnout	239
#50	Flag Pole	101
#269	Flat Foot to Half Toe	237–38
#22	Flexibility Bounce	80
#63	Flexibility Bounce	106
	Flexibility Exercise	97–105
#200	Floor Balance Beam	197
#232	Flying Bird's Nest	215
#292	Forehand Patterning (tennis)	252–53
#49	Forward-Backwards Leg Swings	101
#40	Forward Fall (kneeling)	93
#30	Forward Fall (standing)	86–87
#280	Forward Point and Retract	244
#101	Forward Shoulder Roll	131–32
#75	Four Foot Backward Walk	114
#246	Four-Foot Mix-Up	222
#245	Four Foot Track Walk	221
#79	Frog Hop	116
#348	Glide (skating)	357
#277	Grand Plié	241
#326	Groin Stretch	337
#14	Half Knee Bends, Side	74–75
#62	Hamstring and Groin Stretch	105

Exercise Index

#51	Hand-Held Leg Stretch	102
#108	Handstand	136
#109	Handstand, Kick Up	137
#110	Handstand, wall	138
#207	Hand-Supported Stand-Down	199
#28	Hand Walk-out (standing)	85–86
#324	Hand Walk (parallel)	318
#205	Hanging Traverse	198–99
#106	Headstand	134–35
#107	Headstand, Solo	135
#331	Heel jumps (ski)	340
#332	Heel Shift (ski)	340
#276	Heel-to-Instep Plié	240
#336	Herringbone (ski)	342
#298	High Jump	288–89
#138	High Rung Walking	161
#189	Hill Challenge	187–88
#17	Hip Rotations	76–77
#266	Hip Rotation (Dance)	236
#69	Hip Twists	111
#237	Hopscotch (garage)	219
#149	Hop Toad on a fence	166
#136	Horse and Cart	160
#76	Horse Kick	114
#95	Hub of Wheel	127
#301	Hurdles	290–91
#39	Hydrant (knees)	92–93
#302	Javelin Throw	292
#165	Jump Combo	174–75
#164	Jump Off Backward	174
#181	Jump Over a Dowel	184
#186	Jump Over Steeple (ramp)	186
#252	Jump, Rebounder	224
#86	Jump Rope	119
#88	Jump Rope, Bent Knees	120
#259	Jump Rope, Rebound	228
#87	Jump Rope, Running	120
#278	Jump Series (ballet)	241
#259	Jump Series, Rebounder	227
#162	Jump to Knees	173
#163	Jump to Spraddle	173–74
#253	Jump Turns	224
#259	Jump Turns, Rebounder	227
#126	Keel Crossover	155
#125	Keel Walk, Back	155
#121	Keel Walk, Assisted	153
#124	Keel Walk, Unassisted	154
#340	Kick Turns (ski)	346
#12	Knee Bends	72–74
#285	Knee-Bent Back Extension	245
#284	Knee-Bent Forward Extension	245
#88	Knee-Bent Jump Rope	120
#283	Knee-Bent Side Extension	245
#206	Knee Hang	199
	Kneeling Exercises	90–93
#68	Knee Lifts	111
#257	Knee Pull-Up (rebound)	227
#59	Knee to Armpit, Assisted	104
#35	Knee-to-Nose Kick	91
#198	Knee-to-Nose Stretch, Sitting	197
#42A	Knee to Nose, Supine	94
#57	Knee to Shoulder, Assisted	104
#137	Ladder High Steps	160
#134	Ladder Sides Walking	159
#91	Lateral Knee-Bend Shift	123
#197	Lateral Stretch (wgts.)	195
#118	Layer Cake (stunt)	144
#171	Lean Back on Horse	177
#187	Leap (ramp)	186
#42D	Left Side-Lying Stretch	95
#323	Leg Bob (parallels)	317
#170	Leg Lifts (Horse), Prone	176–77
#267	Leg Rotations	237
#55	Leg Spread, Ear to Knee	103
#52	Leg Spread, Head Down	102
#56	Leg Spread, Held Aloft	103
#44	Leg Spread Side-Drops	98–99
#42	Limbering Series	94
#212	Let-Down	204
#7	Let-Down-Push-Up	33
#201	Limp on Pipe	198
#116	Little Lifts Big (stunt)	142
#4	Lower Back Lift	28
#53	Lower-Back Stretch	102
#157	Machine	170–71
#166	Mantle	175
#190	Military Press	192
#148	Monkey on a Fence	166
#140	Monkey on a Ladder	161
#175	Mount Series A	180
#23	Mouse Trap/Hot Pennies	82–83
#89	One-Arm-Two-Arm Floor Progression	122
#347	One-Foot Balance (skate)	357
#33	One-Foot Balanced Stand	88–89

#351	One-Foot Glide (skate)	358
#160	One-Handed Vault	172
#131	One Legged Wheelbarrow, Track	157
#152	One Legged Wheelbarrow on fence	167
#202	On-On-Off-Off	198
#216	Overhead Pull	207
#11	Overhead Reach (stand)	72
#309	Overhead Reach (swim)	311
#41	Peanut Push	93
#38	Pelvic Tilt, Kneeling	92
#19	Pelvic Tilt, Standing	78
#42E	Pelvic Tilt, Supine	96
#20	Pelvic Tilt, to Toes	78
#183	People Jumping (ramp)	184–85
#234	Pigeon Toes	218
#143	Pigeons on the Fence	164
#208	Pinwheel	200
#214	Pipe, Hamstring Stretch	205
#213	Pipe Plié	204–5
#204	Pipe, Walk and Turn	198
#273	Pliés	239–40
#275	Pliés, Front	240
#274	Pliés, Side	240
#305	Pole Vault	295–97
#199	Prone Arm-and-Leg Lift	196
#61	Prone Back bend	105
#60	Prone Back bend, Assisted	105
#42C	Prone Gluteus Set	95
#196	Pullover	195
#167	Pull-Up, Biceps	175
#265	Pull-Up and Circle	235–36
#168	Pull-Up, Triceps	176
#215	Pump	206
#248	Railroad Ties	222
#287	Raised-Knee Extension	246
#268	Raised Leg Rotation	237
#203	Raised Pipe	198
#288	Raised-Side Extension	247
	Ramp	181–88
#178	Ramp Somersault	182–83
#188	Ramp Turns	187
#32	Ram Push	88
#177	Ramp Walk-Up	182
#256	Rebounder, Apart-Together	226
#258	Rebounder, Jump Rope	227
#254	Rebounder Running	225
#255	Rebounder, Side-to-Side Jumps	225
#346	Recover, Skating	356
#184	Retract Landing Gear (ramp)	185
#191	Reverse Curl (wgts.)	192
#104	Reverse Tailor's Somersault	133
	Riding	321–34
#250	Right-Right-Left-Left	222–23
#42B	Right Side-Lying Stretch	95
#226	Ring Swing	213
#230	Ring, Upside Down	214
#179	Roll Down a Hill	183
#221	Rope Climb	209–10
	Rope, Horizontal	207–8
#222	Rope, Upside-Down hang	210
#263	Round Down and Pull Up	234
#71	Row a Boat	112–13
#133	Rung Walking	159
#299	Running Broad Jump	289–90
#180	Running Jump	183
	Sawhorse	163–81
#176	Scales, Preparation	181
#319	Scissors to Leg Extensions	316
#72	Sealing	113
#156	Seat Lift	170
#297	Serve Pattern	257–58
#304	Shot Put	294–95
#31	Shoulder Push	87–88
#16	Shoulder Rotation, Front	75–76
#15	Shoulder Rotation, Side	75
#261	Shoulder Shrugs	234
#13	Shoulder Shrug Series	74
#105	Shoulder Stand	134
#361	Shoulder Stretch (Myo)	421
#260	Shoulder Twist	233
#295	Shuffle Pattern	255–56
#229	Siamese Twin Swingers	213
#92	Side-Extension Thrust	125
#47	Side Knee-Bend Extension	100
#45	Side Leg Lift	99
#42B–42D	Side-Lying Stretch (limbering)	95–96
#360	Side-Lying Stretch (Myo)	419–20
#281	Side Point and Retract	244
#294	Side Slide	254–55
#81	Side-to-Side Jump	116
#198	Sitting, Knee-to-Nose stretch	195
#218	Sitting Rope, Tug	208
#353	Skating Forward	358
#328	Skiing Fall (Hill)	338
#329	Ski Knee Bends	339

Exercise Index

#	Exercise	Page
#326	Ski March in Place	337
#209	Skin the Cat	201
#82	Skips	117
#327	Ski Walk	337
#343	Sleepwalker Knee Bend	355
#342	Sleepwalker (skate)	354
#21	Snap and Stretch	79
#330	Snowplow	339–40
#356	Snowplow (skate)	360
#339	Snowplow Turn	345
#97	Somersaults	129
#98	Somersaults, Solo	130
#102	Somersaults, Spread Leg	132–33
#99	Somersaults Over, Stop	130
#132	Space Stepping	158
#2	Spine-Down Stretch	27
#52	Spread Leg, Head Down	102
#44	Spread-Leg, Side-Drop	98–99
#325	Spread-Leg Traverse Stairs	318–19
#301	Standing Broad Jump	290
#270	Standing Half Toe To Point	238
#317	Straight Hang and Tuck	315
#155	Straight-Leg Sit-Over	169
#58	Straight-Leg Stretch, Assisted	104
#43	Stretch Sit-Up	98
#42A	Supine, Knee to Nose	94–95
#48	Supine, Knee-to-Nose Kick	101
#195	Supine, Press (wgts.)	194
#8	Swim (warm up)	70
#37	Swing Around	92
#354	Swizzle (skate), Backward	359
#350	Swizzle (skate), Forward	357
#103	Tailor's Somersault	133
#104	Tailor's Somersault, Reverse	133
#174	Team of Horses, Shoulder Stand	178–79
#235	Ten-Past-Ten Walk	218
#36	Thread Needle, Kneeling	91
#29	Thread Needle, Standing	86
#67	Toe Bounces	110
#286	Toe-Rise Extensions	246
#25	Toe Rises	84
#24	Toe Rises, Single	83
#182	Toe-Touch Jump (ramp)	184
#312	Towel, Forward Pull	313
#315	Towel, Leg Pull	314
#316	Towel Leg Pull Balance	314
#313	Towel, Leg Flex	313
#314	Towel, Neck Pull	314
#311	Towel, Shoulder Stretch	312–13
#352	T Position (skate)	358
#123	Track Walk, Back	154
#122	Track Walk, Divided	122
#130	Track Wheelbarrows	156–57
#93	Triple Bike	126
#357	T stop (skating)	360
#318	Tuck and Spread (Parallels)	316
#65	Turned-in Walk	109
#66	Turned-Out Walk	110
#144	Turned-Out Walk on Fence	164
#272	Turn Out	239
	Tumbling	128–44
#89	Two-Arm and One-Arm Floor Progressions	122
#228	Two-Handed Swing Over Pole	213
#227	Two-Handed Twins on Rings	213
#159	Two-Handed Vault, Stretched	172
#158	Two-Handed Vault, Tight	171
#94	Two-Legged Side Thrusts	127
#153	Up-and-Down Obstacles	168
#320	Upper Back Bob (parallels)	316–17
#3	Upper Back Lift (corrective)	28
#222	Upside-Down Hang, Controlled	210
#225	Upside-Down Hang and Climb	212
#230	Upside-Down Hang, Rings	214
#114	VW	140–41
#355	Wag or Wiggle Backward (skate)	359
#10	Waist Twist, Down	71
#308	Waist Twist, Fins	311
#9	Waist Twist, Up	71
#308	Waist Twist Up and Down, Fins	311
#64	Walk	108–9
#77	Walk Hands, Bounce Feet	115
#243	Walking the RR Tracks	221
#233	Walking the Line	217
#119	Walking the Plank	152
#112	Walkover	139
#177	Walk-Up	182
#307	Warm-Ups with Fins	310–11
#194	Weighted Knee Bends	193–94
#135	Wheelbarrow on Ladder	159
#244	Wheelbarrow on RR Tracks	221
#151	Wheelbarrow Troika	167
#78	Wolf in the Garden	115

EXERCISES BY AREA AND BY NUMBER

Abdominal Strength
1a, 1b, 1c, 35, 42a, 42b, 42c, 46, 48, 50, 130, 131, 151, 152, 171, 172

Abdominal Strength
34, 60, 61, 111

Arm Strength
28, 29, 30, 40, 41, 70, 71, 72, 74, 75, 77, 89, 91, 92, 94, 127, 128, 129, 130, 131, 135, 136, 141, 150, 151, 152, 156, 158, 159, 161, 162, 163, 166, 167, 168, 190, 191, 192, 194, 195, 196, 197, 205, 207, 210, 211, 212, 216, 217, 218, 219, 220, 221, 222, 223, 224, 225, 226, 227, 228, 229, 230, 231, 244

Back Strength
3, 4, 5, 35, 39, 49, 169, 170, 199

Back Stretch
22, 52, 53, 56, 57, 59, 60, 61–63, 97–104

Balance
33, 105–110, 119–126, 132, 133, 138, 142–146, 154, 161–163, 174–176, 203, 204, 243, 247, 251, 266–290

Coordination
94, 114, 115, 118, 119, 135, 136, 150–155, 157–164, 173, 174, 175, 180, 182, 188, 208, 209, 237, 243, 245, 246, 249, 251, 254, 258, 259, 296

Eyes
132, 133, 291

Feet
23–27, 33, 64–66, 78, 80–83, 125, 132, 133, 139, 143, 154, 180, 234, 235, 252, 269–289, 296

Flexibility
6, 8, 9, 10, 11, 13, 15, 16, 17, 18, 19, 21, 22, 29, 34, 35, 36, 37, 38, 42A, 42B, 42D, 43, 44, 47,

48, 49, 51, 52, 53, 54, 55, 56, 57, 58, 59, 60, 61, 62, 63, 111, 140, 214, 231, 232

Hamstring
6, 28, 29, 43, 44, 51, 52, 55, 58, 62, 63, 140, 182, 214

Leg Strength
31, 32, 45, 64–96, 158–160, 180–188, 194, 252–259, 266–290

Pelvis
34, 38, 42C, 42E, 54, 69

Pigeon Toes
66, 78, 143, 234

Psoas
2

Turnout
65, 144, 235

EXERCISES BY SPECIALTY OR USING SPECIAL EQUIPMENT

Ballet
260–290

Chin Up
167, 168, 210, 211

Equipment
119–159

Floor Progressions
64–88

Garage Exercises
233–259

Kneeling Exercises
34–41

Ladder
132–141

Parallel Bars (outdoor)
317–325

Partners
114–18

Pipe
200–214

Ramps
177–189

Riding
19, 20, 38, 42E, Chapter 27

Ropes, Rings, Pipe
200–232

Running
306

Russian
89–96

Saw Horse
119–176

Sit and Lie Exercises
42A–42E, 43–62

Skating
342–358

Skiing
326–341, 351

Standing Exercises
8–33

Swim Exercises
307–325

Tennis
291–297

Track
298–305

Tumbling
97–118, 178–189

Warm-Ups
8–22

Weight Bags
190–199

GENERAL INDEX

Abdominals, corrective exercises for, 25–30
Across–the–floor progressions, 107–20
Age, for starting physical activity, 2–3
Ankles, and Myotherapy, 427
Arms, and Myotherapy, 424–25
Arthritis, and Myotherapy, 427
Assessment of child
    age, 2–3
    bones, 6
    build (body), 4–5
    fat, 5–6
    feet, 7–8
    height, 3
    Kraus–Weber Test, 13–17

    letter/guidelines to parents, 56–57, 60–61
    mouth, 6
    posture, 8–11
    Prudden Supplement Test for Optimum Performance, 18
    skin, 6
    teeth, 6
    weight, 3
Asthma, and Myotherapy, 427

Babies
    and swimming, 308–9
    typical day, 19–20
Back, and Myotherapy

flat, 427
pain, 419–21
round, 427
scoliosis, 428
sway, 428
Balance, and Myotherapy, 428
Ballistic stretch, 29–30, 97
Blocks, exercises on, 223
Bones, assessment of, 6
Bowlegs, 10
and Myotherapy, 435
Braces, and Myotherapy, 428
Build (body), 4–5
considerations for physical activity, 4–5
ectomorph, 4
endomorph, 4
mesomorph, 4

Calisthenics, 69
Cancer, and Myotherapy, 428
Cerebral palsy, and Myotherapy, 428–29
Charley horse, and Myotherapy, 429
Chest, and Myotherapy, 425
Colds, and Myotherapy, 429
Competition, self–competition, 57–58
Cross–country running, 304–6
Croup, and Myotherapy, 429

Dance, 228–48
ballet shoes, 230
clothing for, 230
mirror for, 231
movements, 233–41, 278
at barre, 241–47
music for, 230
preparation for, 231
Definition, muscles, 192
Diabetes, and Myotherapy, 429
Discus, 293–94

Dodgeball, 256–58
exercises for, 257–58
Doorway gym, 149
Dropped shoulder, 10–11
Dyslexia, and Myotherapy, 429

Equipment, 149–50
doorway gym, 149
exercises on, 151–215
for home gym, 217–27
ladder, 158
mats, 149
miscellaneous equipment, 150
parallel bars, 147
pipes, 149–50
railroad tracks, 147–48, 151
ramps, 146–47
rings, 213
rope, 207
sawhorse, 146
stairs, 148
for track meet, 287
weight bags, 189–96
Exercise class
clothing for, 66–67
format for, 67
place for, 66, 67
Exercise clothes, 66
foot covering, 66, 82
Exercises
across–the–floor progressions, 107–20
on equipment, 151–88
flexibility exercises, 97–106
kneeling exercises, 90–94
Russian series, 121–27
sitting/lying exercises, 94–96
standing exercises, 81–89
tumbling, 128–44
pair exercises, 141–44
warm–ups, 70–80
See also Exercise index.

Family Life
    child-rearing tips, 262-63
    discipline, 283
    family day, 267
    family projects, 263
        vegetable garden, 263-64
    fathers, 270-74
    mothers, 275-80
    new baby, 261
    parent's wishes for children, 261-62
    siblings, 268
    union for parents, 280-85
Fat
    dangers of, 5
    measuring body fat, 5-6
Fathers, 270-74
Feet
    assessment of, 7-8
    barefoot, value of, 82
    flat, and Myotherapy, 429
    "long second toe," 7-8, 435-36
    tension held in, 7
Figure skating, 351-61
    activities on the ice, 354-60
    clothing for, 352
    lessons, 353-54
    skates, 352-53
Flat back, 9
    Myotherapy for, 427
Flexibility
    ballistic stretch, 29-30, 97
    exercises for, 97-106
    and pulsing, 30
    static stretch, 30, 97
Floor patterns, 217
    exercises on, 217-20
Fractures, and Myotherapy, 430

Girls, 62-64
    failure rates, girls vs. boys, 63-64
    guidelines for mothers, 64
    and physical fitness in schools, 29
    tennis and, 259
Groin, and Myotherapy, 421-24

Handicapped, 378-93
    case examples
        blind children, 385-86, 389-90
        brain injured child, 384-85
        hyperactive child, 383-84
        retarded child, 387-88
    early intervention, value of, 386-87
    exercise program for, 379-82, 391-93
    Special Olympics, 382
Headaches, and Myotherapy, 425-26
Head (forward), and Myotherapy, 430
Height, 3
Hernia, and Myotherapy, 431
Hips, and Myotherapy, 431-32
Home gym (garage/basement), 217-27
    blocks, exercises on, 223
    floor patterns, 217
        exercises on, 217-20
    making of, 217
    railroad tracks, exercises on, 221-23
    rebounder, exercises on, 224-27
Horseback riding, 321-33
    bareback riding, 331
    bridle, 328
    canter, 332-33
    clothing for, 323
    easing horse, 330-31
    gallop, 333
    horse, 325
        feet, care of, 326-27
        grooming of, 325-26
    lessons, components of, 324-25
    mounting horse, 328-33
    saddle, 327
    stable/instruction, what to look for, 322-23

trotting, 331
walking horse, 332

Inflexibility, causes of, 29
Injuries, immediate mobilization, 432–34
Isometric contraction, 155

Javelin throw, 292–93
Jaw pain, and Myotherapy, 434–35

Kneeling exercises, 90–94
Knock-knees, 10
   and Myotherapy, 435
Kraus-Weber Test, 13–17
   failure rates, 19, 45
Kyphosis, round back, 8–9

Ladder, 158
   exercises on, 158–62
Latarjet, Dr., 52–53
Left-handers, tennis and, 258–59
Leg pain
   Myotherapy, 416–19
      sciatica, 420

Mats, 149
Menstrual cramps, and Myotherapy, 437
Milk, skim, value of, 3
Mothers, 275–80
Mouth, as sign of health, 6
Muscles
   muscle stiffness, 69–70
   pain related to, 412, 416
Music
   for dance, 230
   for exercising, 89
   for weight work, 196
Myotherapy, 382, 401, 403, 411–26
   for animals, 439–44
   arms, 424–25
      back pain, 419–20
      shoulder blade, 420–21
   basis of, 412–13
   chest, 425
   conditions aided by
      ankles, pronated, 427
      arthritis, 427
      asthma, 427
      back, flat, 427
      back, round, 427
      back, scoliosis, 428
      back, sway, 428
      balance, 428
      braces, 428
      cancer, 428
      cerebral palsy, 428–29
      Charley horse, 429
      colds, 429
      croup, 429
      diabetes, 429
      dyslexia, 429
      feet, flat, 429
      fractures, 430
      head, forward, 430
      hernia, 431
      hips, 431–32
      jaw pain, 434–35
      knees, knock-knees, 435
      legs, bowlegs, 435
      menstrual cramps, 437
      pigeon toes, 437
      retardation, 437
      shinsplints, 437
      sinus pain, 437
      spasticity, 437
      toes, long second toe, 435–36
      torticollis, 438
   groin, 421–24
   headaches, 425–26
   leg pain, 416–19
      sciatica, 420
   seeking massage, 426

General Index

shoulders, 424
  and trigger points, 412–13, 414
    activation of, 415, 432
    causes of, 414–15
    negative effects of, 415

Natural foods, 5, 265–66
Nutrition
  additives in food, 264–65
  vegetable garden project, 263–64

Oxygen debt, and running, 303–4

Pain, 8
  and muscles, 412, 416
  and stress, 412, 413
  See also Myotherapy.
Parallel bars, 147
  exercises on, 314–18
Parents, physical fitness reports to, 56–57, 60–61
  See also Family life.
Patterning, 125
Physical education
  adding to curriculum, experiment in France, 52–55
  in America, historical view, 21–22, 29
  and high school, 23–24
  historical view, 397–99
  and junior high, 22–23
  and parochial schools, 404
Physical fitness
  Heckler Report, 55
  studies/statistical information, 407–9
Pigeon toes, and Myotherapy, 437
Pipes, 149–50
  exercises on, 197–207
  parallel pipes, 206–7
Pole vault, 295–97
Posture
  bowlegs, 10

  dropped shoulder, 10–11
  flat back, 9
  knock-knees, 10
  protruding abdomen, 9–10
  round back, 8–9
  scoliosis, 11
  swayback, 9
Protruding abdomen, 9–10
Prudden Supplement Test for Optimum Performance, 31–61
  eat sheets, 42–43
  figure measurements, 38–42
  groups, testing of, 44–53
  record keeping, 58–61
  Tests 1 through 5, 32–35
  vital capacity, checking, 36
  weight assessment, 36–37
Pulsing, 30

Railroad tracks, 147–48, 151
  exercises on, 152–57, 221–23
Ramps, 146–47
  exercises on, 181–88
Rebounder, exercises on, 224–27
Recovery, running, 301
Repetitions, 69
Retardation, and Myotherapy, 437
Rings, 213
  exercises on, 213–15
Rope, 207
  exercises on, 207–12
  horizontal rope, 207–8
  two ropes, 210–12
  vertical rope, 208–10
Round back, 8–9
  and Myotherapy, 427
Running, 298–306
  assessment of child, 299
  cross-country running, 304–6
  guidelines for teaching, 300–301
  oxygen debt, 303–4
  race, 302–3

reach, 301
recovery, 301
Russian series, 121–27

Sawhorse, 146
  exercises on, 164–81
Scoliosis, 11
  and Myotherapy, 428
Shinsplints, and Myotherapy, 437
Shot put, 294–95
Shoulders, and Myotherapy, 424
Sinus pain, and Myotherapy, 437
Sitting/lying exercises, 94–96
Skiing, 334–50
  dry ski school, 336–37
  equipment for, 335–36
  frostbite, 348–49
  manners on lift-line, 347
  pre–skiing exercises, 337–43
  racing, 349–50
  on the snow activities, 345–47
  trails, behavior on, 347–48
Skin, as sign of health, 6
Skin diving, 319–20
Spasticity, and Myotherapy, 437
Stairs, 148
Standing exercises, 81–89
Standing straight, practicing, 232–33
Static stretch, 30, 97
Stress, and pain, 412, 413
Stretching, 69
  See also Flexibility.
Summer camp, 362–77
  adaptations of program, to different types of camps, 374–77
  assessment of children, test for, 367–68, 373–74
  daily program, 368–69
  diet, 369
  results of program, 370–72
  stress of program, children's reactions, 372

Swayback, 9
  and Myotherapy, 428
Swimming, 307–20
  babies and, 308–9
  pre–swim exercises, 310–19
  skin diving, 319–20

Teachers, 399–405
  program for classroom teachers, 400–402
Teen fitness, 403
Teeth, as sign of health, 6
Tennis, 249–56
  backhand, exercises for, 253–54
  eye exercises, 251
  forehand, exercises for, 252–53
  and girls, 259
  shuffle pattern, 255–56
  side slides, exercises for, 254–55
  southpaw, 258–59
  value of, 249–50
Toes, and Myotherapy, 435–36
Torticollis, and Myotherapy, 438
Track meet (backyard), 286–97
  activities for, 288–92
  discus, 293–94
  equipment for, 287
  javelin throw, 292–93
  pole vault, 295–97
  shot put, 294–95
Trigger Point Injection, 412–13

Warm–ups, 68–80
  exercises, 70–80
  purpose of, 68
Weight, 3
Weight bags, 189–96
  exercises with, 192–96
  making of, 190
  work sheet for workouts, 196
Weight–training, 189–90
  limitations of, 189

A000021690532